The
Dynamics
of Anxiety
& Hysteria

The
Dynamics
of Anxiety
& Hysteria

An Experimental Application of
Modern Learning Theory to Psychiatry

Hans J. Eysenck

Transaction Publishers
New Brunswick (U.S.A.) and London (U.K.)

Published in 2002 by Transaction Publishers, New Brunswick, New Jersey by arrangement with the estate of Hans J. Eysenck. Originally published in 1957 by Routledge & Kegan Paul.

This book is printed on acid-free paper that meets the American National Standard for Permanence of Paper for Printed Library Materials.

Library of Congress Catalog Number: 2002020280
ISBN: 0-7658-0959-1
Printed in the United States of America

Library of Congress Cataloging-in-Publication Data

Eysenck, H. J. (Hans Jurgen), 1916-
    The dynamics of anxiety and hysteria : an experimental application of
    modern learning theory to psychiatry / Hans J. Eysenck.
        p. cm.
    Includes bibliographical references and index.
    ISBN 0-7658-0959-1 (pbk. : alk. paper)
    1. Hysteria. 2. Anxiety. 3. Learning. I. Title.

RC532 .E9 2002
616.85'24—dc21   2002020280

To the memory of

C. L. HULL

A theory in science is a policy rather than a creed.

J. J. THOMSON

CONTENTS

LIST OF FIGURES

LIST OF FIGURES

LIST OF FIGURES

LIST OF PLATES

xiii

INTRODUCTION

T HIS book is the fifth in a series of monographs in which I
have reported experimental studies and theoretical work
carried out by members of the Psychological Department
of the Institute of Psychiatry, which is a school of the University
of London, a constituent part of the Post-Graduate Medical
Federation, and associated with the Maudsley and the Bethlem
Royal Hospitals. In the first two volumes, *Dimensions of Personality* and *The Scientific Study of Personality*, our concern was in
the main with the dimensional analysis of personality, with
psychiatric nosology, and with taxonomic methods and studies
generally. *The Psychology of Politics* carried this work forward by
making certain deductions from our general theory on to the
field of attitudes and sentiments, and by showing the inter-
connections between personality and political activities. *The
Structure of Human Personality* served to review the literature, in
so far as it could be said to be of an experimental or at least
empirical nature, and thus put the work previously reported
into its proper setting. In this book an attempt has been made
to go beyond classification to a study of dynamics; to pass from
nosology to aetiology, from description to causation. As the
title will indicate, however, our efforts have been restricted to
a rather narrow field; no attempt has been made to deal with
psychotic disorders, for instance. This task is reserved for a
later publication.

In looking for explanatory concepts and mechanisms to
account for the observed phenomena of hysteria and anxiety,
it was inevitable that recourse was had to the principles of
modern learning theory. Of all the branches of psychology, the
study of conditioning and learning is much the most advanced,
the most relevant, and also the most readily applicable to our
problem, and it will be seen that the experiments and theories
of Pavlov, Hull, Tolman and the other great figures of learning

I

theory have an immediate connection with the molar aspects of human behaviour usually dealt with by psychiatrists and students of personality. In the past, theories to account for these phenomena have usually centred upon the contribution of S. Freud and the work of other psychoanalysts. I believe that this approach has by now sufficiently demonstrated its fundamental failure to generate testable hypotheses, to make possible modifications in human conduct, and to account for the results of experimental work; it therefore appears desirable to return to another approach, which is historically linked with the name of Pavlov. This book constitutes an effort to help in this process of reorientation, and to show that those Freudian observations which constitute a lasting contribution to psychiatry can be accounted for in terms of a Pavlovian theory as easily as, but perhaps more rigorously than, in terms of a psychoanalytic one.

As the purpose of this book is constructive rather than critical, I have spent little time on a detailed critique of other approaches, but have rather concentrated on the development of the theoretical model which constitutes the main contribution of this book, and the experimental studies which have been carried out to test deductions made from that theory. Being in any case somewhat antifloccinaucinihilipilificationistically inclined by nature, and having given some space in previous books to points of disagreement, I followed this path all the more willingly by recalling the dictum that a bad theory in science is never killed by criticism, but only by a better theory. Whether the theory here presented is in fact a better one is not a matter on which I would like to be dogmatic; theorizing in science is an uncertain business at the best of times, and never more so than in the early stages of development of a science. Metaphors regarding the relations of later generations to earlier views in matters scientific have varied all the way from 'standing on the shoulders of giants' to being 'the louse on the head of the astronomer', and no doubt the reader will select an appropriate one to suit his taste. To indicate the tentative nature of the hypotheses put forward, I have included in the last chapter a discussion of various criticisms to which the general theory here put forward is subject; this should have the added advantage of enabling reviewers to pass straight from the Introduction to the Conclusion without having to read the intervening parts.

INTRODUCTION

On one point I have to seek the reader's indulgence. Köhler, in that most brilliant and least read of psychological classics *Die Physischen Gestalten in Ruhe und im Stationären Zustand*, wrote two prefaces, addressed to psychologists and physicists respectively, in view of the fact that his book dealt with matters pertaining to both their fields of study. (As a consequence, neither psychologists nor physicists appear to have dared to come near the book.) Similarly, this book is addressed to two groups of readers who are somewhat dissimilar in interest, background training, and allegiance. On the one hand, I am hoping that it will be read by psychiatrists and clinical psychologists interested in theories and facts relating to the genesis of neurotic disorders; on the other hand, I am hoping that it will be read by physiologists and experimental psychologists interested in the integration of a diversity of experimental results in terms of learning theory, with a consequent repercussion on learning theory itself. This interaction and integration of diverse fields of study usually treated in isolation appears to me an absolute necessity if psychology is ever to become more than a collection of chapter headings in elementary textbooks, and I find it difficult to believe that this integration can be achieved in any other way than by reference to the central concept in psychology, namely, that of personality.

Unfortunately, these different groups of prospective readers cannot be assumed to share a common background of knowledge, and it has been necessary to include details about conditioning, learning theory, and various perceptual effects which, while probably new to psychiatrists and many clinical psychologists, will be all too familiar to experimental psychologists. Conversely, details about clinical syndromes, psychiatric theories, and the dimensional analysis of personality, while familiar to psychiatrists and clinical psychologists, may require at least brief recapitulation for experimental psychologists. While I have relied much on the quotation of primary source material, most readers will probably find some topics treated at undue length and in a rather elementary fashion, while other topics are treated too briefly and at too advanced a level. The specific topics falling into these two categories are likely to differ for different readers; in the absence of a unified background among readers a unified treatment of subjects becomes impossible. It is to be hoped that in the future a *rapprochement* may occur between these various groups; until then the writing of books such as this inevitably entails compromises of the kind mentioned, and I can only apologize for the imperfections.

It is always a pleasure to pay debts of gratitude, and there is a long list of friends and colleagues to whom thanks are due for the part their thinking and their experimental work have played in the writing of this book. M. Shapiro has been particularly active in trying to develop a theory of brain-damage on a Pavlovian basis, and it will be obvious how much my thinking owes to his theoretical and experimental work. G. Granger has widened my understanding of physiological processes in visual perception, and both on the theoretical and the experimental side I am indebted to him for very significant contributions. A. Petrie and her work on the effects of leucotomy and other brain-operations have furnished a very important stepping-stone in the development of my theory. P. Slater and A. E. Maxwell, from the statistical section of the Department, have made a considerable contribution by suggesting new methods of analysis and by supervising computations; the same may be said of A. Lubin who introduced canonical variate analysis in this Department. R. Nixon supervised the curve-fitting in the conditioning data. S. B. G. Eysenck made an invaluable contribution by her large-scale experimental and statistical analysis of neurotic and psychotic behaviour. P. Broadhurst, in charge of the animal laboratory of the Department, provided important evidence regarding the Yerkes-Dodson law; his work on the inheritance of emotionality has influenced my thinking, but could not be included in this account. R. Payne and Gwynne Jones have discussed many of the problems which arose in the course of the development of this theory with me, and I am indebted to them for their suggestions, help, and advice; in addition they and A. Yates have carried through a number of very important therapeutic experiments on the results of which I have placed much weight. C. Franks has been in charge of the conditioning laboratory of the Department, and without his contribution a central part of this book would have been missing. D. Trouton, combining the training of psychiatrist and psychologist, has been of considerable help in connection with our drug experiments. W. D. Furneaux, of the Nuffield Research Unit, has made a major contribution by his theoretical and experimental work in the field of cognition and his development of new techniques of intelligence testing; only a portion of this contribution has been used here. J. Tizard, P. Venables, and N. O'Connor, of the M.R.C. Unit, have contributed several important experiments. H. Brengelmann has carried out interesting and relevant work in the perceptual field. I. Martin, J. William, R. Beech, D. Campbell, J. Field, K. Star, A. Broadhurst, and F. Goldmann-Eisler all made contributions on the experimental side, as did J. Inglis and V. Meyer on the theoretical. Last but not least, I wish to thank the sixty or so former Ph.D. students in the Department, those 'mute and inglorious Miltons', without whose devoted work our knowledge would be much less firmly based than in fact it is. Others formerly part of the Department, now outside it, whose contribution I wish to acknowledge are H. Himmelweit, A. Heron, and B. Oppenheim. Most of our research has depended on mechanical and electronic apparatus of various kinds, and thanks are due to S. F. R. Mable, the Chief Technician, and his staff for their devoted work. I am also indebted to Mr. P. Jacobs, who took the photographs which enliven this book.

Much of the work here reported has been made possible by grants from the Rockefeller Foundation, the Nuffield Foundation, the University of London Research Fund, the Medical Research Council, the U.S. Office of Naval Research, and the Bethlem Royal and Maudsley Hospital Research Fund. To all those responsible for the allocation of these funds I am much indebted.

Finally, I wish to record my thanks to my psychiatric colleagues for their patience and forbearance. Much of the work done in the Psychological Department, and many of the theories put forward by its members, must have seemed to them contrary to psychiatric tradition, improbable, unintelligible, and downright perverse. They have borne the burden with patience and Christian forbearance, only occasionally complaining that the psychologists seemed to have adopted the quotation from Goldsmith's *Good Natured Man* as their motto: 'Measures, not men, have always been my mark.' Perhaps this bifurcation of interests mirrors the bifurcation of functions of psychologists and psychiatrists; in any case, how boring would life be if we all thought and did alike! And should we not bear in mind the words of the Bible: 'Omnia in mensura, et numero, et pondere disposuisti'?

Permission to reproduce drawings and figures was kindly granted by the following: H. Kimpton (Fig. 11); *J. exper. Psychol.* (17, 18, 19, 33); *Brit. J. Psychol.* (23, 30, 31, 32, 39, 40); *J. ment. Sci.* (41, 42, 43); *Genet. Psychol. Monogr.* (48, 49); *J. psychosom. Res.* (54, 55, 56); H.M.S.O. (57).

H. J. E.

Institute of Psychiatry,
  Maudsley Hospital,
    7th December, 1956.

Chapter One

THE DIMENSIONAL ANALYSIS
OF ANXIETY AND HYSTERIA

THE function of science may be stated very broadly to be twofold. It attempts to *describe* phenomena, and it attempts to *explain* them. This is not in any sense an absolute distinction; explanation is no more than a very extensive method of description. The law of gravitation explains the falling of unsupported bodies, the movements of the planets, the swing of the pendulum, and many other phenomena, but at the same time it is itself merely a general descriptive formula derived from the facts it then explains. There is thus a certain circularity in all scientific reasoning, but this circularity is not objected to as long as its basis is broad enough. In other words, if we are only dealing with one or two facts, 'explanation' derived from description is tautological. When the facts are very numerous the tautological aspect of explanation vanishes and it becomes generally predictive and scientifically important.

In the field of abnormal behaviour, we can distinguish the same two aspects in the endeavours of psychologists and psychiatrists to deal with the observed phenomena. Classical psychiatry was largely concerned with the description of symptoms and the establishment of syndromes; it seldom ventured far beyond the descriptive realm. Psychoanalysis, on the other hand, attempted to explain the causes of syndromes and symptoms, and for that reason seemed to consider itself justified in calling its approach 'dynamic'.

The general outcome of all this work cannot, by any stretch of the imagination, be called impressive. On the descriptive side, even a cursory glance at modern textbooks will show a remarkable lack of agreement between different groups of psychiatrists. Indeed, even within any one group it will usually be found that there are grave inconsistencies in the views put forward. Thus, the same author may on one page treat syndromes as separate disease entities, while on another page he may put forward a view implying rather the existence of quantitative continua. It is small wonder that psychiatric diagnoses show very little reliability (Eysenck, 1952), or that many psychiatrists have come to despair of this type of description as being at all useful in their day-to-day work.

Nor has the 'dynamic' approach fared any better. Here also disagreement on even the most elementary and fundamental facts is such that it is very doubtful whether any agreed and settled theory may be said to exist at all (Blum, 1953). Here also inconsistencies arise within the writings of any particular author or school. Worst of all, the initial promise of psychoanalysis to improve or cure the mentally ill has not been fulfilled after over 50 years of widespread endeavour. A review of all the available evidence by the present writer disclosed the sad fact that when comparing the effects of psychotherapy with various estimates of spontaneous remission rates, there appeared to be no difference between cures accomplished (Eysenck, 1952).

What, it may be asked, has gone wrong? Why has the achievement both of classical and of dynamic psychiatry so clearly belied its early promise? The answer, or so it seems to the present writer, must lie in the method adopted by psychiatrists. By and large they tend to appeal to intuition, clinical insight, and experience in formulating their views, and to reject experimental methods and statistical analyses. This does not seem to be a feasible position. No one would deny the importance of clinical experience and insight in the *formulation* of hypotheses and theories; indeed it is difficult to see any other breeding-ground for these vitally necessary parts of scientific progress. It is a grave error, however, to assume that the *formulation* of a hypothesis constitutes an acceptable *proof* for that hypothesis. It is to achieve such a proof that experimental and statistical analyses are essential. The clinical method, so called, is an excellent method for suggesting ideas, but its usefulness ends at that point. It is a grave defect of post-Kraepelinian psychiatry that it has rested content with theories and has eschewed the hard and difficult task of proof. This is all the more astonishing as Kraepelin himself had instituted the use of psychological experiments in psychiatry and demonstrated their fruitfulness. Yet, what he said over 50 years ago still very much applies today:

'However much our creative confidence may be diminished by difficulties and disappointments, and however many of our great problems may prove to be insoluble in their present form —nevertheless, our experience has already shown beyond doubt that the psychological experiment is not only a useful but an indispensable part of our scientific background. It is all the more important because in psychiatry, more than in any other branch of medicine, interpretation and system building are regarded more highly than simple observation. In our psychiatric case conferences we constantly find a superabundance of individualistic brilliance, an undisciplined arbitrariness which finds sufficient room for its games only because as yet the slow advance of real science has not narrowed down the possibilities sufficiently. Nearly every psychiatrist assumes the right —some even seem to regard it as an obligation!—to begin by constructing his own psychological system on the basis of rough-and-ready observations of patients, of animals, or even by reference to literary studies. What representative of internal medicine would dare to proclaim a new system of physiology which did not base itself on facts laboriously acquired and tested in the laboratory?'

In many ways the work which the writer has reported in this and previous volumes is nothing more than a continuation of the work so well begun by Kraepelin and his students. Previous volumes, in particular *Dimensions of Personality* and *The Scientific Study of Personality*, have dealt with the descriptive aspects of abnormal behaviour; the present book constitutes an attempt to deal with some of the aetiological, or causal, problems thrown up in these earlier books. The present chapter is devoted to a brief review of the present position in the descriptive, nosological, or taxonomic field; the remainder of the book will then proceed from this foundation to a discussion of explanatory concepts and their application to certain parts of the descriptive scheme. As this chapter is largely a review of previous work, no effort will be made to prove in detail the various points made; for such proofs the reader is referred to previous publications. We shall rather present the results achieved together with certain illustrative material, and briefly mention the statistical and experimental methods used.

The first issue to be raised is that of *continuity*. It used to be argued by analogy with physical diseases, that the syndromes of psychiatry, such as hysteria, constitute separate disease entities possessing separate diagnostic, prognostic, and aetiological features. While this view is not very widely held today, the nomenclature and the systems of diagnosis employed by psychiatrists still make use of it, and it is rare to find an outright refutation of this notion. Nevertheless, this view is quite untenable, both on clinical and experimental grounds. Functional psychiatric disorders are not 'diseases' at all, in the sense that malaria or cancer or haemophilia may be said to be diseases which a person may be said to have or not to have. There are no qualitative differences between so-called normal people and those diagnosed as suffering from anxiety state or hysteria. The difference is a quantitative one, just as is the difference between the average person and the dullard with an I.Q. of 70 is quantitative. The medical notion of mental disease entities is not, in fact, entertained seriously by most psychiatrists, and it is proposed, therefore, that it should formally be relinquished.

In its place we must put an entirely different notion, namely that of a number of separate dimensions or continua, the interaction between which gives rise to the so-called syndromes of classical psychiatry. What these continua are and how they can be established is an important problem which will be illustrated by references to a second problem, namely, that of the identity —or lack of identity—of the neurotic and psychotic continua.

As is well known, classical psychiatry regards neurotic and psychotic disorders as being essentially different, i.e. as lying on two independent, orthogonal continua. Psychoanalysts, and some other modern psychiatrists, on the other hand, believe, as Myerson (1936) puts it, that 'neuroses span the bridge between ... normal mental states and certain psychotic states'. In other words, they believe that there is a single continuum from normal through neurotic to psychotic, so that a person suffering from neurotic disorders might be considered as a mild psychotic, or a person suffering from psychotic disorders as a severe neurotic. The two hypotheses may be illustrated as in Figs. 1 and 2.

This problem is of obvious and fundamental importance to

psychiatry, and its treatment in the literature brings out particularly clearly the failure of the so-called clinical method to supply any kind of proof one way or another. A perusal of several hundred books and papers dealing with this question discloses that the opposing arguments can, in fact, be reduced to the following: 'My clinical experience suggests that there is a continuum between neurotics and psychotics', and, 'My

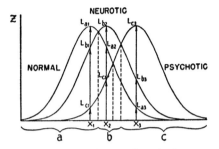

FIG. 1. One-dimensional hypothesis of personality organization.

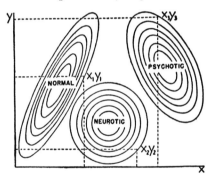

FIG. 2. Two-dimensional hypothesis of personality organization.

clinical experience suggests that there is no continuum between neurotics and psychotics'. Admittedly, other arguments are occasionally brought forward, such as the fact that patients can be found who seem to have *both* neurotic and psychotic symptoms, and who are difficult to diagnose as either one or the other. Such observations, while factually correct, do not provide an argument either way, however. On the one-dimensional hypothesis such people would be postulated to lie between points X_2 and X_3 in Fig. 1. On a two-dimensional hypothesis, they would be postulated to lie between points X_2 and Y_2, and X_3 and Y_3 in Fig. 2. Thus, both fact and argument are irrelevant to the discussion. Clearly, then, the clinical method has failed to provide any plausible solution to our problem. Where clinical experience contradicts clinical experience, clinical experience cannot be the criterion. If we wish to escape from an eternal *impasse* of this kind, we must adopt a more systematic experimental-statistical approach.

One possibility of doing this is by means of a statistical study of the relationships between symptoms actually observed in a representative group of psychiatric patients. Such a study is available in the work of Trouton and Maxwell (1956), who made use of a set of 45 symptoms whose presence or absence was rated by the Psychiatrist-in-Charge on 819 male functional patients at the Maudsley Hospital, aged between 16 and 59 years. The variables included are shown in Table I. Tetrachoric correlations were calculated between them, and a factor analysis performed.

TABLE I

Item Sheet Analysis: Variables Included in the Factor Analysis

Number of
Item in
Factor
Analysis

1		Age (16–39) vs. (40–59).
2		Psychotic vs. non-psychotic (i.e. neurosis and personality disorders).
3	Family History	Family history of psychosis.
4	of Psychiatric	Family history of neurosis.
5	Disorder	Family history of abnormal personality (e.g. psychopathy, alcoholism).
6		Unsatisfactory early life.
7		Unsatisfactory adolescent adjustment.
8	Previous Adjustment	Work position falling and/or frequent unemployment due to instability of patient.
9		Lacks confidence when in society.
10		Unsatisfactory home life as an adult.
11		Neurotic traits in childhood.
12		Hysterical symptoms, life-long or episodic.
13		Obsessional symptoms, life-long or episodic.
14	Previous	Anxiety symptoms, life-long or episodic.
15	Symptoms	Definite mood variations before present illness.
16		Energy output low, lacks effort for success and achievement.

12

Number of Item in Factor Analysis		
17		Symptoms of over 12 months' duration before admission.
18	Causes and	Gradual onset of illness.
19	Onset of	Constitutional causes important or dominant.
20	Illness	Precipitating psychological and social (environmental) causes unimportant.
21		Functional disturbances in systems other than the nervous.
22		Retarded activity.
23		Overactive, excited, manic or hypomanic, non-manic euphoria.
24		Agitated.
25		Impulsive and/or aggressive.
26	Symptoms	Socially withdrawn.
27	of Present	Compulsive acts and/or obsessional thoughts.
28	Illness	Motor disturbances (e.g. posturing, grimacing, and catatonic disturbances).
29		Depressed.
30		Anxious.
31		Mood disturbances (inappropriate or rapidly changing).
32		Suspicious.
33		Irritable.
34		Suicidal feelings, intentions, or serious attempts.
35		Schizophrenic type of thought disorder.
36		Psychogenic impairment of thought or memory.
37		Delusions of guilt, self-reproach, unworthiness.
38		Ideas of reference.
39		Delusions (other than those included in 37 and 38).
40		Hallucinations.
41		Severe insomnia at any time during illness.
42		Gross disturbance of weight and/or food intake.
43		Hypochondriacal attitude towards illness.
44		Denial, indifference or unawareness of symptoms.
45	Outcome in Hospital	Recovered or much improved at time of discharge.

A plot of the two main factors, or dimensions, relevant to our argument is given in Fig. 3. It will be seen that we are dealing with two quite independent clusters of items. One cluster is made up of items like 'life-long or episodic anxiety', 'neurotic traits in childhood', 'unsatisfactory early life', 'life-long or episodic hysterical symptoms', 'anxious', 'symptoms of over twelve months' duration before admission', 'unsatisfactory adolescent adjustment', 'family history of neurosis', 'life-long or episodic obsessional symptoms', 'low energy output', 'bad work record', and 'precipitating enviromental causes important'. All of these are strongly reminiscent of the usual descriptions of neurotic illness and leave little doubt that here we are dealing

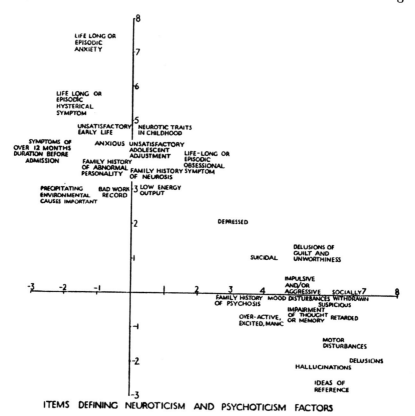

ITEMS DEFINING NEUROTICISM AND PSYCHOTICISM FACTORS

FIG. 3. Items defining neuroticism and psychoticism factors.

with a factor which has often been called 'neuroticism' in the literature (Eysenck, 1947).

Let us now look at the other factor, which is quite independent of the first. Here we find items like 'delusions', 'hallucinations', 'ideas of reference', 'motor disturbances', 'mood disturbances', 'impairment of thought or memory', 'retardation', 'suicidal', 'socially withdrawn', 'suspicious', and 'family history of psychosis'. There is a marked clustering here of items

14

traditionally regarded as characteristic of psychosis, and this factor, therefore, appears to give considerable support to the conception of 'psychoticism', also found in the literature (Eysenck, 1952). More important, however, than this verification of the existence of these two factors is the demonstration that they are *orthogonal*, that is to say, situated at right angles, and quite independent of each other. It would be very difficult indeed to square this picture with the demands of the Freudian or 'unidimensional' theory. According to that theory, we should have found one single factor corresponding to 'degree of abnormality'. The results are therefore completely in accordance with the demands of the two-dimensional type of theory, and suggest strongly that it would be more fruitful to assume the truth of this view.

Certain points are brought out in this figure which may make it of additional interest. The symptom 'depression', for instance, can be seen to be related almost equally strongly to the psychotic and the neurotic factors. This suggests that by itself the presence of depression can tell us nothing about the question of whether the patient's disorder is of a neurotic or psychotic nature; the symptom is equally compatible with both hypotheses. This fact, of course, has been known for a long time; it is interesting, however, to see it brought out so clearly in the analysis.

Before going on to a different type of experiment, it would seem necessary first to deal with an objection frequently made of this kind of proof. What comes out of the analysis, it is suggested, is only what was put into it in the first instance, and if psychiatrists filling in the item sheet hold the view represented in the figure, then their prejudices and biases could have sufficiently swayed their judgment to give rise to data which would support the view originally held. Such a danger undoubtedly exists whenever recourse is had to subjective estimates (Eysenck, 1953). However, in the present case, there is little doubt that the great majority of psychiatrists taking part in the study held views opposed to the one illustrated in Fig. 3; in other words, if the issue was prejudiced it was prejudiced in a direction opposite to the final outcome.

Nevertheless, we are still relying on subjective data, and it seems advisable to try to attempt an alternative proof through the use of somewhat more objective data. Also the method of factor analysis has sometimes been criticized because of its failure to provide an estimate of significance of factors, and the impossibility of calculating rather than estimating factor scores for individuals. Both these difficulties are avoided in the method of canonical variate analysis. As this method has not been widely used in psychology, a discussion of its *rationale* may be of interest.

We may re-state the problem as follows. Let us give q tests to persons psychiatrically allocated to three groups: normal controls, neurotics, and psychotics. Let there be n persons in each group, and let these be equated for intelligence, age, and other relevant parameters. The one-dimensional hypothesis would be satisfied if it were found that in the q-dimensional space generated by the tests, the points indicating the mean positions of the three groups were collinear. The two-dimensional hypothesis would be satisfied if variation extended significantly in more than one direction, so that the three points formed a triangle. A statistical test of significance would of course be required to indicate whether or not the observed departure from collinearity was significant or not. This may appear to be a very formal way of approaching problems historically considered nearly always in semantic terms, but it is difficult to see how any advance can be made in this field without the exact statement of hypotheses, together with the conditions necessary for their testing.

The two alternatives have already been presented in diagrammatic form, Fig. 1 showing the one-dimensional hypothesis, Fig. 2 the two-dimensional one. Distributions around the means of each group are indicated on the ordinate in Fig. 1, and by contour lines in Fig. 2. These figures are taken with slight modifications from Lubin (1950), whose discussion of the statistical problems involved has formed the basis of our approach in this paper.

The statistical procedures appropriate for the solution of problems such as those indicated above are of relatively recent development, and not frequently used by psychologists. As a group, they come under the heading of 'multivariate analysis', and several systematic expositions are available (Wilks, 1932; Kendall, 1946; Bartlett, 1947; Tintner, 1950; Lubin, 1951). In the simplest case, when we are concerned with membership in one of two mutually exclusive groups, such methods as Hotelling's T^2 (1931), Fisher's linear discriminant function (1936),

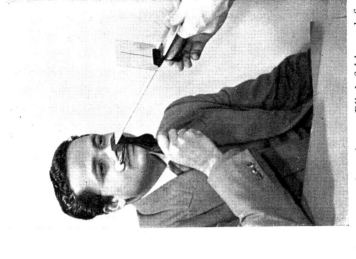

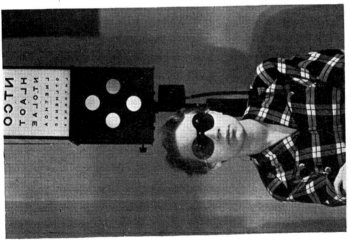

1. Visual acuity test. Letters above subject's head are seen in mirror. Blink-fold used for occluding one eye.

2. Giles's near-point rule, for the measurement of accommodation.

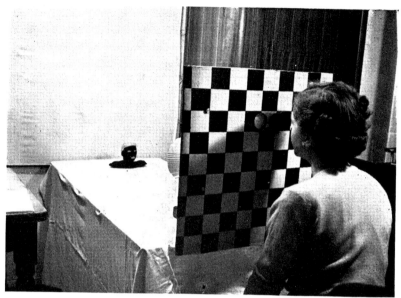

3. Object recognition test. Figure on table is exposed for brief periods through monocular tachistoscope.

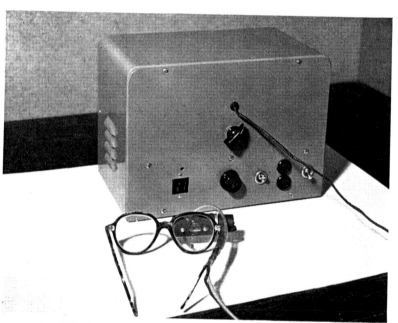

4. Conditioning apparatus for eyeblink reflex. Note polythene tube for application of air-blast to cornea, and light-sensitive cell on spectacle frame for registration of eyeblink.

and Wilks' special case of the lambda criterion (1932) are available. When there are three or more mutually exclusive groups, the simpler formulae can easily be adapted. In the same way in which one can find that linear function of variables which gives the biggest t-ratio for the difference between two group means, it is also possible to find a linear function of variables that maximizes the F-ratio for more than two groups —the multi-group or canonical discriminating function (Fisher, 1938; Letestu, 1948; Rao, 1948; Tukey, 1949; Lubin, 1951). Alternatively Hotelling's (1936) 'most predictable criterion' method may be used, or multivariate analysis of variance (Bartlett, 1938, 1947; Roy, 1939; Rao, 1946; Wilks, 1946; Tukey, 1949) called by Rao 'analysis of dispersion'.

The method of dispersion analysis has been applied to problems of a psychiatric nature only three times. Its first application was made in 1949 by Rao and Slater to differences between neurotic groups; they failed to disprove the one-dimensional hypothesis in this field, probably because of their reliance on ratings instead of objective tests. The second application was made in 1950 by Hamilton in his work on the personality of dyspeptics; he also failed to find significant latent roots other than the first. A third application, by Lubin (1951), dealt precisely with the problem we are considering; his results, as summarized by Eysenck (1952), indicated the strong probability that the two-dimensional hypothesis was correct, but his choice of tests was too restricted to make the conclusion very compelling.

More convincing is another experiment more recently reported by Eysenck (1955). Twenty normal controls, 20 neurotics, and 20 psychotics were tested; all were male with ages ranging from 20 to 40 years. The normal group consisted of soldiers from a reallocation centre. The abnormal groups were chosen from in-patients at the Maudsley Hospital, psychiatric diagnoses determining their allocation to the neurotic or psychotic category. All S's were given the Nufferno test of intelligence. This test, which is of the familiar letter series type, has been developed at this Institute by W. D. Furneaux (1952), and has been used extensively on large groups of the population, as well as on psychiatric patients. It is a 'level' test, especially constructed so that the influence of speed should be as small as possible. A more detailed discussion and description of

17

the test and the psychological principles underlying it has been given elsewhere by Eysenck (1953). Differences among the three groups on this test were quite insignificant, the neurotic group being very slightly brighter than the normal or the psychotic group. The following four tests, among others, were given to all three groups:

(1) *Visual acuity.* The test used consisted of an ordinary Snellen chart with reversed type, which was placed immediately behind the *S* who observed the image of the test-type in a distortion-free ophthalmic mirror at a distance of 3 metres. The right eye was tested first, with the left eye occluded, and after a short pause the left eye was tested with the right eye occluded. After a further pause, binocular visual acuity was tested. The *S*'s acuity was expressed as a Snellen ratio, but for computational purposes the ratios were converted to scores on a 9-point scale and a total score obtained by summing the scores for monocular and binocular acuity. High scores on this test denote superior visual acuity (Plate 1).

(2) *Object Recognition Test.* This test was designed by Brengelmann (1953) and has been described in detail in Eysenck, Granger, and Brengelmann (1957). Essentially, the procedure is as follows. An object on a table is exposed monocularly for varying periods by means of a photographic shutter arrangement. The *S* is required to describe what he sees and also to determine whether what he sees is two- or three-dimensional. There are three exposures of $\frac{1}{100}$ of a sec., five of $\frac{1}{25}$, two of $\frac{1}{5}$, two of $\frac{1}{2}$, two of 1, three of 3, and three of 5 sec. The score used for this investigation is the number of exposures required to recognize the three-dimensional nature of the test objects. (There are two objects in all, one the bust of a man's head, the other two pairs of spectacles. Cf. Plate 3.)

(3) *Mental speed.* The test here used, together with its rationale, has been discussed in detail in Eysenck (1953). The test used is the Nufferno Speed Test (Furneaux, 1955). This consists of a series of very easy letter series problems, in which the *S*'s task is to find solutions as quickly as possible. The actual score used is a logarithm of the time taken over the task. From theoretical considerations and much unpublished work carried out at the Institute, it appeared likely that psychotics would be found very slow in comparison with normals and neurotics.

(4) *Accommodation.* A review by Granger (1953) of perceptual

functions suggested that anomalies of accommodation would be found more frequently in psychiatric patients than in normal S's. The test used here was the Near-Point Rule developed by Giles (1945). This consists of a metal rule about 40 cm. in length, one end of which fits into a holder which is pressed against the face of the S. A card bearing test-type is fitted into a clip which slides along the rule. A 'blur point' is established by moving this card toward the S, and a 'recovery point' by moving it away from him. Details regarding the application of this test may be found in Eysenck, Granger, and Brengelmann (1957). Low scores on this test may be interpreted as indicating superior amplitude of accommodation. The particular score chosen here is that of recovery for the left eye (cf. Plate 2).

The technique of discriminant function analysis used on the data obtained is very much like that of analysis of variance, but being in matrix form requires the calculation of several matrices. First, the total product-sum matrix (G) was computed for the four variables, then the between-groups product-sum matrix (B), the difference between these giving us the within-groups product-sum matrix (W). (The latter was checked by an independent procedure.) Hamilton (1950) and Rao and Slater (1949) proceeded to maximize the general distance function (D^2); we followed instead Lubin's (1950) method of maximizing the square of the correlation ratio, given by

$$R^2 = \left\{ \frac{\text{deviance between groups}}{\text{total deviance}} \right\}$$

In essence, our problem is this. We wish to find a set of weights in order to derive from our four tests a composite score for each S such that the square of the correlation ratio (R^2) between that composite variate and the three groups is at a maximum. Hence, if we take $R^2 = \acute{u}Bu/\acute{u}Gu$, following Lubin (1950), we arrive at the equation $(G^{-1}B - R^2I)u = 0$. (In this expression, G and B have already been defined, u is the column vector of weights and $\acute{u}$ is its transpose. I is the unit diagonal matrix.) The values of R^2 which satisfy this equation are the latent roots of the non-symmetric matrix $G^{-1}B$, each root having a corresponding latent vector u. Obtaining $G^{-1}B$ involves calculating the inverse of the matrix G and post-multiplying it by B. This results in the non-symmetric matrix BG^{-1} from which the latent roots and vectors are extracted using an iterative method for non-symmetric matrices. As the rank of $G^{-1}B$ is always one less than the number of groups (or of tests, whichever is the smaller) only two latent roots were found.

Having obtained these two latent roots, we apply tests of significance, using Bartlett's chi-square test for the significance of the canonical roots: $X^2 = -\left(N - 1 - \dfrac{q + c}{2}\right) \log_e (1 - \lambda)$, where λ is the root whose significance is being tested, $q =$ number of tests, $c =$ number of groups, and $N =$ number of S's. $\lambda_1 = \cdot543944$, which is significant at beyond the $\cdot001$ level, and $\lambda_2 = \cdot155406$, which is significant at the $\cdot02$ level. Both roots are therefore significant, and the two-dimensional hypothesis is supported. The correlation ratio (R) between the three groups and the two variates is $\cdot84$, a not unreasonably low figure when the unreliability of the criterion is borne in mind.

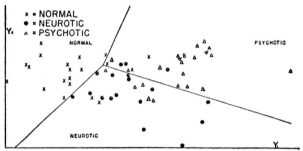

FIG. 4. Variate scores and group segregation using visually fitted lines.

The next step in the procedure consists in computing variate scores for each S on both variates. This is done in the following way. The latent vectors furnish us with two sets of weights to apply to the scores, so that two measures can be calculated for each S, one for each canonical variate. The scores, Y_1 and Y_2, are found by multiplying the score of an S by the appropriate weights and running them over the four tests. A plot of these scores is given in Fig. 4, where normals are represented by crosses, neurotics by dots, and psychotics by triangles. Two methods can be used to segregate the three groups, and thus determine each S's proper status according to his test behaviour. The first method makes use of the Rao quadratic discriminant function to calculate maximum likelihood functions for each S, then allocating him to the most likely of the three groups. This procedure gives 65 per cent of correct classification, as shown in Table II. The second method used fits the discriminant lines visually; these lines are shown in Fig. 4. The number of correct classifications is considerably higher, amounting to 75 per cent, as shown in Table III.

TABLE II

Classification by Discriminant Function Based on Test Scores Compared with Classification Based on Psychiatric Diagnosis

	Test			
Diagnosis	C	N	P	Total
Control	16	3	1	20
Normal	6	10	4	20
Psychotic	2	5	13	20
				60

TABLE III

Classification by Visually Fitted Discriminant Lines Based on Test Scores Compared with Classification Based on Psychiatric Diagnosis

	Test			
Diagnosis	C	N	P	Total
Control	15	2	3	20
Neurotic	0	15	5	20
Psychotic	0	5	15	20
				60

One or two points may call for discussion. A misclassification rate of 25 per cent may seem rather high, particularly when we have in mind the practical application of the method to clinical and selection problems. It seems unlikely, however, that even a set of perfect tests would materially reduce this figure. As Fraser (1947) has shown, an unselected 'normal' group contains between 10 per cent and 30 per cent of persons suffering from severe and often incapacitating symptoms of psychiatric disability; it is only because of the absence of appropriate psychiatric facilities that the persons appear as nominally 'normal'. The test battery would correctly class them in the neurotic or psychotic sectors, but from the point of view of this analysis they would appear to be misclassified.

As regards neurotics misclassified as psychotics, and *vice versa*, the adequacy of the criterion must also be doubted. A review of the reliability of psychiatric diagnoses (Eysenck, 1952) has shown that agreement between psychiatrists, even on major classifications, is far from perfect, and in view of this known deficiency of the criterion the amount of misclassification found is surprisingly small. That this interpretation of the findings is essentially correct is indicated by the following. Two neurotics, marked 'A' and 'B' in the diagram, were placed by the test scores right in the centre of the psychotic cluster. Both were readmitted to the hospital later on, and both had their diagnosis changed from a neurotic to a psychotic one—'schizophrenia' in one case, 'paranoia' in the other. (This change was of course quite independent of the test results: the analysis had not even been completed when it occurred.)

Another point concerns the interpretation and position of the two variates Y_1 and Y_2. The variates are similar, in some of their properties, to Hotelling's principal components in factor analysis. Their position is partly determined by the chance selection of tests, and would not remain invariant under change of some of the tests in the battery. It follows that they usually cannot be interpreted psychologically, any more than can Hotelling's principal components or Thurstone's centroid factors without rotation. Such a 'rotation' in the case of canonical variates is equally permissible, provided it is used to illustrate rather than 'prove' a psychological theory. We can shift our origin and redraw our variates anywhere in the two-dimensional space defined by the original variates, provided that the variates remain orthogonal. Such a rotation has been carried out in an attempt to show that the results of this analysis are compatible with the writer's theory regarding the existence of 'neuroticism' and 'psychoticism', a theory hitherto largely dependent on factor-analytic support. The original variates, Y_1 and Y_2, cannot be interpreted as corresponding to these factors as their position is not invariant. The new variates, Z_1 and Z_2, are shown in Fig. 5; Z_1 corresponds to the factor of 'neuroticism', Z_2 to that of 'psychoticism.'

Similar results, on a much larger scale, were reported by S. G. B. Eysenck (1956), who used 123 normal subjects, 53 neurotics, and 51 psychotics. Six tests were applied to the subjects, including the Maudsley Medical Questionnaire, a Word Association Test, a Static Ataxia Test, a Psychogalvanic Reflex Test, a Manual Dexterity Test, and an Expressive Movement Test of the Luria type. All these tests were found to discriminate at a high level of significance between the various groups.

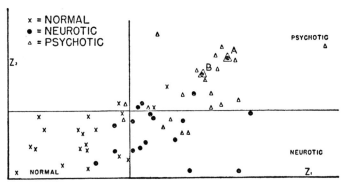

FIG. 5. Rotation of axes of canonical variate solution into psychologically meaningful form.

Using the method of statistical analysis that has been described already, Eysenck obtained the results reported in Table IV. Having demonstrated the significance of both latent

TABLE IV

Latent Vectors

	X_1	X_2
1. Expressive movements	$- 0.450,045$	$-0.116,244$
2. Manual dexterity	$1.000,000$	$1.000,000$
3. P.G.R.	$0.015,541$	$0.072,806$
4. Static ataxia	$- 0.272,682$	$- 0.316,893$
5. Maudsley Medical Questionnaire	$- 0.774,271$	$0.394,398$
6. Word association	$- 0.217,552$	$0.125,206$

Latent Roots

$\lambda_1 = 0.437,605;$ $\lambda_2 = 0.172,877;$ $\lambda_1 + \lambda_2 = 0.610,482$

Diagonal entries of matrix $G^{-1}B = 0.610,484$

Hence λ_1 is *71.7 per cent* of the variance and λ_2 is *28.3 per cent*.

Significance of the Roots

$$X^2 = - \left(N - 1 - \frac{q + c}{2} \right) \log_e (1 - \lambda)$$

$R_1{}^2 = \lambda_1 : X^2 = 127.507$ which is significant at the 0.1 per cent level.
$R_2{}^2 = \lambda_2 : X^2 = 42.026$ which is significant at the 0.1 per cent level.
Total λ_1 and $\lambda_2 : X^2 = 169.533$ which is significant at the 0.1 per cent level.

roots, i.e. having demonstrated the necessity of postulating two dimensions in the description of neurotic and psychotic patients, Eysenck, as a final step, computed scores for each subject on both canonical variates as well as the misclassification for each group. Use was made of the Rao quadratic discriminant function analysis.

'The method is lengthy but the principle is quite straight-forward. The latent vectors gave two sets of weights to apply to the scores, so that two measures could be calculated for each

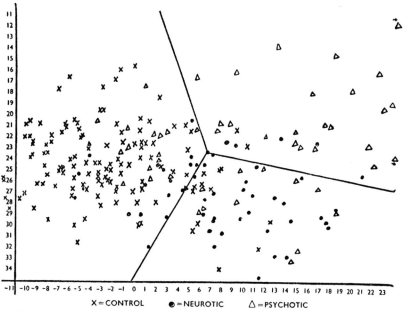

X = CONTROL   ● = NEUROTIC   △ = PSYCHOTIC

Fig. 6. Variate scores and group segregation using minimum likelihood solution.

subject, one for each canonical variate. These scores, Y_1 and Y_2, were found by multiplying the score of a subject on the tests by the appropriate weights, and summing them over the six tests. Having thus found a composite score for each person on both canonical variates, his position with respect to each axis was plotted, and these co-ordinates were then used in a Rao quadratic discriminant function analysis.

'This implies the use of a formula to ascertain the likelihood of a subject belonging to each group. In Fig. 6 each subject was given a position, using crosses to denote controls, dots to denote neurotics, and triangles to denote psychotics. To find the best line of demarcation between the groups, the likelihood scores for borderline cases of the three groups were found, the first lines of demarcation being judged by eye. The likelihood (L_{ij}) of the ith person belonging to the jth group is given by the equation (Lubin, 1950):

$$L_{ij} = 2 \log_e (n_j) - \log_e/C_j/ - d_{ij}C_j{}^{-1}d_{ij}$$

where n_j = number of people in the jth group,
 C_j = covariance matrix for that group,
 d_{ij} = a (1×2) vector giving the deviations of the ith subjects' scores from the mean scores for the group concerned.

'The borderline cases, of whom there were some thirty, each had their likelihood scores calculated from the formula above, one for each of the groups irrespective of that to which he was allocated by diagnosis. The best lines of demarcation were thus found.

'In this way it was possible to reclassify the subjects according to their calculated likelihood scores, and the results of this appear in Table V. From these figures it will be seen that 29 per cent of the subjects were misclassified. Furthermore, if another line is drawn (by eye), in order to find the amount of misclassification between neurotics and psychotics (i.e. leaving out the rather large control group), the misclassification between them is only 21 per cent.'

TABLE V

Test Score Diagnosis

	Psychiatric Diagnosis			
	Controls	Neurotics	Psychotics	Totals
Psychotics	2	5	23	30
Neurotics	12	29	11	52
Controls	109	19	17	145
Totals	123	53	51	227

We may summarize our data and say that whether we use psychiatric symptom ratings or objective psychological tests, and whether we use factor analysis or canonical variate analysis, the answer is the same: two continua, factors, or dimensions are required for the description of neurotic and psychotic disorders, and the hypothesis of a single continuum is

25

rendered somewhat untenable. It would, of course, be possible by the introduction of a number of unlikely *ad hoc* hypotheses to render the facts not completely incompatible with a modified form of the one-dimensional theory, but not without relinquishing those parts of that theory which make it attractive and which give it its unique simplicity.

In searching for a dynamic theory of anxiety and hysteria, then, we may dismiss psychotism from our search, and concentrate rather on neuroticism. Within the neurotic field at least, is it possible to apply a uni-dimensional hypothesis and regard different syndromes and symptoms as differentiated from each other merely in terms of different degrees of severity of illness? Again, the answer must be 'no'. There is considerable evidence, which has been reviewed in great detail in *The Structure of Human Personality* (Eysenck, 1953), that the traditional psychiatric syndromes in the field of neurosis are generated by two factors, continua or dimensions; namely, those of neuroticism and of extraversion-introversion. As Jung was the first to point out, hysteria is a syndrome typically found in the extraverted neurotic; psychasthenia is a syndrome typically found in the introverted neurotic. (The term psychasthenia has become obsolete in recent years and the writer has suggested the term 'dysthymia' as denoting the neurotic syndrome characterized by anxiety, reactive depression, and/or obsession-compulsion features. This term will from now on be used to describe the introverted neurotic.) Results from a factor-analytic study of symptom-ratings on 700 neurotics give the picture shown in Fig. 7 (Eysenck, 1947); they illustrate the position adequately.

This descriptive two-factor pattern of neuroticism or emotionality on the one hand, and extraversion-introversion on the other, is not exactly a modern discovery. It is already apparent in Galen's humoral doctrine, particularly in the form given it by Kant and Wundt. (An excellent discussion of these earlier studies is given by Roback, 1931.) Wundt grouped the four temperaments according to two principles, contrasting the quick (extraverted) with the slow (introverted), and the strong (emotional) with the weak (non-emotional). In his terminology, therefore, the hysteric would emerge as being choleric and the dysthymic as being melancholic. The non-neurotic extraverts and introverts would appear, respectively, as the sanguine and the phlegmatic.

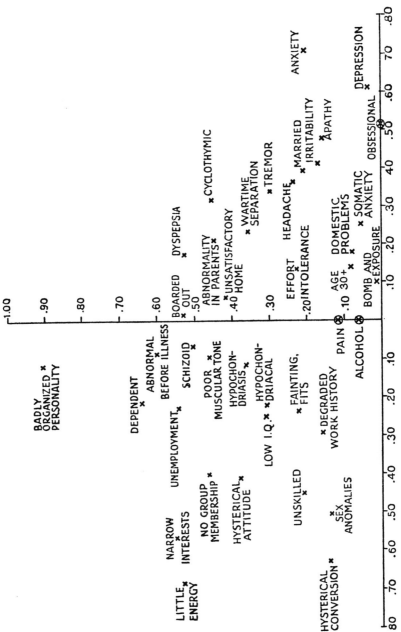

Fig. 7. Items defining neuroticism and extraversion-introversion factors.

THE DYNAMICS OF ANXIETY AND HYSTERIA

In more modern times a more explicitly dimensional theory of temperament has been advanced, particularly by Jordan, by Gross, and by Jung. Descriptively this general theory has been strengthened very much by a large number of extensive experimental and statistical studies which the writer has summarized elsewhere (Eysenck, 1953). Table VI shows some of the differences between extraverts and introverts which have

TABLE VI

	I	E	Reference
Neurotic syndrome:	Dysthymia	Hysteria; Psychopathy	Eysenck, 1947
Body build:	Leptomorph	Eurymorph	Eysenck, 1947
Intellectual function:	Low I.Q./Vocabulary ratio	High I.Q./Vocabulary ratio	Himmelweit, 1945; Foulds, 1956
Perceptual rigidity	High	Low	Canestrari, 1957
Persistence:	High	Low	Eysenck, 1947
Speed:	Low	High	Foulds, 1952
Speed/Accuracy ratio:	Low	High	Himmelweit, 1946
Level of aspiration:	High	Low	Himmelweit, 1947; Miller, 1951
Intra-personal variability:	Low	High	Eysenck, 1947
Sense of humour	Cognitive	Orectic	Eysenck, 1947, 1956
Sociability	Low	High	Eysenck, 1956, 1957
Repression	Weak	Strong	Eriksen, 1954
Social attitudes:	Tender-minded	Tough-minded	Eysenck, 1954
Rorschach test:	M% High	D High	Eysenck, 1956
T.A.T.	Low productivity	High productivity	Foulds, 1953
Conditioning	Quick	Slow	Franks, 1956, 1957
Reminiscence	Low	High	Eysenck, 1956
Figural after-effects	Small	Large	Eysenck, 1955
Stress reactions	Over-active	Inert	Davis, 1948; Venables, 1953
Sedation threshold	High	Low	Shagass, 1956
Perceptual constancy	Low	High	Ardis & Fraser, 1957

been demonstrated experimentally. This table is by no means exhaustive, but it will give the reader a general idea of the kinds of test used in this connection.

A typical research illustrating the relationships between extraversion-introversion, neuroticism, and the various psychiatric diagnoses has been reported by Hildebrand (1953). He tested 25 anxiety states, 10 obsessionals, 10 reactive depressives, 25 hysterics, 20 psychopaths, and 55 neurotics with a mixed diagnoses, making a total of 145 patients. He also tested 25

28

normal soldiers, and as this proved to be a rather unsuitable group, the present writer tested a further 20 normals. (The original normal group was made up of soldiers from a reallocation unit. Soldiers tend to be sent to these units for different disciplinary reasons, and many of them are, in fact, borderline cases of psychopathy and hysteria. From what is known about this group, therefore, it would be expected to be unusually extraverted in its behaviour. This had, in fact, been noted before on several occasions when samples from this population were tested. The second normal group will be referred to as N_2 as opposed to the old normal group, which will be referred to as N_1; it was made up of civilians from whom there was no reason to expect any particular deviation from average behaviour in the direction of either extraversion or introversion. Intelligence tests were given to these various groups without showing any discrimination between them.)

A large battery of tests was given to the subjects, including various questionnaires, a sense of humour test, an aesthetic preference test, tests of suggestibility and static ataxia, qualitative performance in the Porteus Maze test, a persistence test, and a measure of body build. All in all, 22 tests were selected and correlations run between them for all the group, excluding the normals, the hysterics, and the anxiety states; these groups were retained as criterion groups. A factor analysis was then carried out by means of Lawley's maximum likelihood method, and three main factors extracted. These factors were identified respectively as those of neuroticism, extraversion, and intelligence. If these identifications were correct, then factor scores on the extraversion factor should differentiate between hysterics and anxiety states, while factor scores on the neuroticism factor should differentiate between the normal and the neurotic groups. Both these predictions were verified and Fig. 8 shows the actual factor scores of the various groups in the experiment. As predicted, the three dysthymic groups (anxiety states, reactive depressives, and obsessionals) have high scores on introversion and neuroticism; the extraverted neurotic groups, i.e. the hysterics and psychopaths, have high scores on neuroticism and extraversion, with the mixed neurotics having high scores on neuroticism and intermediate scores on extraversion. The extraverted normal group (N_1) is indeed found in the extraverted normal quadrant, while the other normal group (N_2)

has high scores on normality and is intermediate with respect to extraversion. The results of the experiment are very much in line with the hypothesis.

Descriptively, then, there appears to be some reason to suppose that psychiatric diagnoses can be translated into dimensional terminology along quite objective lines. It is suggested that precise description, in terms of a small number of

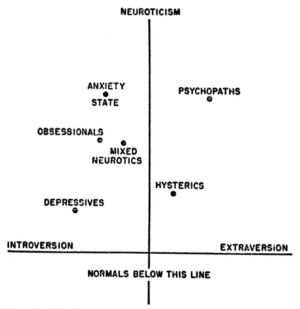

Fig. 8. Position of various clinically diagnosed neurotic groups on two continua as determined by factor scores.

dimensions, is preferable both theoretically and practically to description in terms of an ever-increasing list, or catalogue, of specific diagnoses. It is not suggested that the three dimensions of psychoticism, neuroticism, and extraversion-introversion, with which we have been dealing so far, are the only ones which play a part in abnormal behaviour; it is highly probable that further research will succeed in unearthing other major dimensions. It is clear, however, that the dimensions discovered so far cover a good deal of the ground, and justify a more detailed study in order to throw light on the causal relationships.

The methodology of such further work may require a brief

discussion. Ideally we would wish to measure the precise degree of neuroticism and extraversion of our subjects by means of a large battery of objective tests. We would then test our theories by submitting selected groups of extraverts and introverts, or people high and low respectively on neuroticism, to the experimental tests suggested by our hypothesis. Unfortunately, this is not a practical procedure because few subjects are willing or able to spare the time required. Consequently, one of two substitutes had to be adopted. One of these substitute methods makes use of psychiatric diagnoses as a method of selection, i.e. we may take dysthymics on the one hand, and hysterics and psychopaths on the other, as examples of our introverted and extraverted groups respectively. (Bearing in mind, of course, that those groups would also have high scores on the neuroticism.) This method has obvious disadvantages; psychiatric diagnoses are not very reliable, and different psychiatrists often have different notions of the nature of hysteria, psychopathy, or dysthymia. While these difficulties are great, they are not insurmountable. In selecting extreme cases, psychiatric reliability tends to be higher than when covering the whole range. Different views of the nature of the defining symptoms of a given disorder can often be overcome by a detailed discussion prior to the beginning of the experiment. The method is a makeshift one but it is too useful to be given up completely.

An alternative which suggests itself is the use of questionnaires whose factor loadings on neuroticism and extraversion are known. In the Hildebrand study, for instance, Guilford's D and C scales and the Maudsley Medical Questionnaire had loadings of about ·8 on the neuroticism factor; Guilford's R scale had a loading of approximately ·6 on the extraversion factor. The writer (Eysenck, 1957) has, on the basis of findings such as these, elaborated two brief but very reliable questionnaires which may be used as reasonable criteria for the selection of groups located towards extremes of one or the other of our two factors. The use of questionnaires in this connection also has obvious disadvantages, many of which have been discussed by the writer elsewhere (Eysenck, 1953).[1] Nevertheless, when

[1] There are three widely used, well conceived and constructed sets of questionnaires in the personality field which claim to measure a variety of traits. It has been shown that the Guilford series gives rise to second-order factors closely related to extraversion-introversion and neuroticism (Eysenck, 1953), and that the M.M.P.I.

THE DYNAMICS OF ANXIETY AND HYSTERIA

carefully constructed, questionnaires may give useful information which it would not be wise to disregard completely. Most
of the studies reported in the following chapters have made use
of one or the other of these two methods; occasionally, the
methods have been combined (diagnoses + questionnaires).
Such a combination or 'double screening' procedure overcomes
some of the disadvantages attaching to either method when
used singly. It is probably the most satisfactory alternative
available at the moment to selection by means of a whole
battery of tests.

One additional method is available to us in selecting contrasting populations for the testing of hypotheses relating to the
nature of extraversion and introversion. This method consists
in the comparison of patients with brain-damage and others
not so afflicted. The behaviour of brain-damaged patients and
patients who have had leucotomy operations performed on them
strongly reminds the observer of the behaviour of extremely
extraverted and even hysterical and psychopathic individuals.
The change from the former, often strongly introverted, personality of such patients is certainly startling, and many clinical
reports and accounts exist to bear out this general observation.
Most of the experimental work relevant to this general propo-
sition has been carried out by A. Petrie (1952, 1953, 1956),
partly in collaboration with Le Beau (1954, 1956). The details
of this work are very complex, but the guilding principles are
essentially simple. They may be stated as follows: If a given
operation is predicted to produce a certain shift on a given
personality continuum, *then all tests which are significantly associated with this personality continuum should change in a predictable
direction.* To prove therefore that there is a shift in the direction
of greater extraversion after pre-frontal lobotomy, we would
have to administer a battery of, say, six tests before, shortly
after, and a year after operation. These tests, if properly chosen
from factorial studies as good measures of extraversion, should

by suitable manipulation can also be scored so as to measure these two second-
order factors (Eriksen, 1955; Franks *et al.*, 1957). The third system, that of
Cattell's 'sixteen personality factor questionnaire' (Cattell *et al.*, 1949), has also
been analysed recently (Cattell, 1957) with a view to discovering second-order
factors, and it is reassuring to find that he too ends up with extraversion-introversion and a neuroticism factor, as well as another factor which might be identified
with psychoticism. Thus there appears to be some degree of agreement in this
field, rather along the lines adumbrated by the writer (Eysenck, 1953).

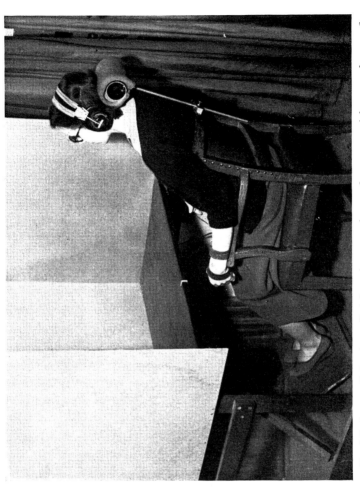

5. Eyeblink conditioning. Subject in sound-proof room, with ear-phones for transmission of conditioned stimulus, special glasses for transmission of un-conditioned stimulus (puff of air) and registration of eyeblink. Note attach-ments on hand for registration of PGR.

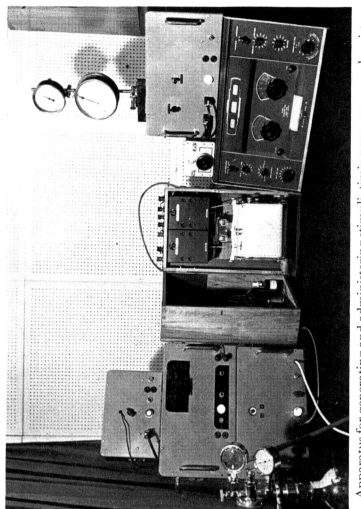

6. Apparatus for generating and administering stimuli, timing sequences, and register-ing responses, in conditioning experiment.

all show a change in score in the direction of greater extraversion. The same applies to changes in neuroticism, psychoticism and intelligence, all of which have been investigated by Petrie.

The main results of this work have been summarized by Petrie (1952), and by Le Beau (1954) in his book *Psychochirurgie et Fonctions Mentales* in the form of three main conclusions:

(1) The observed changes in behaviour do not depend entirely on the amount of brain tissue removed. Extraversion, for example, increases after an operation involving the convexity, but there is no indication of any such increase after cingulectomy. Indeed, after this operation, the small changes which are observed point, if anything, to an increase in introversion. As regards psychoticism, the difference is equally impressive; after cingulectomy, all the tests which serve as a measure of psychoticism show a decreased score, whereas after operations involving the convexity, there is no such diminution.

(2) The observed changes support the theory favouring localization of different functions in different parts of the frontal lobes. Le Beau gives a figure in which changes in the different personality factors are related to operations involving different Brodman areas. He adds as a warning that one is not justified in concluding from a schematic diagram such as this that there exists in these zones mental functions exactly corresponding to the observed personality changes. Nevertheless, he concludes, there is here a demonstration of a certain specificity, and he makes a further point that the psychological test results agree, to a remarkable extent, with clinical observations of post-operative syndromes.

(3) A comparison of selective operations and of leucotomies demonstrates also the existence of a quantitative factor, as far as the convexity is concerned; this quantitative factor is related both to the degree of neuroticism and, even more strongly, the increase in extraversion after operation.

This relationship between brain-damage and extraverted behaviour has been discussed by the writer in detail before (Eysenck, 1952), as have been the many qualifications which must be added to this general statement to make it square with the facts (cf. Yates, 1954). Nevertheless, even allowing for the influence of many other factors additional to those under discussion, it is a tenable hypothesis that among many other effects brain damage produces in general a tendency towards more extraverted behaviour patterns. If this be admitted, and the evidence from both clinical and experimental studies is certainly strong, then we would expect any general theory of extraversion to be able to predict this fact also, and conversely, we would be able to use brain-damaged patients as examples of extraverted patients to be contrasted with non-brain-damaged subjects who on the average would be predicted to be more introverted. This use of brain damage as an extraverting factor is very tentative, but we shall see that the experiments to be summarized in the next chapters tend to bear out the theory on which this use has been based.

We have very briefly and inadequately indicated the rough picture produced by our taxonomic or descriptive studies; we must now in the next chapter turn to an equally brief and inadequate discussion of those general psychological laws which we propose to apply in order to explain the facts summarized in Table VI, and to predict further phenomena associated with extraversion and introversion respectively. The rest of the book will then be devoted to a discussion of the experimental results achieved in this connection.

Chapter Two

LEARNING THEORY AND HUMAN BEHAVIOUR

As pointed out in the Introduction, the main purpose of this book is the twofold one of deriving all or most of the known phenomena regarding extraversion (hysteria) and introversion (dysthymia) from the postulates of a general behaviour theory, and of making deductions from these principles on to hitherto unknown phenomena which can be verified or disproved experimentally. This chapter attempts to present, very briefly and succinctly, an outline of the behaviour theory in question, and to illustrate the process of deduction from it by means of several examples. It may appear a task of supererogation to present the postulate system of this behaviour theory here because this has been done so well by Hull (1940, 1943, 1951, 1952) in his original publications, and by McGeoch and Irion (1952), by Osgood (1953), and by Hilgard (1956), in their various summaries. There are three reasons why the present course was adopted.

In the first place, while psychological readers of this book may be assumed to be thoroughly familiar with the details of modern learning theory, no such assumption seems tenable with respect to psychiatrists, psychoanalysts, anthropologists, or the hypothetical 'intelligent layman', all of whom might be interested in the theory here developed, at least to the extent of giving it a passing glance. It is unlikely that most of these readers would be willing to undertake the considerable labour of acquainting themselves even with the outlined discussions obtainable in the books mentioned above.

In the second place, there are many assumptions and

35

postulates in Hull's behaviour system which are not essential for the theory here presented. Thus, to take but one example, the Hullian theory is a *reinforcement* theory in the sense of postulating that the learning of repeated stimulus-response connections only takes place when drive reduction reinforces or rewards the response in question. This postulate distinguishes Hullian theory from so-called contiguity theories such as Guthrie's or Tolman's, which do not make this assumption. There has been much argument about the place of reinforcement in learning theory and experimental evidence has been produced to throw some doubt on the universality of the reinforcement postulate. Yet the deductions from our own theory are not dependent on this particular postulate, and critics of reinforcement theory would be able to accept our deductions, if these be otherwise considered reasonable, as easily as can adherents of reinforcement theory. In order to avoid the rejection of our deductions on the basis of the rejection of *irrelevant* Hullian postulates, it seemed desirable to give a brief account of those parts of behaviour theory which are, in fact, relevant to our deductions, mentioning other postulates only in order to round off the historical presentation.

In the third place, the Hullian system, even when purged of certain postulates which are not absolutely essential for our deductions, is still subject to criticism on two grounds:

(*a*) There are internal contradictions, some of them caused, at least in part, by Hull's failure to specify clearly enough his meaning, others definitely implying logical contradictions. The most serious example of this, as we shall see, occurs in connection with his development of the theory of inhibition, and we have found it necessary to propose a rather different formula to the one given by Hull himself.

(*b*) There is experimental evidence which fairly decisively negates certain assumptions made by Hull, and where these assumptions are relevant to our own deductions, it has been found necessary to change Hull's theory in the direction of making it conform to experimental facts. As we shall see later, this has been necessary particularly in respect to Hull's so-called 'work' theory of inhibition, which is peripheral in nature. The evidence has forced us to return to the Pavlovian notion of central inhibition, and as this point is crucial to our system of deductions, it has been necessary to present some of the evidence.

This chapter, therefore, is included in order to give readers unfamiliar with modern learning theory an inkling of the constructs used, their method of combination, and the way in which observable phenomena are derived from the theory; in order to indicate which are the essential parts of the theory from the point of view of the deductions made, and which are the parts which can be jeopardized without damage; and in order to rewrite some of the Hullian postulates to make them logically consistent, and more in line with recent experimental evidence. The concepts used and some of the deductions given by way of exemplification have been illustrated by reference to results from our own laboratory. This has been done not so much because these results are better than those usually quoted in the literature, but simply because the methods and types of apparatus illustrated here will be used in later chapters by way of proof of certain deductions following from our own postulates. Thus, for instance, the process of conditioning and extinction is illustrated not in terms of the usual salivation of Pavlovian dogs, but in terms of our own work with the conditioned eye-blink reflex, the reason being that in our experiments with hysterics and dysthymics, we have relied largely on the conditioned eye-blink for evidence in respect to the deductions made from our typological postulate. This eye-blink experiment is introduced here rather than later in order to save space and avoid duplication.

In a similar way, the particular phenomena used in this chapter to illustrate deductions from Hullian theory (the work decrement, the effects of massed practice, and reminiscence effects) have been chosen from the very large number of possible experimental demonstrations because these are the phenomena which we have used in our experimental work to test the predictions made from behaviour theory in conjunction with our typological postulate. Other possible derivations and phenomena are mentioned in passing, but very detailed discussion would go well beyond the limits of a chapter such as this. The same is true of the presentation of alternative theories, and a detailed discussion of the experimental evidence in the light of published criticisms. The reader who wishes to go into these matters in sufficient detail to form an independent opinion will perforce have to go to the original literature and make himself thoroughly familiar with the theories and the experiments constituting modern learning theory. It is one of the writer's cherished hopes in writing this book that it may serve as a stimulus to psychologists and non-psychologists alike to make themselves more familiar with what is undoubtedly the central and most highly developed part of modern psychology, in order to be able to discover for themselves the rich opportunities of application and of research given by this system.

Modern behaviour theory, particularly in the form which Hull has given it, can best be understood as an attempt to integrate two great experimental schools each of which has concentrated its efforts on one particular type of experiment. These two schools are that of Pavlov, employing the conditioning type of experiment, and that of Thorndike, making use of trial-and-error learning. In turn these two schools are connected with certain semi-philosophical doctrines going back over many years and known respectively by the terms *associationism* and *hedonism*. Pavlov, following the associationists, considered the principle of *contiguity* as the most basic one in the modification of conduct; Thorndike, following the hedonists, considered the law of *effect* the most basic one in the modification of conduct. It was left to Hull, Tolman, and other modern learning theorists to try and reconcile these two great principles.

Large numbers of philosophers from Aristotle, through Hobbes and Locke, to Hartley, Hume and Mill, have discussed the problems of learning, memory and thought in terms of the association of ideas; this association might be based on contiguity alone, or alternatively, similarity and other factors might be admitted. Little advance was possible while philosophical discussion and accidental observation were the only tools of investigation and while unsubstantial 'ideas' constituted the hypothetical elements between which, through the action of association, connections were being formed. It was left to Pavlov to substitute for subjective and unobservable ideas, measurable and objective stimulus-response connections and to show in his conditioning experiments how a law governing the formation of these connections could be experimentally investigated.

Pavlov's fundamental conditioning and extinction techniques are almost universally known. A particular stimulus which reflexly, or from a lengthy period of previous learning, causes a particular response, is selected for investigation; this stimulus is known as the UCS, or unconditioned stimulus. Also selected is a neutral stimulus known as the CS or conditioned stimulus, the main property of which is that it does not produce the response in question. Thus a puff of air delivered to the cornea of the eye might be the UCS for the eye-blink response; a tone delivered over ear-phones might be the CS. Before the experiment starts, the experimenter would make sure that the tone itself did not produce an eye-blink, but that the puff of air invariably did so. In a typical Pavlovian experiment the CS would be paired a number of times with the UCS until finally the CS alone, and without the accompaniment of the UCS, would be capable of producing the response. In other words, by pairing a number of times the sound with the puff of air, we would finally arrive at a point where the sound alone would produce the eye-blink.

Details of the procedure used in our laboratories and representative results will now be given. The experiment takes place in a sound-proof or, at least, sound-deadened room, as disturbing noises from the outside may have serious effects on the experiment. The experimental room is divided in two by means of a curtain, the experimenter and all the apparatus being in one part, the subject all by himself in the other, without any disturbing visual stimuli of any kind, excepting a small red light which the subject is instructed to fixate throughout the experiment. The subject is given ear-phones which are padded to exclude any slight noises made by the apparatus and the experimenter, and which transmit the CS, which is a pure tone delivered to both ears at a frequency of 1100 cycles per second for a duration of 800 m.sec. (All time intervals are accurately controlled by means of an electronic timer.)

The subject also wears a spectacle frame, the right lens of which has a small aperture into which a plastic polythene tube is fitted. Air supply from a compressed air cylinder is puffed into the eye through this tube by means of an electrically operated valve. This UCS consists of an air puff lasting 500 m.sec. delivered at a pressure of 65 mm. of Mercury through the 2·5 mm. internal diameter polythene tube at approximately 2 cm. from the right eye. The eyelid movements are recorded by means of a photo-electric cell attached to the same spectacle frame as the polythene tube. This photo-electric method of recording eyelid movements is particularly suitable for working with nervous subjects and patients since it does not require any electrodes or artificial eyelashes to be attached to the eyes of the subject, and the subject does not have to keep his head rigidly still. The method has been described in detail elsewhere (Franks & Withers, 1955); briefly it makes use of a small photo-electric cell and linear amplifier, the amplifier EMF being used to drive the pen of a recording milliammeter. This milli-ammeter is equipped with several channels so that eyelid move-ments, the occurrence of the CS and the UCS, as well as recordings of the P.G.R. and other autonomic reactions, all appear on the same record. The apparatus and setting are shown in Plates 4, 5, and 6.

The procedure used would be as follows: Before the con-ditioning session is begun, each subject is given three tone stimuli. These are followed by three air puffs, and these in turn are followed by three more tone stimuli. Sufficient time is allowed to elapse between the conditioned and the uncon-ditioned stimuli to eliminate any possibility of learning through contiguity. Subjects who give reactions to the last three tone stimuli are excluded from the conditioning study in order to eliminate the possibility of pseudo-conditioning or original sensitivity to the tone. (The term pseudo-conditioning refers to a phenomenon in which the conditioned stimuli produce such a marked increase in the sensitivity of the subject that he now reacts to stimuli to which he did not react previously, and which had not been paired with the conditioned stimulus.)

The conditioning session consists of 30 reinforced trials, i.e. trials in which the puff and the tone are paired; these are randomly interspersed with 18 test trials or acquisition trials in which the tone only is given so as to make possible the measure-ment of the amount of conditioning that has taken place. After the acquisition trials, 10 extinction trials are given, i.e. trials during which the tone is never reinforced by the puff of air, and during which, as Pavlov had shown, conditioned reflexes become deconditioned, unlearned, or extinguished.

Hearing thresholds are obtained for both ears simultaneously for the frequency of 1100 cycles per second, and all subjects excluded whose hearing thresholds are below − 20 db. The red light which the subject has in front of his eyes at a distance of about 3 feet, has 6·3 v. and 0·5 amp. The subject is instructed to look at it whenever it is on, and the experimenter switches the light on five to ten seconds before any stimulus is delivered and switches it off a few seconds afterwards. This procedure reduces strain in the subject and ensures that his eyes are open during the critical period just before any stimulus is delivered, without having to tell him to keep his eyes open; it also reduces

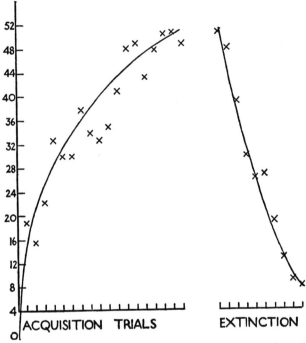

FIG. 9. Acquisition and extinction of conditioned eyeblink reflex.

eye movements and spontaneous blinking during this critical period.

A conditioned response is recorded whenever the record shows a deflection of 1·27 mm. or more during a latency of between 156 and 625 m.sec. after the onset of the CS. The subject is under the impression that his ability to relax is being studied and a passive attitude is encouraged throughout.

Under these conditions the results shown in Fig. 9 are obtained. The curves shown in this figure represent the average records of 94 normal persons of average intelligence, both male and female, who underwent the experiment. (By normal we shall here and in the future mean persons who had never, to the best of our knowledge, had a nervous breakdown or a psychotic episode; who had never sought help or advice from a psychiatrist; who had not been boarded out from the Army or dismissed from a job on the grounds of any form of neuro-psychiatric disorder. These are very crude criteria, and even so it is quite probable that a small number of our subjects would have been rejected if a more detailed investigation could have been made into their past lives. For the purpose of group comparison, however, the criteria seemed sufficient, particularly as success in differentiating such normals from other groups would be achieved in spite, and not because of, any deficiency in our criteria. We considered the possibility of excluding subjects from the normal category in terms of clinical impression, or behaviour during their visit to the laboratory; thus, for instance, it might have been advisable to exclude one subject who fainted on accidentally seeing some apparatus, or another one who, when left alone in a room for a few minutes, disconnected all the leads in the apparatus and connected them up again in random fashion. We considered that the element of subjectivity which such a method of selection would introduce would not be adequately balanced by any advantage in the definition of normality of our experimental group which might be secured.)

The properties of the acquisition and extinction curves shown in Fig. 9 demonstrate regular features which are observed in all such work. Acquisition trials show a negatively accelerated curve tending towards, but not in 30 trials reaching, an asymptote. The extinction curve is negatively decelerated and approximates, but does not reach, zero.

What is the theoretical interpretation of curves such as this? Pavlov assumes that each reinforced trial increases the power of conduction in the central nervous system of certain links between the conditioned stimulus and the response; the condition responsible for this increase he considers to be the temporal contiguity of the CS and the UCS. This increase in conductivity of the connecting link, which he likens to the connection made in a telephone exchange, he calls *excitation*, so that the growth in the acquisition curve in Fig. 9 may be taken to represent a growth in excitation or excitatory potential in the synapses of the central nervous system, or whatever other part of the cortex is taken to be the physiological and neurological locus for this molar concept of excitation.[1]

The decrease in responsiveness shown under conditions of extinction is credited by Pavlov to the action of *inhibition*. This is a rather complex concept in his theory and takes on a number of forms. Fundamentally he seems to have had in mind two rather distinct forms of inhibition which he calls external and internal inhibition. External inhibition arises when during the process of conditioning, some loud noise or other distracting stimulus interferes in the experiment. When this happens the conditioned response is weakened or made to disappear completely. Conversely when such an extraneous stimulus interrupts the process of extinction, the extinguished reflex may suddenly revive for a very brief period. This is called 'disinhibition' or the (external) inhibition of an (internal) inhibition. (Modern learning theorists tend to look for an explanation of 'disinhibition' in terms of the change of stimulus pattern and the different gradients of the stimulus generalization of excitatory and inhibitory potentials.) However that may be, external inhibition is clearly similar in nature to the common-sense concept of distraction, and does not appear to be anything like as mysterious as the concept of internal inhibition.

This is how Pavlov introduces this concept: 'In the second type of inhibition, which may be termed *internal* inhibition, the positive conditioned stimulus itself becomes, under definite conditions, negative or inhibitory; it now evokes in the cells of the cortex a process of inhibition instead of the usual excitation.

[1] Regarding the notion of an actual physical *locus* in the cortex corresponding to the hypothetical link, reference may be made to an experiment by Culler (1938). First of all this investigator conditioned some dogs to contract the right semitendinosus muscle in response to a tone. He then exposed under complete anaesthesia the left cerebral cortex for direct stimulation. As long as the conditioned reflex existed the semi-tendinosus muscle also reacted to direct electric stimulation of a small spot not more than 2 square millimetres in area located on the anterior ectosylvian gyrus 20–25 mm. from the motor point for the semi-tendinosus muscle. *When the conditioned response to the tone was extinguished so was the response to stimulation of this spot, and when the former response was reinstated so was the latter.* No other area with these properties was found in the cortex, and dogs tested before conditioning did not show any evidence of semi-tendinosus contraction on stimulation of the anterior ectosylvian area.

Conditions favouring the development of conditioned reflexes of the negative or inhibitory type are of frequent occurrence, and these reflexes are met with not less frequently than reflexes of the positive or excitatory type. The most striking difference between external and internal inhibition is that, whereas . . . external inhibition is produced on the very first application of an extra stimulus, internal inhibition, on the other hand, always develops progressively, quite often very slowly, and in many cases with difficulty.'

What are the conditions under which this internal inhibition develops? One of them, as we have already seen, is experimental extinction, or the repeated application of a conditioned stimulus which is not followed by reinforcement. The obvious objection that we may be dealing here, not with another process, but simply with the natural decrease of the excitation established in the original conditioning experiment, is met by Pavlov by the experimental demonstration of what is known as *spontaneous recovery*. If, after the reflex has been conditioned and extinguished, a few hours are allowed to elapse, then it will be found that without any further conditioning at all, the conditioned reflex can be produced again by the CS. This suggests the dissipation in time of some form of inhibition which has held the excitatory potential in check. A similar kind of reasoning applies also to the phenomenon of disinhibition. Neither can be explained simply in terms of the growth and decay in time of excitatory potential.

One of the conditions determining the rate of experimental extinction, and thus the growth of internal inhibition, is the length of time elapsing between successive repetitions of the stimulus without reinforcement. 'The shorter the pause the more quickly will extinction of the reflex be obtained, and in most cases a smaller number of repetitions will be required.' Thus, what we will repeatedly encounter under the name of 'massed practice', as opposed to 'spaced practice', appears to be conducive to the growth of inhibition.

Other types of inhibition mentioned by Pavlov are conditioned inhibition, inhibition of delay, differential inhibition, and inhibition with reinforcement. In conditioned inhibition, 'a positive conditioned stimulus is formally established . . . by means of the usual repetitions with reinforcement. A new stimulus is now occasionally added, and whenever the combina-

44

tion is applied ... it is never accompanied by the unconditioned stimulus. In this way the combination is gradually rendered ineffective, so that the conditioned stimulus when applied in combination with the additional stimulus, loses its positive effect, although when applied singly and with constant reinforcement it retains its full powers ... The action of the additional stimulus can be tested ... by applying it in combination with some other positive conditioned stimulus with which it has never previously been associated. In such a case the inhibitory properties of the additional stimulus become clearly revealed, the result being the immediate diminution in the positive reflex response. This is true not only in the case of homogeneous reflexes, but also in the case of heterogeneous reflexes, and the inhibitory effect may extend even to the unconditioned reflexes themselves.'

Closely allied to the concept of conditioned inhibition is that of differential inhibition. Pavlov claims that stimulus-response connections formed during conditioning are not restricted to the actual stimuli employed but show what is called *stimulus generalization*. Thus a dog which has been conditioned to respond with salivation to a touch on the thigh would also respond with salivation to a touch on other parts of the body; in other words, the original stimulus generalizes to other similar stimuli. This stimulus generalization is found to follow a *gradient*, in the sense that the farther away a new stimulus is from the original conditioned one on the stimulus continuum, the less is the response elicited. In one experiment the dog involved gave 53 drops of saliva when touched on the thigh of the hind leg, 45 when touched on the pelvis, 39 when touched in the middle of the trunk, 23 when touched on the foreleg and 19 when touched on the front paw. (The original conditioning experiment had been done on the thigh of the hind leg.)

Pavlov also showed that by means of *conditioned inhibition* it was possible to abolish this stimulus generalization; thus by constantly reinforcing the touch on the thigh, but never reinforcing the touch on the shoulder, the animal would finally inhibit his response to the touch on the shoulder while still responding to the touch on the thigh. This differentiation between similar stimuli Pavlov labelled 'differential inhibition'.

Inhibition of delay is involved when a lengthy time interval is made to intervene between the beginning of the CS and reinforcement. Thus, in what are known as *delayed reflexes* the CS may occur half an hour before the UCS is applied and the reinforcement given. After a period of training the animal will inhibit salivation of the CS until the time for the reinforcement has nearly arrived. Pavlov's proof for the existence of inhibition during this period lies again in the demonstration of the possibility of disinhibition; when, during this half hour period between the application of the CS and the UCS, some external stimulus is applied, the salivation begins immediately.

A last type of inhibition which Pavlov calls 'inhibition with reinforcement' is perhaps the most interesting and important of all. 'The cortical cells under the influence of the conditioned stimulus always tend to pass, though sometimes very slowly, into a state of inhibition.' After a very large number of repetitions with reinforcement, Pavlov found that conditioned reflexes failed to occur. In other words, when the constant strengthening of the conditioned reflex in the orthodox manner has continued too long, finally it produces complete extinction. That this is due to inhibition Pavlov tries to show in the following manner: When an effective positive CS is applied shortly after the application of the CS which has just lost its positive properties, the resulting reflex suffers diminution. Similarly, when one among a number of CS has lost its positive effect, its disuse in the experiment leads to an increase in the effect of the remaining stimuli.

The two types of inhibition which Pavlov distinguishes as external and internal can, with advantage, be termed spatial and temporal inhibition, and an illustration of the hypothetical cortical action underlying them is given in Fig. 10. The *law of temporal inhibition* might be put like this: 'Whenever a stimulus-response connection is made in the central nervous system, both positive (excitatory, facilitative) and negative (inhibitory, obstructive) changes occur in the neural media responsible for the transmission of the impulse. The former type of change is responsible for conditioning and learning and makes easier the passage of the neural impulse linking stimulus and response; the latter type of change is responsible for unlearning and extinction and makes more difficult the passage of the neural impulse linking stimulus and response. Excitatory and inhibitory changes obey different laws; thus inhibition quickly dissipates with time, whereas excitation does not.' This formulation accounts for most of the facts of internal inhibition, though not all; we shall have to wait for a discussion of Hull's theories before we can understand such a phenomenon as that of inhibition with reinforcement.

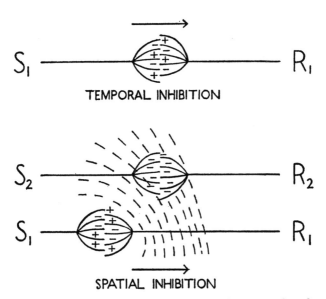

FIG. 10. Schematic representation of temporal and spatial inhibition.

Spatial inhibition, as can be seen from Fig. 10, is quite different from temporal inhibition. In the latter, a simple repetition of neural impulses going through a set of neurones produces certain changes in these neurones and synapses and alters more or less permanently their properties of transmission. In the case of spatial inhibition, two sets of stimulus-response connections occur simultaneously, or so close in point of time that the stimulus traces of the one overlap with the occurrence of the other. Under these conditions the earlier S–R connection interferes with the later one to a degree dependent on the amount of energy involved in both. This interference is of a purely momentary character and has no long-term properties. Where temporal inhibition may be likened to the popular concept of *fatigue*, spatial inhibition may be likened to the concept of *distraction*.

This notion of 'cortical fatigue' is certainly one which Pavlov favours. 'The development of inhibition in the case of conditioned reflexes which remain without reinforcement must be considered only as a special instance of a more general case, since the state of inhibition can develop also when the conditioned reflexes are reinforced. The cortical cells under the influence of the conditioned stimulus always tend to pass, though sometimes very slowly, into a state of inhibition. The function performed by the unconditioned reflex after the conditioned reflex has become established is merely to retard the development of inhibition . . . The fundamental fact in all these experiments, which repeats itself time after time, is the transition sooner or later into inhibition of the state of the cortical elements acted upon by the conditioned stimulus. So as concerns all the experimental evidence at our disposal up to the present, this transition must be regarded as depending on a functional exhaustion of the cortical elements as a result of their activity in response to a stimulus. Such an exhaustion would obviously be dependent upon the duration and intensity of this activity. On the other hand it is also obvious that the process of inhibition cannot be regarded as identical with such functional auto-destruction of the cortical elements, since a state of inhibition which is initiated in an active cell spreads to other cortical elements which were not active and which were not therefore functionally exhausted . . . Hand in hand with the exhaustion of the cortical elements there goes of course their recovery. We should expect, therefore, that the inhibition which appears to stand in some kind of relation to functional exhaustion of the cortical elements should disappear with functional recovery. This expectation fits the case of spontaneous recovery of extinguished conditioned reflexes, which after some interval of time return to their normal strength.' However, Pavlov realized the limitation of the fatigue theory in accounting for all the effects of inhibition. 'It is obvious that only certain cases of the development or disappearance of inhibition can be brought into relation with a supposed functional exhaustion and recovery of the cortical elements, and we cannot interpret in this fashion the cases of permanent and unvarying inhibitions in which the activity of the cortex is so rich —for example, all cases where an established inhibitory conditioned stimulus evokes an inhibition of the cortical elements directly and without a preceding phase of excitation—as, for instance, in the case of differentiation and conditioned inhibition.'

Pavlov was not happy with the concept of external inhibition, and returned to it again under the title of *induction*. This 'concerns the reinforcing effect exerted by one process upon the other, both in respect to the cortical points directly excited or inhibited and those into which the excitation or inhibition had irradiated. This effect will be referred to as *induction*—a term introduced by E. Hering and C. S. Sherrington. Induction is mutual, or reciprocal, excitation leading to increased inhibition and inhibition leading to increased excitation. The former is referred to as "the phase of negative induction" and the latter as "the phase of positive induction", or, briefly, "negative" and "positive" induction respectively.'

An example of negative induction or spatial inhibition will be taken from the work of Ischlondsky (1930, 1949), who has done much to popularize this concept and apply it in the psychiatric field. He takes as his starting-point the common observation that the pain which a person may suffer in the dentist's chair can often be relieved by strong muscular exertion, such as gripping the edge of the seat. This he interprets as a typical case of negative induction in which the positive stimulus, i.e. the gripping of the chair and the consequent increase in receptor activity, *inhibits* the second stimulus-response activity, i.e. the pain responses consequent upon stimulation from the dentist's drill.

Realizing that a more experimental approach was required, Ischlondsky objectified the three variables involved. Instead of the dentist's drill he employed an algesiometer, a kind of thumbscrew device, in which a turn of the screw presses a steel point into the skin of the subject so that the setting of the algesiometer is monotonically related to the amount of pressure exerted on the skin of the subject. The pain threshold was measured objectively by observation of changes in the size of the pupil. As is well known, painful stimuli produce strong excitation of the sympathetic nervous system as a result of which the pupillary muscle contracts and the pupil becomes dilated. Ischlondsky made use of this dilation as an objective index of the pain threshold and found it to be closely related to verbal reports of pain by his subjects. He objectified the pressure of the patient on the edge of the chair by giving his subjects a dynamometer which they had to press to predetermined settings. Having thus objectified the three variables he proceeded to measure the pain threshold of his subjects as a function of the effect of physical effort exerted upon the dynamometer. According to the theory of negative induction a strong primary stimulus (strong pull on the dynamometer) should produce a greater inhibitory effect on the pain stimulus (raise its threshold higher) than would a weak pull on the

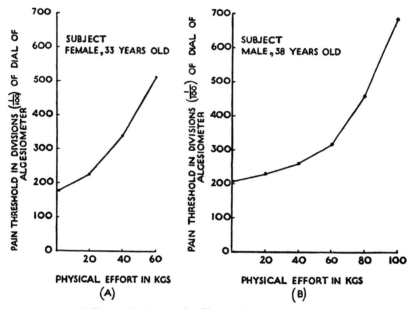

FIG. 11. Effect of physical effort (dynamometer pull) upon pain threshold, as example of spatial inhibition.

dynamometer. Some of his results are shown in Fig. 11, and it will be seen that the results bear out the hypothesis.

Pavlov left the problem of the relationship between what we have called *temporal* and *spatial* inhibition open, and later workers have tended to concentrate almost exclusively on temporal inhibition to the exclusion of spatial inhibition. In Hull's system, for instance, temporal inhibition emerges as I_R (reactive inhibition), while spatial inhibition is largely omitted from systematic consideration. We shall return to this problem in a later chapter.

In his development of learning through association by contiguity Pavlov neglected the important question of motivation almost entirely. He did note that no, or very little, conditioning took place when his dogs were not in a state of hunger, because in that case the unconditioned stimulus itself fails to produce salivation. He did not, however, go on from this observation to elucidate the role that motivation plays in learning generally.

Like the investigation of the forces of association, the study of motivational drives has strong historical roots, particularly in the philosophy of *hedonism*. To the hedonist, the search for pleasure and the avoidance of pain are the great drives which determine individual and social conduct, and which form the basis of social interaction and organization. Like the theory of association, that of hedonism goes back at least to Plato and Aristotle; it received its classical modern statement in the work of Hobbes and Bentham, and was formally introduced into experimental psychology by Thorndike (1898, 1911, 1932, 1949) on the basis of his trial-and-error experiments with cats escaping from puzzle boxes. He named this principle the *law of effect*, and although originally it was only one of several principles it later on became for him by far the most important law in terms of which to interpret animal and human learning. His statement of the law of effect was as follows: 'Of several responses made to the same situation, those which are accompanied or closely followed by satisfaction to the animal will, other things being equal, be more firmly connected with the situation, so that when it recurs, they will be more likely to occur; those which are accompanied or closely followed by discomfort to the animal will, other things being equal, have their connection with the situation weakened so that, when it recurs, they will be less likely to occur. The greater the satisfaction or discomfort the greater the strengthening or weakening of the bond.' Thorndike is careful to give an independent definition of satisfiers and annoyers in terms which are independent of subjective experience and report: 'By a satisfying state of affairs is meant one which the animal does nothing to avoid, even doing such things as to attain and preserve it. By a discomforting state of affairs is meant one which the animal avoids and abandons.'

The law of effect, like the law of association by contiguity, has received a very considerable and searching degree of experimental investigation, and this is not the place to duplicate such reviews as those by Waters (1934), Postman (1943), and others.

We will, instead, go on to consider Hull's attempt to integrate in a formal system these two laws, thus making good the one-sided nature of theories emphasizing only one or the other. In stating his views we must note first of all that Hull, like Tolman and other modern learning theorists, makes a sharp and clear-cut distinction between terms and concepts which are often used interchangeably by earlier writers. These two concepts are those of *habit* and *performance*. In discussing this differentiation, it will be useful to introduce some of the symbols which Hull has so liberally used in his writings, because we shall use these symbols throughout the remainder of the book. The reason for preferring symbols to words is a very simple one. Such a term as 'habit' has many different meanings to different people; thus we use it equally to refer to the *habitual act* itself, as when we say that a person has a habit of smoking or chewing gum; or we use it to refer to the *underlying modification of the nervous system* which, under appropriate circumstances, is in part responsible for the habitual act to occur. It is important to make distinctions such as this, and as ordinary English words cannot easily be used in highly specialized senses, the employment of symbols is almost mandatory.

Hull defines habit ($_sH_R$) as a stimulus-response connection developed through a number of reinforced repetitions (N); performance, or the evocation of this habit in an observable and measurable form, he symbolizes by $_sE_R$. He also uses the concept of *primary drive* (D), which is a term to cover such states as food deprivation, sex deprivation, oxygen deprivation and so on.

These three terms are combined to give the most fundamental law of behaviour, namely $_sE_R = {_sH_R} \times D$. In other words, *habits only issue in observable behaviour when they are acted upon by drives.* Intuitively, this will not appear as an unreasonable kind of statement. A person may have developed a habit of eating fish and chips, or snails, or birds' nests, but he will only translate this habit into action when a drive (hunger) is present.[1]

Concepts such as $_sE_R$, $_sH_R$ and D are what is known as inter-

---

[1] Tolman (1932), Hull's best known opponent, gives a very similar formula, viz. B = f(C, M), where B (performance) is considered as a joint function of the organism's cognitions C and its motivational states M. White (1943) has tried to make Tolman's theory more specific, and has suggested that cognitions and needs combine in a multiplicative manner to determine response strength. There is thus considerable agreement regarding this fundamental formula.

vening variables or hypothetical constructs (McCorquodale & Meehl, 1948). They cannot themselves be observed or measured, and we clearly need observable and experimentally manipulable variables in terms of which to study hypothetical relations expressed in general laws such as the one mentioned above. Roughly speaking, there are two sets of variables which we need to study: on the one hand the antecedent conditions or input variables, i.e. those on the stimulus side; and on the other, the consequent conditions or output variables, i.e. those on the response side. As regards the latter, Hull specifies three main variables which can be used as indicators of $_sE_R$. These are reaction latency $(_st_R)$, or the *speed* with which a learnt response follows a stimulus; reaction amplitude (A), which denotes the *strength* of the learned reaction; and the number of non-reinforced responses to extinction (n).

Among antecedent conditions the important ones are the number of reinforced S–R connections (N); the drive conditions (C_D), such as the number of hours an organism has gone without food, etc.; the intensity of the stimulus (S); and the amount of reward (w), which might be the actual weight of the food given as reinforcement.

Hull's aim is to formulate a set of equations which will link the antecedent conditions (stimulus conditions) with the consequent conditions (response conditions) through a number of hypothetical constructs. These constructs fall into groups which have distinguishable properties. We have already encountered habits and drives; we have also encountered reaction potential. In addition to this we have what may be called S–R conditions such as V (stimulus-intensity dynamism) which is a hypothetical construct produced by stimulus intensity (S), and K (incentive-reinforcement) which is produced by w, the amount of reward offered. (Neither V nor K will play any further part in our development; they have only been mentioned for the sake of completeness. In experimental work they are usually kept as constant as possible, unless, of course, the experiment is directly concerned with S and W as independent variables.)

We must now, however, introduce two further concepts which play a very important part in Hull's theory, and which are of considerable importance also in the application of behaviour theory to personality. These are the concepts of reactive inhibition (I_R) and conditioned inhibition $(_sI_R)$. We will first briefly give Hull's own theory regarding these two types of inhibition, then quote some of the criticisms which have been made of it, and lastly suggest an improved formulation which will be used in our own deductions. Reactive inhibition is closely similar to Pavlov's internal inhibition, or as we have called it, *temporal inhibition*. It is a kind of neural fatigue, produced whenever a response occurs, and as such acts as a barrier to repetition and directly inhibits reaction potential. It also, however, has a second aspect because of the discomfort and pain associated with fatigue generally. These act as *drives* and consequently produce reinforcement whenever I_R is reduced through inactivity. However, we have seen in the general statement of Hull's fundamental law that *whenever a stimulus-response sequence is followed by reinforcement then that stimulus-response sequence becomes associated more firmly*. In the present case, the reinforcement (the cessation of the pain generated by the reactive inhibition produced by an S–R sequence) follows the *cessation* of that S–R sequence, so that the reinforcement applies to the state of rest or non-activity of the specific S–R sequence which had originally generated the I_R in question. Thus after a number of repetitions of the S–R sequence during which I_R is built up, a rest causes the fatigue-like I_R to dissipate, and this dissipation of I_R acts as reinforcement for the non-active state of this particular S–R connection. Thus we get the concept of $_sI_R$ or conditioned inhibition, i.e. the notion of *a habit of not responding*. I_R is a drive which dissipates with rest and therefore produces a non-permanent reduction in $_sE_R$; $_sI_R$ is a habit and therefore produces a permanent reduction in $_sE_R$. Hull makes $_sI_R$ and I_R summate to produce a general state of inhibition $(\bar{I}_R)$ and integrates them with his general formula in the following manner:

$$_s\bar{E}_R = (D \times {}_sH_R) - (I_R + {}_s\bar{I}_R)$$

or, more briefly,

$$_s\bar{E}_R = {}_sE_R - {}_F\bar{I}_R$$

($_s\bar{E}_R$ symbolizes the effective reaction potential, i.e. the reaction potential after inhibition has been subtracted from $_sE_R$).

It will be fairly clear why Hull is postulating two kinds of inhibition. We have already noted in our discussion of Pavlovian work that some inhibition effects are only temporary and dissipate quickly with rest. Other inhibition effects are very long-lasting and do not dissipate. Now, clearly, concepts of a given class must have similar properties, as otherwise their class character is too ill-defined to make prediction possible. While Pavlov realized the problem, he did not succeed in finding a solution to it. Hull was able to do so by a simple and straightforward application of his general principle according to which habits multiply with drives to produce reaction potential. By making I_R a drive dissipating in time, he also ensured in terms of his system the creation of $_SI_R$ as a habit *not* dissipating in time. We thus have two inhibitory variables possessing the required properties and fitting in with the two great classes of concepts, i.e. drives and habits, postulated by Hull.

Hull tried to find an appropriate antecedent condition for the development of reactive inhibition in the amount of work done, stating his general position in the following words: 'The net amount of functioning inhibitory potential resulting from a sequence of reaction evocations is a positively accelerated function of the amount of work (W) involved in the performance of the response in question.' In seizing upon this 'work' explanation of reactive inhibition, which had originally been advanced by Mowrer (1943) and Miller (1941), Hull was enabled to keep his theory 'peripheralist' in contradistinction to the Pavlovian concept of inhibition, which is central.

Hull's theory of inhibition has been subject to a considerable degree of criticism (Koch, 1954). Part of this criticism relates to logical contradictions within the theory itself, others relate to the failure of empirical studies to agree with parts of the hypothesis. Taking the latter first, we find that a number of studies have reported failure to find increased inhibition with an increase in W. Ellis (1953) has discussed the matter in some detail and has pointed out the complexity of the issue involved. (Cf. also an excellent review of 'The influence of work on behaviour' by Solomon, 1948.) Empirically, the position appears to be that sometimes predictions made on the basis of the Miller-Mowrer work hypothesis are verified, but that usually they are not. On the whole the evidence suggests that this part of the inhibition theory should be dropped. (Cf. Trotter, 1956, for a careful experimental refutation of the original Mowrer-Miller argument, as well as a considered criticism of their methodology.)

Related to the experiments on the work hypothesis of inhibition are studies dealing with the peripheral nature of inhibition altogether. It has been shown that reactive inhibition can be generated by perceptual tests involving the minimum of physical effort; an example of this is the Tsai-Partington pathways test in which the subject is given a piece of paper covered with numbers and instructed to trace a line with his pencil from one to two, then from two to three, and so on. The major part of the test consists in the perceptual search for the next number; the muscular movement of tracing the line is slight, and only occurs after the interval of rest during which visual search goes on. Strong reactive inhibition is generated in this test in spite of the almost complete absence of W (Ammons, 1955).

Again it has been shown that inhibition can be transferred from the right hand to the left hand in certain performance tasks, and although a slight part of this inhibition may be due to common muscular innervations such as those involved in standing in front of the desk, or making following movements with the head, there is little doubt that the major part of the inhibition accruing is of central rather than of peripheral origin (Ammons, 1951; Grice & Reynolds, 1952; Irion & Gustafson, 1952; Kimble, 1952; Rockway, 1953).

A third line of argument stems from the work of Hovland and Kurtz (1951), who showed that if a subject does difficult mental work of another kind just before committing a list of nonsense syllables to memory, *more* reminiscence for that list follows than if he did not do this mental work previous to learning, or was permitted a rest between the mental work and the learning task. It is difficult to see how a 'work' theory of the crude 'foot-pounds' type could be applied to mental work of the kind here used, or how a peripheral explanation is applicable. The same comment applies to a fourth type of experimental evidence, namely that related to 'stimulus satiation' in spontaneous alternation behaviour (Dennis, 1939; Montgomery, 1952; Glanzer, 1953).

Even in Pavlov's own work, findings such as that of disinhibition appear fairly crucial in deciding that a peripheral hypothesis is not really warranted by the facts, and that a hypothesis postulating more central inhibitory effects must be used. The term central in this connection means *anywhere within the central nervous system from a point separated by at least one synapse from the receptor organ on the one side, to a point separated by at least one synapse from the effector organ on the other.* It is quite possible, of course, that additional to this central type of inhibition such factors as muscular fatigue, receptor adaptation, and so forth play a part in many of the phenomena discussed under the heading of 'inhibition'. Behaviour is complex and usually determined by more than one factor; it is the task of the experimentalist to try and sort out the various influences present.

In saying that inhibition is a central phenomenon we do not mean to suggest that it is not affected by such determinants as amount of work done, or strength of stimulation. Presumably the total amount of inhibition generated is determined by the number of fibres involved in an activity, the number of synapses crossed, and other factors of a similar kind. An increase in the amount of work done, or an increase in sensory stimulation, presumably involve a larger number of fibres and a larger number of synapses; in this way some of the experimentally demonstrated phenomena usually explained in terms of the work hypothesis on a peripheral conception of inhibition, can also find an explanation in terms of our central theory. (Solomon, 1948, suggests a purely *stimulus* theory of inhibition by making use of the concept of response-produced kinaesthetic stimulation. Such a theory is ruled out by the same experiments which rule out the 'work' theory as a very likely explanation of the facts.)

On the theoretical side, critics have pointed out quite rightly that Hull has not been consistent in his treatment of I_R as a drive variable and sI_R as a habit variable. In his general formulation he postulates that drive and habit variables interact multiplicatively to produce sE_R. Yet he makes I_R additive with sI_R to produce $\dot{I}_R$. This is not admissible in terms of his own theory, and neither is the fact that he subtracts both the drive (I_R) and the habit (sI_R) from sE_R to form $s\bar{E}_R$. As a habit, sI_R should subtract from sH_R, as Osgood (1953) has suggested; in his formulation, I_R would, however, still summate algebraically with sE_R. This solution does not seem radical enough in view of the fact that I_R is conceived as a *drive* by Hull, and a drive can hardly be subtracted from a performance construct.

Gwynne Jones, in an unpublished paper, has suggested a solution more in line with Hull's own general system. In his formulation he groups positive drive (D) with negative drive

(I_R) and positive habit ($_sH_R$) with negative habit ($_sI_R$), so that the final formula reads:

$$_s\bar{E}_R = f(_sH_R + {_sI_R}) \times f(D) + I_R)$$

At this point and before expanding the formula it may be advisable to alter one of the symbols used. I_R has certain traditional connotations, i.e. that of being peripheral, of being dependent on the amount of work done, and of summating algebraically with conditioned inhibition, which makes the use of the symbol in the present context inadvisable. We shall therefore from now on refer to positive drive as D_+ and to I_R, conceived of as a central phenomenon having drive properties of a negative character, as D_-. We can now expand our formula and obtain the following statement:

$$_s\bar{E}_R = f(D_+ \times {_sH_R}) + f(D_+ \times {_sI_R}) + f(D_- \times {_sH_R}) + f(D_- \times {_sI_R})$$

Each of the four terms in this equation contains the product of a drive and a habit, and these products are additive and produce effective reaction potential $_s\bar{E}_R$. It should be noted, of course, that D_- is a negative drive, i.e. a drive leading to the *cessation* of activity, and that $_sI_R$ is a negative habit, i.e. a habit of *not* responding. Thus while $D_+ \times {_sH_R}$ would give rise to a positive $_sE_R$, $D_- \times {_sH_R}$ would give rise to a negative performance, i.e. a failure to react. Similarly, $D_+ \times {_sI_R}$ would produce a failure to react. Of particular interest in this connection is the last term in the equation. Both D_- and $_sI_R$ have a *negative* sign, so that their product should be positive, i.e. a negative drive in conjunction with a negative habit should produce a positive reaction. The phenomenon of disinhibition may be tentatively thought to fall under this category, and other evidence is quoted by Gwynne Jones in his paper.

The whole scheme of antecedent conditions, hypothetical constructs, and consequent conditions is shown in Fig. 12. A few of the symbols appearing in this figure have not yet been discussed, namely, $_sO_R$ and $_sL_R$. These symbols refer to oscillation and reaction threshold respectively, and introduce two important considerations into the determination of the effective reaction potential. Behavioural oscillation ($_sO_R$) is introduced by Hull to account for the fact that reaction potentials ($_sE_R$) vary from moment to moment. Reaction threshold ($_sL_R$) refers to the fact that $_sE_R$ has to reach a certain size (rise above the threshold) before leading to measurable reaction. Adding these to $_s\bar{E}_R$ gives us the momentary effective potential ($_s\tilde{E}_R$) which is indexed by the three outwardly observable consequent conditions already discussed.

This, in very brief outline and leaving out a very large number of qualifications, corollaries, and less relevant postulates, is the behaviour system which we shall use in making our deductions

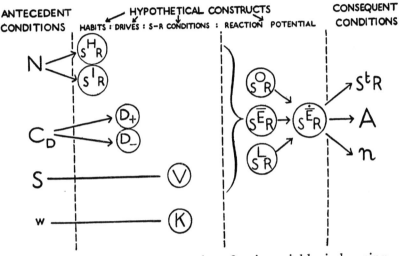

FIG. 12. Schematic representation of main variables in learning theory used to account for personality differences.

or personality theory. Before doing so, however, we may consider for a moment the changes that take place in behaviour as learning proceeds, and see to what extent experimental facts bear out these deductions. Let us take first of all the first term in our equation, i.e. $D_+ \times {_sH_R}$. If we assume that D_+ remains constant during a learning task and that $_sH_R$ grows towards a pre-determined asymptote at a negatively accelerated rate, determined by the number of reinforcements received, we obtain a typical growth curve similar to that shown in Fig. 9. Quite a different type of curve is produced by another term in the equation, namely, $D_- \times {_sH_R}$. Kimble (1949, 1952) has extended Hull's theory by a detailed discussion of the growth of reactive inhibition and in rough outline we shall follow his argument. According to him, D_- grows with each repetition

59

until it reaches a level at which it balances D_+. At this point $(D_+ \times {}_sH_R) + (D_- \times {}_sH_R) = O$, and behaviour $({}_s\bar{E}_R)$ ceases. This cessation of behaviour may be called an *involuntary rest pause* (I.R.P.), and during it a certain portion of D_- dissipates. When enough inhibitive drive has dissipated, activity begins again, and more D_- is accumulated, until the critical level where $D_+ = D_-$ is reached again, and another involuntary rest pause supervenes. Thus, in terms of these two parts of the equation, performance should continue in fits and starts, the

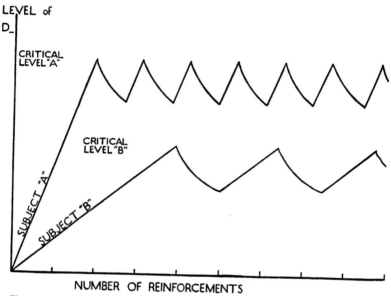

Fig. 13. Schematic representation of mode of action of reactive inhibition.

fits and starts beginning at the point where D_- for the first time reaches the level of D_+ (cf. Fig. 13).

These involuntary rest pauses, as we have noticed before, act as reinforcement to the resting state and generate ${}_sI_R$, or conditioned inhibition. Conditioned inhibition, as a habit, grows in precisely the same fashion as ${}_sH_R$, i.e. in a negatively accelerated manner until it approaches its asymptote. Being a negative habit it acts in the opposite direction to ${}_sH_R$, and as both are multiplied by the same set of drives (D_+ and D_-), the final level of performance will be determined by the levels of the respective asymptotes of ${}_sI_R$ and ${}_sH_R$. Around this final level there will be a certain amount of fluctuation due to the fits and starts introduced by the term $D_+ \times {}_sH_R$, as explained above, and to ${}_sO_R$.

The last term in the equation, i.e. $D_- \times {}_sI_R$, multiplies two negative variables and therefore has a positive outcome which should be set against the $D_- \times {}_sH_R$ term. We thus have a very complex system of determinants for even quite simple learning and performance tasks, and we must now turn to examine some of the documented phenomena in this field to determine whether, in fact, these behave in conformity with our general formula. In doing so we shall start with a set of phenomena often referred to as the *work decrement*.

The reason for this choice is as follows. Our general theory is one of performance rather than of learning, and conceptual analysis becomes much simpler if we take as our object of study a task already practised so much that ${}_sH_R$ and ${}_sI_R$ can be presumed to have come very near to their respective asymptotes. By thus choosing a task practised to such an extent that learning does not occur any more to a significant extent, we simplify our analysis and are able to illustrate certain deductions more clearly than would be possible by the choice of a more complex type of example.

Studies of the work decrement have been very numerous, partly because the results of study of the effect of repetition on complex learning activity were so very different from those of repetition on simple muscular tasks. The latter, which may be exemplified by the pulling of a dynamometer or ergograph in time to a metronome, typically show a rapid decrement with zero performance as the asymptote; this asymptote is approached more-or-less quickly according to the strength of pull required and the muscular endowment of the subject. The findings with respect to mental tasks, however, are quite different (Robinson, 1934), and curves representing long, continued performance on such tasks have certain peculiarities which we are now able to deduce from learning theory. Curiously enough, this task has not previously been performed by learning theorists. One possible reason for this neglect may be related to the Mowrer-Miller work theory of inhibition adapted by Hull and criticized in this chapter. If we accept the work hypothesis of inhibition, then it would be very difficult to explain the differences between muscular work and mental work. If we accept the central theory of inhibition (advocated in this chapter) and use it to account for the phenomona referred to as the *work decrement,* leaving muscular fatigue of a largely peripheral nature to account for the decrement observed in muscular work, then no difficulties arise from the different properties shown by these two types of tasks.

Let us start out then with a simple, largely mental, task having only a relatively slight muscular accompaniment, such as writing as quickly as possible the letters abc, abc, abc, . . . The writing of these letters has been practised so much that we may assume $_sH_R$ and $_sI_R$ to have come very close to their respective asymptotes. D_+ will have a certain size while D_-, at the beginning of the experiment, will be zero. Thus we start at a certain level of performance which is determined by the size of D_+ and the respective asymptotes of $_sH_R$ and $_sI_R$. During the first minute or so of practice, D_- will be growing until it reaches a critical level where it is equal to D_+ and begins to enforce involuntary rest pauses. Let us discuss the period before this critical period is reached. As D_- grows it interacts with $_sH_R$ to produce a decrement in performance, and with $_sI_R$ to produce an increment. As $_sH_R$ is stronger than $_sI_R$, the total effect would be a slight decrement. However, this effect theoretically should be more than compensated by another effect, namely, the extinction of $_sI_R$. We have seen that conditioned inhibition is reinforced by the involuntary rest pauses occurring when D_- equals D_+. During the period now under consideration, i.e. while D_- is growing but has not yet reached the level of D_+, no involuntary rest pauses occur to reinforce $_sI_R$ and, in accordance with the laws of learning, $_sI_R$ being un-reinforced, undergoes extinction. This extinction of conditioned inhibition, which has been experimentally demonstrated by the writer elsewhere (Eysenck, 1956), should produce a steep rise in performance, counterbalanced only to some extent by the slight decrease, predicted previously, due to the growth of D_-.

Thus, our theory would predict an initial spurt lasting until D_- equals D_+ and the involuntary rest pauses again occur to reinforce $_sI_R$. This initial spurt then is the first prediction made from our theory, and there is ample evidence in the literature that on well-practiced tasks, such as those under consideration, initial spurts are nearly always observed. The explanation for these spurts has usually been given in terms of what Pavlov calls 'mentalistic concepts', such as freshness, lack of fatigue or boredom, interest, and so on. The position taken here is that these concepts, and the mental states corresponding to them, are the products of the laws of performance, just as much as are the objective facts of the work curve. What is seen in the work curve as a 'spurt' is subjectively reported by the subject as 'interest'; what is seen in the curve as a decrement is reported subjectively by the subject as 'boredom'. Both spurt and interest are due to the failure of D_- to build up rapidly and produce the involuntary rest pauses which form a reinforcement for $_sI_R$. Both decrement and boredom are due to the effects of D_- and $_sI_R$.

We now come to our second prediction. We have followed the course of work to the point where D_- equals D_+ and where our theory demands the occurrence of short involuntary rest pauses. Two predictions can be made. The first prediction is that performance should now decline because:

(a) $_sI_R$ is again being reinforced and therefore approaches again its asymptotic level, thus impairing performance;

(b) the involuntary rest pauses produce a decrement in performance.

Performance is usually integrated over certain periods of time, such as one minute or ten minutes, and the loss in performance due to involuntary rest pauses will clearly lead to a decrement in total performance as so integrated. Thus, on both accounts we would predict a decrement in performance following the point where D_- equals D_+, and where the initial spurt ends. Such declines are reported almost universally from studies of protracted mental work. We would predict this decrement to continue until $_sI_R$ has approached its asymptote again; from that point onwards the only changes in the level of the curve should be those introduced by the involuntary rest pauses produced by D_-. Again, the long maintained, even rate of performance, continuing for sometimes as long as 24 hours, has been commented on by many investigators. This prediction, too, would therefore appear to be borne out.

So far our theory has made considerable use of the involuntary rest pauses 'bootlegged', as it were, by an organism in whom D_- has reached a critical level. It would clearly be highly desirable to find experimental proof of a more direct kind for

63

the existence of these rest pauses. Particularly important in this connection has been the work of Bills (1931, 1935, 1936, 1943), who states his hypothesis very clearly: '(1) . . . The failure to find large and rapid decrement in mental work, such as is found in muscular work, is due to the fact that the subject gets frequent short rests which give sufficient opportunity for recovering from accumulated fatigue and thus cover up or stave off decrement. (2) The fact of a more or less rhythmic fluctuation in the degree and direction of attention has long been recognized on the subjective side, and it is reasonable to suppose that some corresponding form of fluctuation in performance level would be found as soon as a sufficiently refined technique should be devised for investigating it. (3) The consideration of a refractory period in nerve operations, especially the recent findings of Forbes pointing to the existence of a cumulative refractory period, of greater length than the single phase, suggests that a corresponding recurrent gap in the mental activity ought to occur. (4) Granted the existence of such recurrent periods of lowered mental functioning it would be natural to expect that they would have an important bearing on the occurrence of error and would yield important information about the cause of errors.'

Bills used five different types of mental work, such as colour naming, naming opposites, addition and subtraction, getting his fifty subjects to carry out 7 min. of work on each of 8 days. All responses were verbal, and errors were timed and noted. Bills called the involuntary rest pauses we have been discussing 'blocks', and he defines them as 'pauses in the response equivalent to the time of two or more average responses'. Summarizing these experiments, Bills concludes that 'perhaps the most striking results . . . is the evidence of rhythmic blocking. For all S_s under all conditions of practice and fatigue this rhythm tends to strike an average rate of one block every 17 sec. Individual differences are great . . . some S_s block every 10 sec. and some every 30 sec.' He also noted that 'there is a constant tendency for errors to occur in conjunction with blocks, suggesting that the cause of errors lies in the recurrent low condition of neural functioning, which the blocks reveal.' Altogether his main conclusions offer a striking support for the hypothesis of involuntary rest pauses when he summarizes his findings by saying that: 'In mental work involving considerable homogeneity and continuity, there occur with almost rhythmic regularity blocks, or pauses, during which no response occurs.' [1]

A third deduction from our general theory might be phrased like this: involuntary rest pauses are produced by the accumulation of negative drive up to the level of positive drive prevailing at the time. If these rhythmic accumulations could be prevented by introducing official rest pauses at the time when normally involuntary rest pauses or 'blocks' would have appeared, then these experimenter-produced rest pauses should have the effect of allowing D_- to dissipate. By thus preventing the accumulation of sufficient D_- to produce involuntary rest pauses, the latter should be obliterated from the record. Bills (1936) has reported one such experiment in which he finds indeed that the introduction of experimenter-produced rest pauses, equalling those normally appearing as 'blocks', resulted in the almost complete disappearance of the 'blocks' from the subject's record. Several other writers have verified Bills' conclusion regarding the existence and importance of 'blocking' in continuous work (e.g. Philip, 1939; Maillaux & Neuberger, 1941; Warren & Clark, 1937; Freeman & Wonderlic, 1935).

A fourth deduction from our principles may be made in terms of a general rule formulated by Poffenberger (1927) as follows: 'The more nearly the work involves the continuous exercise of a single function, the more will output of work decrease; and the more varied the functions involved in the work, the less will output of work decrease.' Robinson and Bills (1926), in a well-known experimental study, put the same hypothesis slightly differently: 'It is the broad principle of refractoriness of response that gives the basis for interpreting the influence of homogeneity of work upon the magnitude of the work decrement. The fewer the part-activities involved in continuous work, the shorter will

---

[1] Another author who has been much preoccupied with fluctuations in mental output is Philpott (1932, 1950); he and his students have published some 50 theses and papers, which have been well summarized and reviewed by Warburton (1957). Philpott's main conclusions from all this work were: (1) Curves of output are non-random; (2) Curves contain periodic rhythms; (3) Rhythms in grand total curves tend to be constant in phase. He also argued that these rhythmic fluctuations were of geometric (logarithmic) rather than of arithmetic periodicity. Unfortunately most of the data on which this work was done were expressed as deviations from a moving average, a procedure subject to the Slutzky-Yule effect and thus generating an artificial oscillatory series. Data free from this effect appear to produce regular arithmetic rhythms, thus reinforcing the results of Bills, Robinson, and the other authors quoted above. A repetition of much of Philpott's pioneering work with proper statistical safeguards would appear overdue.

be the time-intervals between the successive stimulations of each of these activities and, within a given time range, the more frequent will be those successive stimulations . . . the degree of refractoriness is a function of both the recency and the frequency with which an activity is called into function.' In other words, more negative drive will be produced by quick and immediate repetition of an activity, because the interpolation of other activities would allow time for D_- to dissipate in part, or in its entirety, before the activity was performed again.

In their experiment Robinson and Bills produced an increase in heterogeneity by making their subjects write either ab, ab, ab, . . .; abc, abc, abc, . . .; or, abcdef, abcdef, abcdef, . . . Twenty-four subjects were used altogether, each writing for 20 min. on each of 6 days. Conditions were rotated and the expected results were found; the more homogeneous the conditions of practice, the greater was the work decrement. A similar result was found when 18 subjects had to read aloud twenty times running letters from a card containing one hundred letters. Different degrees of heterogeneity were produced by having 2, 4, 8, 16, and 24 different letters on different cards, and rotating the order of cards for the different subjects.

The fifth deduction from our general theory may be made in terms of what is sometimes called the 'common element theory of transfer'. If two tasks are made up in such a way that something which they may have in common can be experimentally controlled, will there then be any relation between the amount in common and the amount of transfer of work decrement? If we practise writing adg, adg, . . ., thus producing a large amount of D_- for this particular combination of letters, will this produce a decrement on our performance in tasks, such as writing acfi, acfi, . . .; adji, adji, . . .; adgi, adgi, . . ., in proportion to the number of letters each of these tasks has in common with the original one? Results reported by Bills and McTeer (1932) show clearly that the more elements there are in common between constant and altered tasks, the more deleterious is the influence of the former on the latter. There is a direct and consistent relation between the number of elements common to the two tasks and the amount of decrement transferred from the variable to the standard.

Here then we have five deductions from our general theory, all of which are confirmed by experimental study of the work decrement. It is true that the experiments were carried out, and the results known, before the theory was put forward in its exact form, but it should be noted that Hull in presenting his theory did not refer to studies of the work decrement at all, and that a rather similar theory to that advanced here underlay the experiments done by Robinson, Bills, and the other psychologists we have quoted. Where we now talk about 'inhibition' they framed their hypotheses rather in terms of 'refractoriness' (Dodge, 1917, 1928, 1931; Robinson, 1926, 1934; Bills, 1931, 1943). Nevertheless, these two concepts are very closely related in possessing similar qualities and generating similar predictions. However that may be, the results quoted may be taken as giving strong support to the theory here put forward.

We must now turn to a slightly different set of phenomena, namely, those of massed practice as opposed to spaced practice. When we practise an activity which is relatively new to us, i.e. one in which neither $_sH_R$ nor $_sI_R$ are anywhere near their respective asymptotes, then it clearly follows from our general theory that massed practice should be less effective, other things being equal, than spaced practice, because while both types of practice generate D_-, spaced practice enables this accumulated D_- to dissipate after each unit of practice before the next unit of practice occurs. Consequently, if the distribution of practice is properly arranged, D_- can be prevented from ever reaching a high enough level to equalize D_+, and in this way not only do we prevent the occurrence of involuntary rest pauses but also retard the growth of $_sI_R$ through withholding, to a large extent, the reinforcing conditions which are necessary for its growth. The literature on this point is too great, and the number of adequate summaries easily available too large, to make it worth while to quote experimental support for the truth of this generalization. Under appropriate conditions, massed practice is nearly always found to be inferior to spaced practice (McGeoch & Irion, 1952).

There is one interesting deduction from this line of argument, however, which is rather less well known and which enables us to carry out some rather interesting experiments. If we take the same task and get one group to practise it under massed conditions (M group), while another group practises it under distributed practice conditions (D group), then our theory would lead us to expect a better performance on the part of the D

67

group. But now suppose that we introduce a long rest pause and re-test both groups after this pause. Our D group, not having any considerable amount of D_ to dissipate, would perform at roughly the same level at which performance was terminated by the rest pause. The M group, however, having accumulated a considerable degree of D_ before the rest pause, should have dissipated all, or most of, this negative drive potential during the rest pause, thus starting off at a higher level than that at which performance was stopped by the rest pause. This phenomenon of improved performance after rest is called *reminiscence*, and its experimental verification constitutes an important support for our general theory. (The re-emergence, after a day's rest, of the conditioned reflexes which had been extinguished may be considered an early adumbration of the phenomenon of *reminiscence*.)

A demonstration of this phenomenon, in the form in which it has been used in our experimental work upon personality functions, may illustrate this point. The task used is the so-called pursuit rotor, shown in Plates 7 and 8. It consists of a rotating bakelite disc, somewhat resembling a gramophone turntable. A small metal disc is set flush into the bakelite turntable near its outer rim so that it rotates at a speed of one rotation per second in front of the subject, who is standing facing the apparatus and looking down on it. In his right hand the subject holds an articulated rod with a metal tip; his instructions are to follow the rotating disc with this rod and to try and keep the metal tip of the rod in touch with the metal disc. The apparatus is wired in such a way that whenever the tip touches the disc a current is activated which in turn causes an electric clock to move, which records, with an accuracy of 1,000th of a second, the duration of the contact. There are two such clocks, and an automatic switch throws the one into the circuit and the other out of the circuit every 10 sec. The experimenter writes down the setting on the face of the clock which has just been taken out of the circuit, thus making a record of the exact time during the 10 sec. period that the subject was 'on target'. The clock then automatically resets itself, and when it is thrown into the circuit again the experimenter records the setting of the other clock. In this way it is possible to get a 10 sec. by 10 sec. record of the continuous activity of the subject. Fig. 14 shows the actual performance on this task of two groups of subjects, one

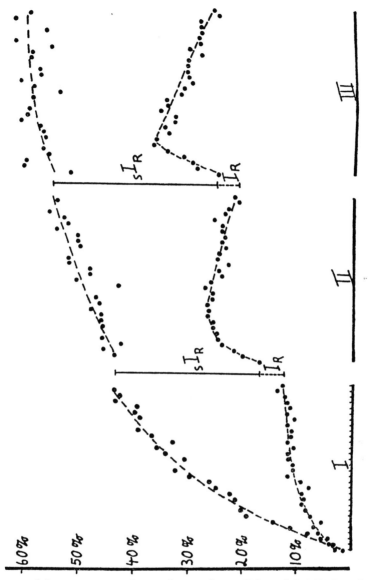

FIG. 14. Measurement of reactive and conditioned inhibition by comparison of massed and spaced practice groups performance on pursuit rotor.

working under conditions of massed practice (the lower set of curves) and one working under conditions of distributed practice (the upper set of curves).

The M group consisted of 50 male university students whose records are averaged in the figure. The task consisted of three sets of 30 consecutive 10 sec. performances, separated by 10 min. rest pauses. Reminiscence phenomena can be seen clearly in the part of the curve marked I_R; they are demonstrated by the improvement of the first 10 sec. period of practice after the rest over the last 10 sec. period of practice before the rest.

The set of curves in the upper half of the figure, which reports the average scores of 25 subjects, consists of 10 sec. trials, separated by 30 sec. rest periods. Each 10 sec. period was preceded by $2\frac{1}{2}$ sec. of practice during which no score was kept. This was done in order to make comparable the 10 sec. period of work in this group with corresponding 10 sec. periods of work in the other group where practice was massed, i.e. continuous. For the massed group each 10 sec. period would begin with the subject already in the middle of his task. If, in the distributed group, the subjects were instructed to begin work at the beginning of the 10 sec. period, then at least a second or two would be lost in his getting the stylus on to the turntable, beginning to move it, etc. The $2\frac{1}{2}$ sec. periods preceding each trial were not scored but, nevertheless, furnished a chance to practise for each subject, and were therefore included in an estimate of the total amount of time spent in practice by the subjects in the D groups. For this reason, therefore, there are only 24 trials for the D group to compare with 30 trials of the M group. This ensures that the amount of time of practice for the two groups would be identical in each of the three periods of practice (300 sec. = 30 × 10 sec. = 24 × $12\frac{1}{2}$ sec.).

One further exception should be noted—the D group started by having three 10 sec. consecutive trials. This was done in order to make comparison possible between the M and D groups with respect to their ability on the task. Statistical analysis failed to show any reason why the null hypothesis should be rejected. After 300 sec. practice and again after 600 sec. practice, the D group was given a 10 min. rest, exactly as had the M group.

Two points will be obvious from the diagram. One is the superiority in learning and performance of the D group over the M group; this is in accordance with our hypothesis. The other phenomenon is the occurrence of conditioned inhibition, i.e. the relatively permanent decrement produced by the massing of practice. It will be seen that at no time after the first 10 min. rest period does the M curve reach the level of the D curve. This is as would have been predicted in terms of our theory, and the data reported will therefore be considered as supporting the theory. The reader will also notice the spurt in the M curve immediately following each rest pause. This can be explained in precisely the same terms as the initial spurt in the work curve, discussed on a previous page; as pointed out there, during the first 50 or 60 sec. of practice, D_- is building up to the point of equality with D_+, and the failure of involuntary rest pauses to occur during this time and to reinforce $_sI_R$ leads to the partial extinction of conditioned inhibition. It might be predicted also that if we had switched our M group from massed to spaced practice after the first or the second rest period, then this process of the extinction of $_sI_R$ would have continued unabated until the M curve had reached the D curve. Denny *et al.* (1955) have in fact shown that this is so.

These few deductions, as well as the conditioning phenomena, discussed at the beginning of this chapter, present only a small sample of the facts summarized and predicted by Hullian behaviour theory. It would be tempting to go on and quote further examples of the usefulness and value of this theory; however, our concern here is rather with the application of the theory to the study of personality, and, consequently, other phenomena (except where they are mentioned in passing in the remainder of this book) will not be discussed. It need hardly be emphasized that no adequate understanding of learning theory can be gained from reading the small number of selected examples given here, and the reader is referred again to the detailed discussions by Osgood (1953), by Hilgard (1956), and by McGeoch and Irion (1952).

Chapter Three

PERSONALITY AND LEARNING
THEORY : CRITICAL

As Allport (1937) has demonstrated in his textbook, there are as many definitions of personality as there are varieties of Heinz products, and there appears to be little point in adding another definition at the beginning of this chapter. There are two types of concepts in science, namely, those which have meaning in terms of the scientific system itself, and those which are merely descriptive of an area of study. Concepts of the first type would be mass, electron, reaction potential, gene and drive; concepts of the second type would be physics, society and personality. It is only with concepts of the first kind that accurate, preferably operational, and if possible quantitative, definitions are possible, and it is only with concepts of this kind that disputes and discussions about proper definitions have any point. The concepts of the second kind have no scientific meaning, are created purely for the sake of administrative or descriptive convenience, and the precise meaning assigned to them is left to the individual writer. Without wishing to argue the point therefore we will proceed to delineate the position which personality study appears to us to hold in the general framework of the biological sciences and the social studies, and to leave the justification for this to a later section of this book.

In a sense it might be said that the position of personality study within psychology is similar to that of psychology within the group of biological and social studies. Fig. 15 may serve as a very schematic and *ad hoc* sketch map of the position. On the one side we see arrayed the biological sciences such as neurology, physiology, morphology and anatomy, with certain others such as biochemistry looming in the background and linking these

72

biological sciences with the more exact ones of physics and chemistry. At the other extreme we have the large field of social studies (we are purposely refraining from calling them sciences because none of them has reached the point in its development where that honorific title can, with any degree of confidence, be bestowed upon it). The main among these are anthropology, sociology, economics and history, with a variety of other fields of study completing the picture.

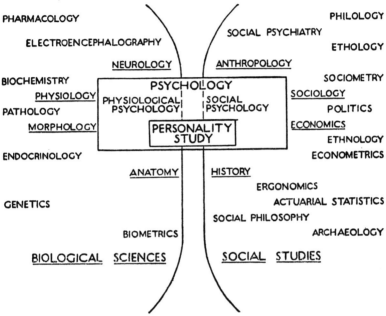

FIG. 15. The position of psychology and personality study in the field of the biological sciences and the social studies.

The importance of psychology, as will be seen from its position in the diagram, lies in the fact that it acts as a bridge between these two great fields. As an optimistic psychologist might say, his subject has one foot firmly in the biological camp and the other equally firmly in the social field, straddling them both like a veritable Colossus, and integrating their respective contributions to the welfare of humanity. Alternatively, as a more disillusioned scientist might express it, psychology with two feet of clay precariously poised in two equally hostile camps, has managed with uncommon agility to sit down between two stools. Whichever of these two similes expresses the truth, there is no doubt that psychology must base itself on the scientifically ascertained facts of biology and must in turn serve as a basis for any fruitful development in the social field.

So far we have talked about psychology as if it were a unified field, but everyone knows this is not so. In fact, psychology is divided in two. On the one hand we have the physiological, comparative and experimental psychologists, their allegiance definitely on the biological side, on the other hand we have the social, clinical and educational psychologists with an allegiance equally firmly on the social side. These two groups of psychologists do not speak the same language, they do not share the same concepts, they do not use the same methods, and it is often doubtful whether they have the same objectives. (In addition, they hardly ever read each other's publications.) Thus the split between the biological and social fields is not really bridged by psychology; it runs right through psychology and divides it into two relatively independent camps.

Perhaps another look at Fig. 15 will make this general view clearer. What characterizes the biological sciences as opposed to the social studies is surely the *segmental* nature of their experiments. The physiologist and the neurologist attempt to study isolated nerve fibres, occurrences at the synapse, or at best the individual reflex arc. The attempt is made to exclude all external influences which might disturb the experiment, and the aim is to vary one condition at a time. Functional laws are thus derived which are of the greatest importance and value, but which are clearly true only as applied to the particular segment under investigation. When we come to the natural unit of study of the psychologist, i.e. the individual person (or indeed, the individual animal; there is no distinction in principle here), these segmental laws are always modified by the eruption of other factors and influences which the experimenter can exclude, but which may play a very powerful part in the actual behaviour of the intact organism. We cannot, therefore, assume necessarily that the laws which hold for the nerve-muscle preparation are also the laws which hold for the behaviour of a given person. Clearly, a broadening is required for the study of the interrelations among different influences and laws. The greater the number of influences taken into account, the farther the field of study moves to the right of the diagram, until we reach the social field where it is no longer even the individual who is the object of investigation, but where we search for general laws accounting for the behaviour of groups. The personality psychologist has to take over the laws which general psychology provides for him, and attempt to account for the complex types of normal and abnormal behaviour with which he has to deal, in those terms; in turn he hands on his generalizations to the social psychologist, who uses them for his ends. In all this there is no systematic breaking point from the simplest segmental type of experiment to the most complex interaction processes among large groups, such as nations. Yet it is advantageous to recognize, on the practical level, that the aims of the physiological psychologist who attempts the quantification of one of Hull's postulates are different from those of the personality psychologist who attempts to account for a hysterical conversion symptom or a schizophrenic hallucination.

It is here that personality study comes into its own. Just as psychology ideally provides the bridge between the biological and social fields, so personality study within psychology provides a bridge between the physiological and social sides. This, to the writer, is its proper function, and this is its proper place. It cannot be denied that in actual fact those who study personality have often failed to attack the subject with due regard to this twofold link. It is the failure on the part of many personality theorists and many experimentalists in the personality field to take the integrative function of their subject seriously which has been primarily responsible for the disjunctive appearance of psychology, and it will be the prime purpose of this book to show (i) that 'bridging operations' of the type suggested are theoretically feasible and experimentally possible, (ii) that operations of this kind are of inestimable value in the advancement of personality study itself, and (iii) that they, in turn, throw much light on problems in both the fields of physiological psychology and social psychology, problems which would otherwise not be susceptible to scientific solutions.

In taking this point of view it becomes incumbent upon us to indicate our position with respect to a dichotomy in the manner of defining personality which has been most clearly expressed by Brand (1954). He points out that there are two quite antagonistic concepts of personality which he refers to as individual-behaviour conceptions and general-behaviour conceptions of personality. This is what Brand has to say about this

75

distinction: 'The designation *individual-behaviour* (or) *general-behaviour* . . . for each variety of definition indicates its essential nature. The choice of designation was difficult, because there are already available such distinctions as *molar-molecular* (Littman, Rosen, 1950) ; *central peripheral*, or *-proximal*, or *-distal* (Brunswick, 1952); or S–O–R, or W–S–Ow–R–W (Brunswick, 1952); or the S–R and the R–R (Spence, 1951), or *inside* and *outside* (McKinnon, 1944). The fact that some definitions say, however, that the study of personality is the study of individual behaviour, whereas others say that the study of personality is not distinguishable from the study of behaviour in general, is the basis for the designation used here. We believe these distinctions to be the most important differences between definitions of personality. The individual-behaviour definitions imply the study of individual behaviour. The general-behaviour definitions imply a study of the commonalities in behaviour and the minimizing of individual differences. Our view is that this distinction, individual-behaviour or general-behaviour, is fundamental.'

This distinction between these two conceptions reflects the distinction between physiological and social psychology. Individual-behaviour conceptions, emphasizing individual differences, uniqueness of personality, holistic methods of observation and descriptively derived units of analysis are opposed by general-behaviour conceptions which emphasize general laws, and deny the need for a special theory of personality with a distinct subject matter and laws within their general behaviour theory.

Brand does the present writer the honour of quoting him as a supporter of both camps, and indeed this is roughly a correct description of the position here maintained. It is possible that, in the long run, the general-behaviour type of view will prevail, and that in the description of behaviour we shall be able to rely completely on the interaction of certain general laws. Regularities in human behaviour will therefore be derivable completely from experimental psychology and the laws of learning theory. Indeed, it is not impossible that these in turn might be derivable from neurology and physiology or even from biochemistry, and, ultimately, from physics and chemistry. However, such a desirable state of affairs appears to be very much in the distant future, and at the moment there appear to exist methods for isolating regularities and invariances of behaviour on a purely descriptive basis, for which no rationale can necessarily be found in the general laws so far produced by psychologists. These observed regularities would therefore constitute a legitimate field of study, and it is invariances of this kind that the individual behaviour conception of personality emphasizes.

How can a view such as this deal with criticisms such as those brought forward by Miller and Dollard (1950) or by Mowrer (1950), who simply say that personality is the learned behaviour of human beings? How are we to maintain our position in the face of Klein and Krech (1951) when they uphold the view of a behaviour theory based on 'the most general regulatory principles which determine a person's responses and account for individual differences among people'? As Brand (1954) summarizes this position: 'Any theory of behaviour is also a theory of personality because the behaviour theory includes laws predicting individual differences in behaviour. Since these laws are based upon the behaviour of many individuals, they would hold for a given person and for every one in general.'

The facts of the matter, unfortunately, are a little more complex. Let us take as a simple example Crozier's formula (1929) for the orientation of young rats on an inclined plane in the dark:

$$\theta = K \log \sin \frac{\lim 55°}{\lim 20°} a$$

The most relevant feature of this formula to which attention may here be drawn is the constant K which is different for different species of rats or even for different individuals within a species. This is not independently determined, and is simply given a value necessary to make the equation fit the curve. As Hull (1945) has been forced to admit in another context, constants of this kind are always required to modify the general laws and the general deductions from those laws which are generated by his theory. To predict the behaviour of an individual, therefore, it would apparently be necessary to know the behaviour of that individual in the particular situation for which a prediction is required before any such prediction can be made. This is an impasse into which some, at least, of the general behaviour theorists appear to be driven.

77

The situation however may not be as bad as all that. Adams (1954), in his discussion of Crozier's formula, has indicated that K '*may* represent an unknown complex of anatomical characteristics, such as centre of gravity, length of femur, and angle of pelvic girdle'. If that were so then K would be derivable *independently* of the actual behaviour of the rat on the inclined plane in the dark, and we would have a genuine case of prediction. This, of course, would merely throw the burden of finding the source of individual differences on to other sciences such as genetics, anatomy, morphology, and so on.

Hull himself seems to have recognized this dual nature and function of constants in psychology. In 1945 he pointed out that 'the natural science approach to behaviour theory presents two major tasks. The first is to make a satisfactory working analysis of the various behaviour processes; this consists in deriving, i.e. deducing, from the primary laws of the system the characteristic observable phenomena of the behaviour process in question as displayed by the modal or average organism under given conditions. . . . The second major task of the natural science approach to behaviour theory concerns the problem of innate behavioural differences under identical conditions between different species and between individuals within a given species. . . . Both types of tasks cry loudly and insistently for completion. But most neglected of all is the relationship between the two approaches.'

An example may make clearer the distinction between constants used in physics, as for instance in the well-known gravitational formula : $s = \frac{1}{2}gt^2$, and formulae such as that given by Gantt (1944) for the growth of the conditioned response $CR = a + b(1 - e^{-cQ})$, where a, b, c are constants for a given dog, CR is the conditioned response in units of secretion, and Q is the quantity of food by which the conditioned stimulus is habitually followed (e is of course the base of the natural logarithms). In the physical formula the term 'g' is an intervening variable which enters into many equations which define it uniquely, and the formula as a whole is of general applicability. The constants a, b, and c in Gantt's formula do not recur in any other formula and vary from one animal to another. This same feature is characteristic of both empirical and rational formulae in psychology, as can easily be seen by inspecting a few representative specimens. This is Ebbinghaus's (1885) 'curve of retention' formula: $b = \dfrac{100\mathrm{K}}{(\log t)^c + \mathrm{K}}$, where b is the amount retained, t is the time elapsed, and c and K are arbitrary constants depending on differences in material learned and in persons doing the learning and retaining. Again, here is the Culler and Girden (1951) formula for learning: $y = \dfrac{be^{\mathrm{A}x}}{c + e^{\mathrm{A}x}}$, where y is a measure of learning, x a measure of practice, c a constant of integration, e the base for natural logarithms, b a limit of attainment, and A *a constant for learner and tasks.*

These are both empirical formulae, but the position is no different when we turn to rational formulae such as Thurstone's (1930):

$$\frac{2p - 1}{\sqrt{p - p^2}} = \frac{\mathrm{K}t}{\sqrt{m}} + \mathrm{Z}$$

where p is the measure of attainment, Z a constant of integration, t time, m a constant reflecting task complexity, and K *a constant reflecting learning ability.*

It is important to realize this distinction which is absolutely fundamental if one wishes to understand the weakness of the point of view advocated by the 'general behaviour' theorists. Ultimately, the difference between a typically physical formula and a typically psychological one is simply this: the physical formula, in its ideal form, deals with objects which, from the point of view of the formula, are homogeneous. The formula: $\frac{1}{2}gt^2$ applies to sticks and stones as much as to pigs and psychologists; when dropped from the Leaning Tower of Pisa, or any other suitable point in space, all these objects fall at the same rate of acceleration. Psychological formulae, however, inevitably deal with animals or human beings which, from the point of view of the formula, are heterogeneous. It is attractive to say, as Mowrer does, that personality is the learned behaviour of human beings, but we must remember that these human beings differ with respect to the rate of acquisition of learned responses, with respect to the strength of their drives, and so forth.

Perhaps an example from Hull's own theory may make this point clearer. Let us, for the sake of argument, accept the general formula proposed in the last chapter, according to which behaviour potential is a multiplicative function of drives and habits, both in their positive and negative forms. This

79

general formula can only give us *individual* predictions if we assume that there are no individual differences in the rate of formation of excitatory and inhibitory potentials, respectively, or in the amount of drive generated under identical stimulation conditions. Now it is well known, and will be documented later on in this chapter, that these assumptions cannot be made, and that considerable individual differences do exist in these respects. Of necessity, therefore, we are forced to introduce a whole host of constants into our formulae if any kind of individual prediction is to be made. This point will become obvious when we look at Hull's formula for $_sH_R$, which reads:

$$_sH_R = M(1 - e^{-Kt})$$

where M is the upper limit of habit strengths, t the number of trials, e the base of natural logarithms, and K *a constant expressing learning rate*. Both M and K differ from person to person, so that prediction of an individual's score depends on previous knowledge of that score. (This point will be dealt with on an experimental basis in a later chapter.) The crucial problem for a personality theory based on these Hullian postulates is, therefore, the same as that posed by Crozier's K. Is it possible to obtain *independent estimates* of the rate of growth of excitory potential, rate of growth of drive strength in response to stimulation, and to the various other factors determining it? The assumption will be made in this book that such independent determination is possible, and evidence will be brought forward to show that this assumption makes it possible for us to predict $_s\dot{E}_R$ *for individuals* with better than chance success. Once this possibility of independent determination is demonstrated, the point at issue between individual behaviour theories and general behaviour theories disappears. Individual differences in behaviour, in personality traits, and in position along the measured dimensions of personality can then be based upon individual differences in the rate of change of the constructs of learning theory. It is in this sense that the writer would like to view the present contribution to this argument.

In the discussion to follow we have dealt with individual differences and those hypothetical constructs which measure rate of learning and performance; we have not dealt with the contents of the learning process, i.e. with those particular acts and ideas which are learned. This topic will be taken up in a

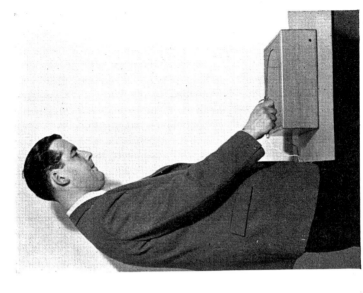

8. Pursuit rotor in action. Tip of rod is in contact with metal disc.

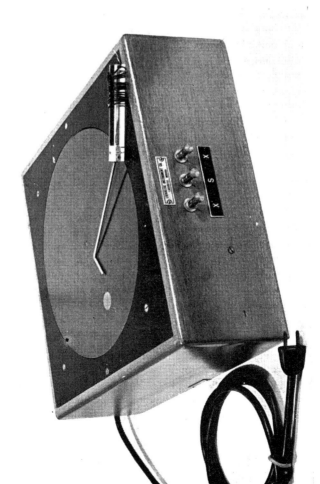

7. Pursuit rotor, with articulated rod.

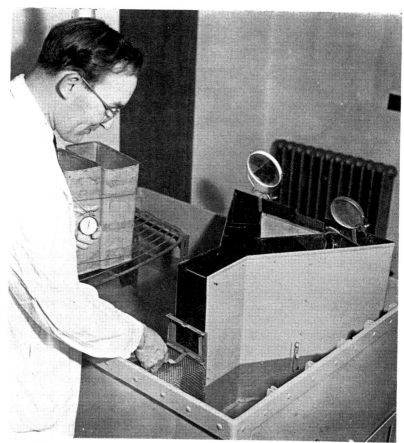

9. Y-maze for under-water swimming discrimination learning experiment. Note starting cage in experimenter's right hand.

later part of this book. It is not treated as fully as its importance deserves, for the very simple reason that the greater part of social psychology, personality psychology, psychoanalysis, and psychiatry has, for the past 30 years, concerned itself almost exclusively with this particular aspect, to the relative neglect of the problems here stressed. The novel contribution we wish to make relates to *function* and not to the *content* of learning, and it is function, therefore, which is emphasized throughout this book.

Abstract discussions are seldom as convincing as experimental demonstrations and, consequently, much of this book will be given over to a discussion of one particular theory and one particular set of experiments aimed at defining the general point of view put forward here. The chief hypothesis to be

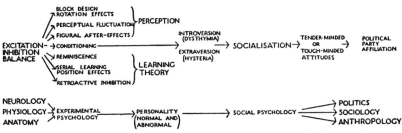

FIG. 16. Schematic drawing representing causal chain from neurology through experimental psychology, personality study and social psychology to sociology.

discussed is shown diagrammatically in Fig. 16, where the writer has traced out the causal chain leading from the concepts of excitation and inhibition, as they appear in some of the biological sciences, through conditioning (concept in experimental psychology); and introversion/extraversion (a concept in personality theory); to social attitude organization and political party adherence (concepts on the social studies side). Of particular importance in this chain is the concept of introversion/extraversion because it provides a link between the biological and experimental psychology concepts on the one hand, and those of social psychology on the other. It gains in importance also from the fact that, as we have seen in a previous chapter, this concept of extraversion/introversion is closely related to psychiatric theories and descriptions—in particular, to the categories of hysteria and psychopathy on the one hand, and the group of dysthymic syndromes on the other.

Before turning to the positive task of developing the general theory along the lines just mentioned, it will be necessary to discuss, at least briefly, several previous attempts to relate learning theory to personality functioning and to point out why these attempts cannot be considered successful, and to what extent they nevertheless constitute important beginnings, the positive contributions from which may be incorporated into a more general theory. Before turning to our own hypothesis, therefore, we shall deal briefly with the work of Mowrer, that of Miller and Dollard, and that of Spence and his associates. This discussion will be brief and will inevitably fail to do justice to the ingenuity and the persuasiveness of these writers. The reader is urged to consult the original publications in order to give these authors a fairer hearing than can be afforded them in a brief chapter such as this, where stress is laid on criticism rather than on appreciation.

Mowrer (1950), and Miller and Dollard (1950), may be discussed together because, although their theories show differences, they both agree on one important point. These men, and their students and disciples, all agreed on the paramount importance of psychoanalytic theory in the description and explanation of human conduct, both normal and abnormal; they see it as their main objective to link up learning theory with the tenets of psychoanalysis, which they appear to accept quite uncritically and unquestioningly.

A brief discussion of the orthodox Freudian theory and its translation into Hullian terms by Dollard and Miller has been given by Mowrer (1953). He first gives an elementary dictionary for translating terms within one system into those of the other; a dictionary which apparently he would be willing to share with Dollard and Miller. 'It is evident, first of all, that what Freud referred to as id corresponds roughly to the *primary drives* as defined by learning theorists. It is likewise clear that what Freud called superego is a product of social conditioning or sign learning. And it is equally evident that the *ego* is that part or agency of the personality which mediates *solution* learning.' He then goes on to account for the development of a neurosis in two stages, the first covert, the second manifest. 'As a result of unduly severe social conditioning (parental discipline), the child's secondary drives (particularly fears) come into conflict with the child's primary drives; and the only successful solution to this conflict which the child can find, in his particular life situation and stage of development, is one which consists of walling off (repressing) the offending primary drives (id forces) and thereby denying them access to the problem-solving (ego) mechanisms. In this way the conflict is ended and the individual is left free, for a time, to direct his attention and problem-solving, instrumental behaviour toward the secondary, socially acquired (superego) drives, i.e. toward being "good". The second stage in the development of a neurosis materializes when the habits (repressions) which have been devised as solutions to the earlier conflict between certain primary and secondary drives become weakened and there is a threatened recrudescence of the conflict. Now new, more elaborate habits or "symptoms" ... have to be instituted, and these give the picture of full-blown, clinically manifest *neurosis*.'

As opposed to this clinical version of Freudian theory as advocated by Miller and Dollard, Mowrer states: 'My own clinical experience leads me to believe that neurosis follows a different course. In Freudian terms, this alternative view is that neurosis arises, not when an excessively severe superego develops and overpowers the ego, thus forcing a repudiation or repression of id forces, but rather when the ego, which is initially under the *complete* sway of the id, remains essentially id dominated and directs repressive action *against the superego* ... this alternative view holds that the neurotic individual is one in whom the primary drives not only have had but still have major control over the problem-solving processes and cause these to be directed toward the blocking, inhibition, or nullification of the secondary, acquired drives of guilt, obligation and fear. The problem-solving activity which is usually referred to clinically as self-protectiveness or defensiveness thus functions in the interest of the primary drives or id, rather than, as Freud posited, in the services of the socially derived forces of the superego.'

The reader will find in this quotation evidence for all the criticisms which we have to bring against this general form of theorizing. Both Miller and Mowrer have shown great ability and meticulous regard for scientific procedure in their work on the development of learning theory. Both appear to have thrown these qualities overboard in dealing with the personality side. Instead of referring to objective fact, experimental verification and empirical correlation, they embrace the speculative and unproven psychoanalytic system, and attempt to bridge the gap between this system and learning theory by what we may refer to as a method of *dictionary construction*. This reliance on non-scientific procedures becomes particularly apparent in relation to those issues which divide the Mowrer theory from that of Dollard and Miller. According to Dollard and Miller, the formula for neurosis might be written in the following way: superego + ego >id. Mowrer's formula, on the other hand, would be id + ego >superego. Here indeed we would seem to have a fundamental and basic contradiction on the personality side which one might expect to lead to a great volume of empirical work and experimental verification. Such an expectation, however, would be disappointed. All that Mowrer, in fact, has to say, as quoted above, is that 'my own clinical experience leads me to believe that neurosis follows a different course'! In a very similar manner there is little in Dollard and Miller's book beyond simple appeal to their clinical experience.

Now it must be clear that scientifically any individual's clinical experience is not acceptable as proof, although it may be suggestive of hypotheses. Where all competent clinicians are agreed on certain issues in terms of their experience, some writers might be prepared to give a slightly higher veridical value to their pronouncements. Wherever, as in this case, there is a complete and fundamental contradiction, it is clear that we need a criterion to judge between these opposed clinical 'experiences'. Such a criterion must, of necessity, be different in kind from clinical experience itself; in fact it must be a criterion deriving from the usual methods of science, i.e. the clear-cut statement of theories, the making of deductions derivable from these theories, and the experimental testing of these deductions. It is not only the fact that neither Miller nor Mowrer follows this course which is so disquieting and so disappointing, it is the fact that neither of them appears to realize the necessity for importing into the field of personality study the same experimental rigor which informs their work in the field of learning theory.

The reader who is disinclined to regard the contradiction between Mowrer on the one hand and Miller and Dollard on the other as being quite as important as is suggested here, may consider for a moment its implication for the treatment of neurotic disorders. According to Mowrer, the aim of psychotherapy would be the strengthening of the superego and the weakening of the id. According to Miller and Dollard, the aim of psychotherapy would be the strengthening of the id and the weakening of the superego. In other words, these two groups of workers, on the basis of their clinical experience, are advocating procedures for the relief of neurotic suffering which are exactly antagonistic to each other! If one of these theories happened to be right and if psychotherapy were, in fact, a method capable of producing any kind of change in human behaviour (an assumption for which there does not exist any empirical evidence), then the adherents of the other theory would, in fact, be making their patients worse, not better. Yet both claim therapeutic successes as evidence for the truth of their respective theories, and use learning theory to explain this putative and suppositious effect. We need only remind the reader that a review of the existing evidence (Eysenck, 1952) fails to confirm the hypothesis that *any* form of psychotherapy produces therapeutic effects in excess of the spontaneous remission rate, so high in neurotic disorders, to see that the attempts of Mowrer, and of Miller and Dollard, are founded on very shifting sands indeed.

There are many other consequences which follow from the failure of learning theorists to take seriously the task of scientific investigation on the personality side, and their tendency to make do with a speculative, imprecise and unverifiable personality theory such as the Freudian. Thus, the ambiguities and contradictions contained in the personality theory are not resolved—they are merely translated into different terms. As Butler (1954) has put it, in an excellent discussion of the matter: 'The translations contribute nothing to our knowledge of psychotherapy. The specifiable referents of the terms of learning theory reside in the experimental situations created by the learning experimenters.

'The behaviour of patients and clients and therapists in psychotherapy is as unspecified as ever it was, and this is very unspecified indeed. What are exact terms in learning theory then become as inexact as their semantic equivalents in psychotherapeutic and personality theory, and the connections between the propositions are connections which can be demonstrated to hold for the other. To put it bluntly, the unification of the domain has by and large been on the semantic level.

Once one has succeeded in finding a certain isomorphism between the propositions of therapeutic theory, the propositions of therapy-based personality theories, and the propositions of learning theories, with some paring down of the former propositions and some relaxation of the latter, one finds himself turning to experiments with animals and finding analogues. These analogues, I might add, have not contributed much, if anything, to learning theory. Why should they when the experimenter started with learning theory, found isomorphisms, and came back to the domain of learning? They do not contribute directly to psychotherapeutic theories because the referents of the terms used in such theories are unknown in any scientific sense.'

While Mowrer and Miller and Dollard have thus laid themselves open to serious criticism by their too easy acceptance of one particular form of personality theory, and of clinical evidence generally as opposed to experimental evidence, it should not be assumed that they have no worth-while contributions to make. Nothing could be farther from the truth. Most modern theories in this field, not excepting the one to be proposed later on, are very heavily indebted to these writers for their demonstration of the existence of learnable drives and, in particular, the role of anxiety in learning.

The reader may remember the role of the primary reinforcement principle in Hull's postulate system. It is clear that many of the drives which activate human beings are not of this nature, and Hull was forced to postulate the existence of secondary drives and secondary reinforcements, i.e. drives and reinforcements which acquire their dynamic properties through learning. As Miller (1951) states in an excellent summary of the literature, 'A learnable drive or reward is one that can be acquired by previously ineffective cues as a result of learning. Thus, if a child that has not previously feared dogs learns to fear them after having been bitten, it shows that fear is learnable. Similarly, if appropriate training causes a previously ineffective token or coin to be used as a reward, we may call it a learnable reward . . . the fact that a drive is learnable, as a reaction to new cues, does not rule out the possibility that it may also be an innate response to certain stimuli. Thus, although fear may be an innate response to pain, it may also be learned as a reaction to many other stimuli. The ultimate test of drive and reward is their ability to produce the learning and performance of new responses.'

Most of the work that has been done in this field has been devoted to a demonstration that fear is a learnable drive, and fear reduction a reward. In a typical demonstration experiment, the experimenter might put a rat in an apparatus consisting of two compartments: one, white, with a metal grid as a floor; the other, black, with a solid floor. These compartments would be separated by a door which could be opened in various ways by the experimenter, or by the rat. In order to teach the rat to fear the white compartment, he is given electric shocks from the grid and allowed to escape into the black compartment. After ten such trials, the door between the compartments is shut, and the rat is put again in the white compartment, but without being given a shock. Under these circumstances, the conditioned fear, or anxiety, produced by the learning trials is so strong that the animal learns to open the door by moving a wheel or pressing a board. Thus through a process of learning, the white chamber has become associated with fear, and now constitutes a drive stimulus (S_D) strong enough to motivate learning in the rat, i.e. to make him solve the problem presented by the varoius mechanisms for opening the door leading from the white to the black compartment.

Miller and Mowrer maintain, on the basis of much research, (1) that learned drives, such as fear, obey the same laws as do overt responses; and (2) that they have the same drive and cue properties as strong external stimuli. The results of experiments 'agree with . . . everyday observations that fear can motivate people to learn a great variety of responses, and that it is sufficiently distinctive so that people can be taught to respond to it with a verbal label that transfers to a variety of new frightening situations'.

This pioneering work of Mowrer and of Miller has produced results widely accepted by psychologists of different theoretical backgrounds, and it has been applied by many people to an elucidation of some of the phenomena of human neurosis in which fear or anxiety plays an important part. Our main interest in this book is not with neuroses, or neuroticism as such, however, and we shall not go any further into details regarding these applications, except to note one point.

One possible and promising hypothesis regarding the main

cause of neurotic disorder postulates a strong innate autonomic lability as predisposing some people towards neurotic tendencies (Eysenck, 1952, 1953). The evidence regarding this theory has been reviewed elsewhere and will not be repeated here; we merely wish to indicate that it is likely that the strength of primary drive is proportional to the strength of learned drives, and that, consequently, conditioned fears are strongest in those people having the strongest innate fear reactions. Thus to take Miller's example of the child learning to fear dogs after having been bitten, we may argue with some show of reasonableness that the fear thus learned is likely to be proportional to the fear and general autonomic disturbances expressed at the time of the original traumatic event.

If we follow Mowrer and Miller in their argument, then it will be obvious that fear or anxiety must be regarded as part of the general drive level of the individual, and it also follows that differences in anxiety or neuroticism will enter into the general Hullian formula for increasing the amount of drive, or D. This, at least, is the argument presented by Spence (1951, 1953, 1954), Taylor (1951, 1956), and other members of the Iowa group. Their argument is given very clearly by Taylor: 'According to Hull, all habits (H) activated in a given situation combine multiplicatively with the total effective drive state (D) operating at the moment to form excitatory potential $E(E = f(H \times D))$. Total effective drive, in the Hullian system, is determined by the summation of all extant need states, primary and secondary, irrespective of their relevancy to the type of reinforcement employed. Since response strength is determined in part by E, the implication of varying drive level in any situation in which a single habit is evoked is clear; the higher the drive, the greater the value of E and hence of response strength. Thus in simple non-competitional experimental arrangements involving only a single habit tendency the performance level of high-drive Ss should be greater than that for low-drive groups.'

In order to conduct experiments in this field and to test deductions from this hypothesis it becomes necessary to have some measure of anxiety in the individual. This was achieved by the constructions of the manifest anxiety scale (MAS) (Taylor, 1953). This scale is a good measure of neuroticism, but it also correlates to some extent with introversion (Franks,

1956; Eysenck, 1957). The theoretical argument advanced by Spence and Taylor would relate that part of the MAS which measures neuroticism to the D variable; there is no obvious relationship between introversion and D. However, it must be clear that any results obtained by a scale such as MAS, which simultaneously measures two orthogonal dimensions, must be difficult to interpret. The effects produced cannot be easily related to any one dimension. If in any 'simple non-competitional experimental arrangements involving only a single habit tendency' (i.e. in conditioning experiments such as the eyeblink experiment described in the previous chapter), performance of subjects scoring high on the MAS should indeed be greater than that of subjects scoring low on the MAS, then it would certainly be possible to argue that these differences were due to a higher D (or neuroticism) in the one group as compared with the other. It might, however, also be possible to argue that the differences in performances were in no way related to differences in D, but were produced rather by differences in extraversion/introversion. Or again it might be possible to argue that both neuroticism and introversion were relevant to the observed differences in performance. Thus the failure of Spence and Taylor to carry out a dimensional analysis of their scale, or to pay any attention to the results of such work carried out by personality theorists, has rendered their experiments ambiguous and difficult to interpret. Results, however much they might be in line with prediction, could equally well be interpreted along quite different lines. Thus Spence and Taylor, very much like Mowrer and Miller, are strong on the side of learning theory but weak in relation to personality theory. This weakness in both cases is related to a failure to take seriously the problems of dimensional analysis posed in the personality field.

Most of the experimental work has been concerned with eyeblink conditioning, and in most cases the experiment has involved the contrasting of groups of low- and high-scoring subjects. In all cases but one, the prediction that anxious subjects would give higher rates of conditioning than non-anxious subjects has been borne out (Spence & Farber, 1953; Spence, Farber & Taylor, 1954; Spence & Taylor, 1951, 1953; Taylor, 1951); even in the one exception while the differences observed were non-significant they were in the expected

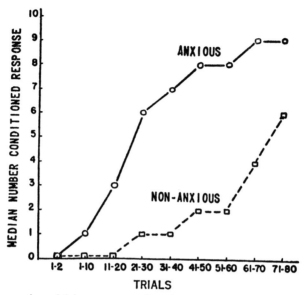

FIG. 17. Acquisition curves showing the median number of conditioned eyeblink responses of anxious and non-anxious groups in successive blocks of 10 trials.

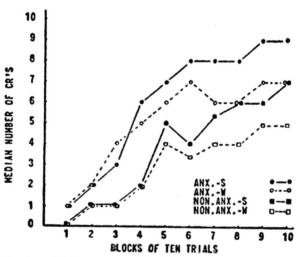

FIG. 18. Acquisition curves showing the median number of conditioned eyeblink responses of anxious and non-anxious groups submitted to strong (S) and weak (W) intensities of air puff.

direction (Hilgard *et al.*, 1951). The hypothesis advanced by Spence and Taylor thus finds some support in the data. Typical diagrams from a few of these studies are given below as an illustration of this work (Figs. 17, 18, 19). It should be remembered that we are comparing *extreme* groups; when the relation is studied over complete, unselected groups it becomes rather more tenuous.

One way of demonstrating the tenuous relation observed between the rate of conditioning and MAS score makes use of product-moment correlations obtained when the entire range

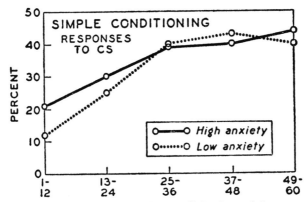

FIG. 19. Course of simple conditioning of the eye-blink for anxious and non-anxious groups.

of scores is used, rather than the two extremes. Relationships tend to be monotonic, although not always linear, with medium-scoring subjects tending to perform like low scorers rather than like high scorers. The correlation observed under these conditions are in the range of ·25 (Taylor, 1956); in other words, only about 6 per cent of the variance is common to the two variables. This relationship is so slight that it is difficult to regard it as very impressive, even if one were entitled to assume that the demonstration of a relation between conditioning and MAS did unequivocally support the Spence-Taylor theory.

It should not be assumed that the relationship between anxiety and conditioning, postulated by Spence and Taylor, constitutes a novel prediction in any sense. Ten years previously Welch and Kubis (1947), and Schiff *et al.* (1949) had demonstrated in a whole series of studies, making use of the conditioned PGR response, that patients suffering from anxiety conditioned very much more quickly than did normals. The differences reported by them were rather more impressive and significant than those found by Spence and Taylor. Historically, the work of Darrow and Heath (1932) constitutes perhaps one of the first efforts to relate condition to personality, and he also obtained results not very dissimilar from those reported by Welch and Kubis, and by Spence and Taylor. Altogether, then, we may say that there is a considerable body of evidence suggesting that students and psychiatric patients suffering from anxiety tend to condition more quickly as far as the protective reflexes are concerned, than do students or patients not suffering from anxiety. The existence of a relationship is clear enough, then, although it does not seem to be a particularly strong one in normal groups; what is not so clear is the relevance of these facts to the theory advanced by Spence and Taylor. The ambiguity is due, as pointed out before, to their failure to perform a proper dimensional analysis on their criterion scale.

A number of studies have also been carried out in connection with predictions made on differences between anxious and non-anxious subjects to be found in experiments involving differential conditioning and stimulus generalization. 'The predictions derived from the theory in this instance are that anxious Ss should exhibit a greater excitatory strength both to the positive (reinforced) CS and to the negative (non-reinforced) CS, and further, that the difference in excitatory strengths of the two stimuli should be greater for the anxious groups.'

Spence and his colleagues (Spence & Beecroft, 1954; Spence & Farber, 1954) have produced some evidence in favour of this prediction, while Hilgard, Jones and Kaplan (1951) have produced some contradictory findings. The additional work of Rosenbaum (1953) and Wenar (1954) does not clarify this position very much, and altogether it cannot be said that this deduction from the Hullian theory has found much support, as even Spence's favourable results are in the main insignificant (cf. Restle & Beecroft, 1955).

We have criticized the Spence and Taylor theory in terms of its failure to investigate the possibility that differences in conditioning might be related to differences in extraversion/introversion rather than to differences in neuroticism. Our own theory, to be developed in the next chapter, leads to the prediction of quicker conditioning in introverts than in extraverts, and we will discuss there the evidence supporting this conception. The evidence to be considered will be found to be in contradiction to predictions made from the Spence-Taylor theory, and, accordingly, the conclusion to be derived from this work will be that Spence and Taylor were in error as far as their general theory is concerned. There is, however, one rather different type of proof, also leading to the same conclusion, which may with advantage be included in this chapter. This proof relates to an underlying assumption of the Spence and Taylor theory which they take from Hull's general system, i.e. the notion that 'total effective drive ... is determined by the summation of all extant need states, primary and secondary, irrespective of their source and their relevancy to the type of reinforcement employed'. If we wish to test this assumption, then it would seem that Spence and Taylor have not chosen a very suitable drive for experimental manipulation. Anxiety is difficult to measure—the reader may like to consult the large body of critical literature which has grown up around the MAS as a measure of anxiety (Franks, 1956)—and it cannot be experimentally manipulated except by the rather clumsy method of differential selection of groups on the basis of questionnaires, or other test scores. A much more direct method would appear to be that of experimentally manipulating drives such as hunger and thirst; if the Taylor/Spence paradigm is at all correct, then we would expect that an increase in hunger and thirst drive would produce an increase in the rate of conditioning.

This deduction was tested in our laboratory by Franks (1957). Allocating student subjects, at random, to a hunger-thirst and a satiated group, he prevented the former from having food or drink for a minimum period of 18 hours, while the other group were given food and drink at regular intervals right up to the beginning of the experiment. Knowledge of the group to which each subject belonged was withheld from the experimenter in order to prevent any possibility of contamination of results. Under these conditions, the theory under investigation would predict the superiority in the rate of conditioning of the hungry over the satiated group. Fig. 20 shows the actual results obtained during the acquisition and extinction periods. At no point are the differences between groups significant and, if anything, the satiated subjects are very slightly superior.

We may deduce from this experiment that the basis of Spence

and Taylor's hypothesis is faulty and that drives do not combine by summation in the way suggested by Hull. If this conclusion be accepted, then there is no reason for assuming that anxiety-neuroticism as an *irrelevant* drive should produce any increase in the rate of conditioning. The results suggest not only a failure of the Spence/Taylor type of deduction, but also the necessity for reconstructing an important part of the Hullian theory. This, however, is not a task which can be attempted in this volume.

To deny that irrelevant drives in the conditioning situation

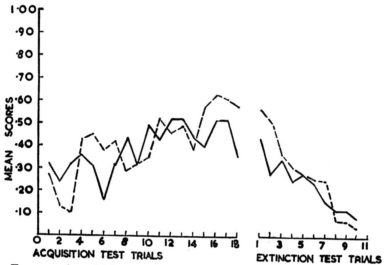

FIG. 20. Acquisition and extinction of conditioned eyeblink reflex in groups with high (——) and low (----) hunger drive.

are responsible for the observed differences in rate of conditioning between introverted and extraverted groups is not to be construed as a denial of the importance of relevant drives in simple and complex learning situations. Degree of hunger affects conditioned salivation, although it does not affect the conditioned eyeblink. However, the clearest statement regarding the influence of drives on learning and performance is probably given in the so-called Yerkes-Dodson law (Yerkes & Dodson, 1908), a law which has been familiar to psychologists for almost fifty years, and which was derived from observations of the behaviour of animals set to learn complex and easy tasks under varying degrees of motivation. It was found that the relationship between motivation or drive on the one hand, and learning or performance on the other, was curvilinear, the optimal drive level usually lying below the highest level used in the experiment and above the lowest level. Thus, when a very weak electric shock was used as a drive, the animal would learn only slowly. When a very strong shock was used, the very strength of the stimulus appeared to interfere with the learning and performance of the animal. Intermediate degrees of shock were found to produce the best results. It was further shown that the level at which the drive was most effective depended on the complexity of the task. The more complex the task, the lower was the optimal drive level; the simpler the task, the higher was the optimum drive level. This was found to be true with both animals and humans (Young, 1936), and, indeed, most people would probably regard this generalization as intuitively evident on the basis of their own experience. A very strong drive, such as fear or anger, might be highly efficient in motivating a simple response like running away or hitting out, but it would probably not be an efficient drive for carrying out some complex and difficult intellectual or manipulatory activity.

A typical demonstration of the Yerkes-Dodson law is contained in the following experiment reported by Broadhurst (1957). The task presented to the animal consisted in making the correct choice of the right or left arm of a Y-maze. This maze, which is illustrated in Plate 9, consisted of stainless steel and was immersed in water, thus forcing the animal to swim through it in order to reach a platform above water level. (Plate 10 shows an animal emerging from the water and climbing on to the platform.) The arms of the Y were provided with doors which could be locked or left unlocked; if the animal chose the incorrect arm of the Y he would be forced to retrace his path because the locked door prevented his escape. Doors were locked and unlocked in random sequence, and the correct (unlocked) path was indicated by being illuminated more brightly than the incorrect (locked) path. Three different ratios of brightness (1:300, 1:60, and 1:15) constituted the three levels of difficulty, and will be referred to as easy, moderate, and difficult.

The drive employed was that of air deprivation; the rats were put into a starting cage which was submerged for varying lengths of time before a rat was released directly into the maze. (Photograph 11 shows the starting cage.) Once in the maze it was forced to swim under water by means of a metal screen which prevented it from surfacing. Photograph 12 shows a rat emerging from the starting cage and touching the metal screen which forces it to stay under water until it has solved the problem and has passed the unlocked door which allows it access to the outer world. Four levels of motivation were used, viz. 0, 2, 4, and 8 sec. delay before release. Proof for the efficacy of this method of drive manipulation was sought in a

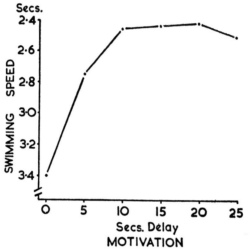

Fig. 21. Speed of underwater swimming of rats as a function of motivation (delay before release in seconds).

preliminary experiment, in which speed of swimming a 4 ft. underwater straightaway was studied as a function of different periods of pre-trial immersion. The results of the experiment are shown in Fig. 21; each point represents the mean time for 20 rats. It will be seen that there is a monotonic and almost linear increase of swimming speed with length of delay until the 10 sec. point is reached; thereafter the curve flattens out and even falls a little at the 25 sec. point. The results of this experiment determined the choice of delay periods in the main experiment, and suggested that periods of delay longer than 8

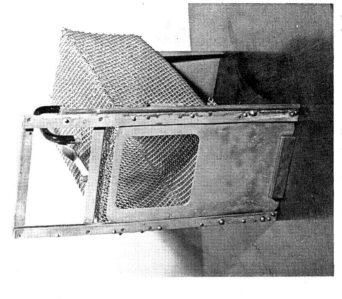

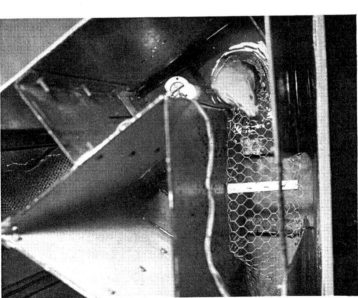

10. Rat emerging from under-water maze. Note lamp on right used to indicate correct path by suitable adjustment of brightness.

11. Starting cage for under-water swimming experiment. Animal is released after variable immersion under water.

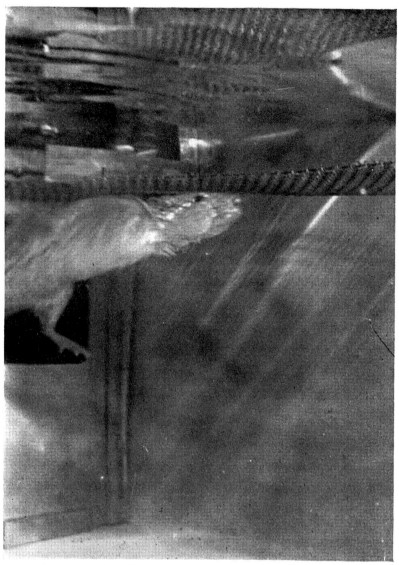

12. Rat emerging from starting cage and beginning to swim under water.

to 10 sec. would introduce complicating factors without a corresponding increase in drive.

Altogether 120 animals were used in the main experiment, distributed at random over the different combinations of drive and difficulty level. The animals were put through the usual pretraining procedure, and were then given 10 trials per day for 10 days—a total of 100 trials—in the experimental situation. A count was kept of the number of incorrect choices, and a

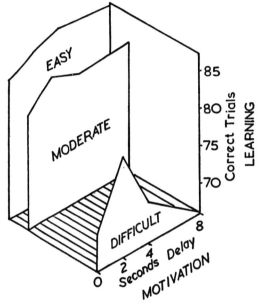

FIG. 22. Results of experiment illustrating the Yerkes-Dodson law. Learning as a monotonic function of difficulty of task, as a curvilinear function of degree of motivation, and as a function of interaction between these two variables.

record made of the time taken by each animal to solve the problem. The results were subjected to an analysis of variance, which confirmed the impression given by the diagrammatic representation of the results in Fig. 22. The easier discriminations were learned more quickly; intensity of motivation showed a curvilinear relationship to efficiency of learning, the 2 sec. delay period being the optimal one; and the optimum motivation for the task decreased with increasing difficulty of the task. Thus this experiment confirmed the basic contention of the

Yerkes-Dodson law, indicating (*a*) the importance of relevant drive to learning, (*b*) the curvilinear relationship between drive level and learning, and (*c*) the interaction between optimal drive level and task difficulty.

The Yerkes-Dodson law refers to drive level in terms of the specification of the stimuli applied to groups of animals or human subjects, i.e. in terms of the amount of shock administered, etc. In view of our more extensive knowledge of individual differences, we would almost certainly be justified in saying that the amount of drive aroused in different subjects by a standard stimulus will vary so that we must add a third dimension to the two envisaged by Yerkes and Dodson. In addition to drive and response complexity as determiners of performance, we must also introduce individual differences in what might perhaps be called 'arousability' or emotionability; thus the emotional, anxious, or neurotic person might react even to a very slight electric shock in a manner suggesting that, for him, this is a very strong drive, whereas a more stable, non-emotional kind of person might be able to accommodate quite a strong shock without allowing it to interfere with his efficient learning and performance habits. To the two dimensions of 'strength of drive' and 'difficulty of problem' contained in the Yerkes-Dodson formulation, we must therefore add the third dimension of 'drive arousability' or of emotionality; this dimension would be predicted to act in the same way as that of strength of drive. A partial confirmation of this view has been furnished by Broadhurst in the study already quoted. He split his population in two by selecting 'emotional' and 'non-emotional' rats from a selective breeding experiment. The test of 'emotionality' used was the Hall (1934) 'open field' test, illustrated in Plate 13; this consists essentially in the measurement of the degree of urination and defecation of the rat when introduced into an 'open field', brightly lit, and without opportunities for hiding and withdrawal. This test has been thoroughly described and investigated by Broadhurst (1956, 1957), and it would seem to be reliable and valid enough for the purpose in hand. The results obtained in part support the hypothesis; emotional animals learn the easy discrimination faster than non-emotionals, and are about equal on the moderately difficult one; similarly, they learn faster under low motivation and are about equal at medium levels. However, under the most intense motivation, and on the most difficult discrimination, they fail to be inferior, as predicted, but show a slight superiority instead.

Work with animals thus only partly supports our attempt to link personality differences (if we may extend the term 'personality' to differences in the emotionality of rats!) with the Yerkes-Dodson law. Work with human beings has been rather more successful, as we shall show. However, in dealing with the considerable body of work reported in this connection, we must return to the Hullian theory. We shall show that it is possible to deduce the Yerkes-Dodson law from Hull's postulates, making use in this connection of certain arguments and deductions provided by Spence, who has also been responsible for some exceptionally elegant and well-designed experimental demonstrations. He does not, however, refer in his published work to the Yerkes-Dodson law, and consequently cannot be held responsible for the deductions here put forward.

Let us look again at the general formula of the Hullian system according to which habit multiplied by drive produces performance. Habit here means a strongly formed stimulus-response connection in the nervous system which mediates a particular response when a particular stimulus is administered. Under the simplest conditions imaginable, we might specify that the subject is presented with a situation in which only one particular response is possible in a given situation, and that this response is the one required to be learned. Simple Pavlovian conditioning provides such a situation; the response of salivation is the only one elicited in the experimental situation by the UCS, and it is this response which is required. Under these conditions *the stronger the (relevant) drive the stronger the performance* —within limits set by the possibly nocuous nature of the stimulus producing defensive reactions in the animal which might interfere with performance. (Cf. the paradoxical results obtained by Venables and Tizard (1956) in their work on schizophrenics.)

Now let us consider a more complex situation in which there are two competing responses elicited in the situation. Thus, an animal confronted with a T maze has two conflicting responses when reaching the point of separation; these responses might be called R responses (tendency to go right) and L responses (tendency to go left). These tendencies are determined

99

by a variety of antecedent conditions which are sometimes, but not always, under experimental control. Thus, early in the learning process, animals tend to prefer turns which point directly towards the feed box, although these may be the wrong turns. Again, when running, the animal prefers those turns which require it to make less acute angles in its movement. Or again, many animals have preference for right or left turning, possibly based on bodily asymmetry. Let us assume that in a situation of this kind the stronger response is the incorrect response. Under these conditions, the stronger the drive the more superior would the incorrect response be over the correct response in determining performance, and the more difficult would it be for the animal to unlearn the incorrect response and to learn the correct one. Substituting individual differences for amount of drive in animals or human subjects, this would lead us to say that a subject in whom a constant, external, applied stimulation produced a greater drive under complex learning conditions, where the correct response was low in the habit-family hierarchy, would have much greater difficulty in learning than another subject in whom the same stimulus situation developed a lesser drive. Thus, in a complex situation of this kind, we would make a prediction essentially identical with the statement of the Yerkes-Dodson law. The term complexity in that law is directly related in Hullian terminology to the number of alternative responses and to the position of the correct response in the habit-family hierarchy. Thus, the Yerkes-Dodson law can be deduced from Hullian learning theory and with it all the consequences discussed above. (Good discussion of this theory will be found, together with supporting experimental evidence, in Taylor, 1956, Farber, 1954, and Child, 1954.)

One element in this general theory still requires discussion, and that is the concept of *drive*. In Hull's theory a variable is considered to have the properties of a drive if '(a) the elimination or reduction in the magnitude of the variable is reinforcing, i.e. leads to the increased probability of recurrence, in the same situation, of the responses that precede the modification of the variable; and/or (b) that the presence of the variable energizes or intensifies whatever reaction tendencies exist in the given situation' (Farber, 1954). Anxiety, as we have mentioned before, has been postulated to have the qualities of a drive by

Mowrer (1939) in a very famous paper entitled 'A Stimulus-Response Analysis of Anxiety and Its Role as a Reinforcing Agent', and experimental work by him, Miller (1951), and many others has since put this notion on a firm basis. According to this theory, which is indeed implicit already in Pavlov, an originally indifferent stimulus, which is presented a number of times in close temporal contiguity with a noxious, painful, or threatening stimulus, ends by causing a state called *anxiety* or *fear*, which is a conditioned form of the pain reaction. 'This state of affairs . . . may then motivate innumerable random acts, from which will be selected and fixated . . . the behaviour that most effectively reduces anxiety' (Mowrer, 1939).

This notion of anxiety as a drive is a central one in Spence's set of deductions. Using the Taylor Manifest Anxiety Scale, which we have discussed in a previous chapter, as a measure of individual differences in anxiety, he predicts, in line with the deductions made from Hull's theory, that *on complex tasks, individuals high in anxiety will learn less quickly than individuals low in anxiety.*

We must now go on to review the experimental evidence relating to the other prediction made by Spence, to the effect that in situations where several incorrect response tendencies are relatively high in the habit-family hierarchy, high anxiety should make for poorer performance than low anxiety. Farber and Spence (1953), Taylor and Spence (1952), Ramond (1953), Osler (1954), Montague (1953), Lucas (1952), Lazarus *et al.* (1954), Hughes *et al.* (1954), Gaier (1952), Deese *et al.* (1953), Castaneda and Pelermo (1955), Buchwald and Yamaguchi (1955), Axelrod *et al.* (1956), Gordon and Berlyne (1954), L'Abate (1956), Heilitzer *et al.* (1956), Beam (1955), and others have reported a whole series of studies. In some of these a kind of verbal multiple-T maze was employed, and it was found that predictions regarding the inferiority of high anxiety subjects was verified. Similar results have been reported with respect to a stylus maze. When high anxiety and low anxiety subjects were matched for total score, significant evidence was found that on the easy choice points high anxiety subjects performed better than low anxiety subjects, while on the most difficult choice points the opposite was true. Quite generally in these studies there are found correlations between difficulty in choice point and amount of difference between high anxiety and low anxiety subjects' performance at the choice point, a finding definitely in line with Spence's theory.

In these studies there is no experimental manipulation of the difficulty or complexity variable; the existence of competing responses is deduced from the fact that a given choice point in a T maze presents above average difficulty in learning of the subject. Lucas (1952), Montague (1953), and others have made a rather more quantitative approach to this problem by varying experimentally the amount of response competition. Thus, for instance, the experimental variable introduced might be the extent to which, in a list of consonants presented in a memory test, some of the consonants are repeated in different locations within the list. Evidence was found to indicate that the greater the number of duplications the greater the inferiority in performance of a high anxiety group. In another experiment serial rote learning was used and the two experimental variables consisted in intra-list similarity and the varying association value of the nonsense syllables used. Both high intra-list similarity and low association value were found to produce a difference in performance between high anxiety subjects and low anxiety subjects in favour of the latter. These, as well as many other studies recently reported, 'do add up to a convincing demonstration that as a task becomes more complex (in the sense of involving conflict among various response tendencies) there is a tendency for high anxiety subjects to show increasingly poor performance in comparison with low anxiety subjects'. This general assessment, made in review of this work in 1954 by Child, might now have to be modified a little in view of the fact that several negative results have been reported; nevertheless, on the whole the evidence is decidedly in favour of the application of the Yerkes-Dodson law to this general field.

In saying this we should, however, remember that proof of the applicability of the Yerkes-Dodson law does not necessarily imply the correctness of Spence's derivation of the law from the Hullian theory. One alternative hypothesis, which would seem to agree quite well with much of the experimental work, has been put forward by Mandler (1952) and Sarason (1956). These writers assume that anxiety produces certain responses which interfere with the efficient learning or performance of complex tasks. Their theory thus presents an alternative to Spence's. Where Spence assumes that anxiety, acting as a drive, *strengthens already existing* response tendencies which are incorrect as far as a solution to the problem is concerned, Mandler and Sarason hypothesize that anxiety *produces interfering responses* which cause a decrement in learning and/or performance. There is no reason to assume, however, that these two sets of theories are in any sense incompatible or antagonistic. The evidence presented in these various studies suggests very strongly that both hypotheses have an element of truth in them and that therefore the Yerkes-Dodson law, as an empirical statement of relationships, may be the result of quite different causal sets of influences. It should not be difficult to devise crucial experiments to assess the relevance of both these different types of theories, because the Hullian theory would lead one to predict that in a complex situation in which the correct response was the predominant one, high anxiety should lead to better performance, whereas on the alternative theory we would predict that high anxiety would interfere with performance in such a situation. Thus it may be surmised that the Hullian theory applies particularly where the development of $_sH_R$ is concerned, i.e. in learning situations where the correct response is relatively low in the habit-family hierarchy, whereas Mandler and Sarason's hypothesis would apply more particularly in relation to $_sE_R$, i.e. the performance of learned habits in which the correct response was high in the habit-family hierarchy.

In this general treatment we are still faced with the problem of the dimensional aspects of the term 'anxiety'. There is no direct evidence on the point, but the writer (1957) has suggested that with respect to complex learning tasks, the relevant portion of the variance of the anxiety scale is that related to neuroticism rather than that related to extraversion-introversion. This hypothesis then would relate neuroticism directly to the Yerkes-Dodson law as a kind of multiplicative personality variable interacting with the objective drive stimuli. The evidence in favour of this interpretation is largely indirect. It arises partly from the studies already reviewed, partly from such findings as the inferiority of neurotics as compared with normals, matched for sex, age, and intelligence, on complex motor tasks such as those involved in manual and finger dexterity (Eysenck, 1947, 1952). Such differences in performance could be rationalized in terms of the Yerkes-Dodson law and might be regarded as a prototype of a whole group of performances of a complex nature in which neurotics have been found inferior to normals. This point is an important one, as, if the reasoning is correct, we could regard a large variety of empirical tests of neuroticism as being rationally based and therefore as occupying a much higher status in the hierarchy of test procedures than they would do if justification for their use were merely empirical.

One last word should perhaps be said regarding the apparent contradiction in some of the theorizing summarized above. Basing ourselves on the Franks experiment with the hunger drive, we have postulated that in conditioning *drives do not summate in the manner postulated by Hull* to provide a general fund of libidinal energy. Yet in our discussion of complex learning we have made use of the general multiplicative theorem linking drive and habit to performance. The reason for this apparent contradiction is twofold. In the first place, the drives manipulated in the conditioning situation appear to be *irrelevant,* and irrelevant drive, as Franks has shown, does not appear to affect performance. In the complex learning situation, however, anxiety must be regarded as a very *relevant* drive, directly interacting with performance. Thus the main difference would appear to be with respect to the *relevance or lack of relevance* of the drive under consideration, namely, anxiety.

Another difference which must not be overlooked is this. In conditioning we are dealing with a type of response acquisition which is largely confined to the autonomic nervous system, and which, as Mowrer (1950) and many others have shown, shows properties in certain ways different from those appearing in ordinary learning. Complex learning on the other hand is mediated largely by the central nervous system and is much more dependent for its motivation on drive reduction. As Mowrer has argued, the Hullian formulations involving *drive reduction* apply to learning rather than *conditioning,* and the facts briefly reviewed here would certainly seem to lend some support to this general belief. (This point will be discussed much more thoroughly in a later chapter.)

We are now in a position to summarize the main conclusions of this chapter. We have argued that the type of application of learning theory to personality study which is offered by Mowrer, and by Miller and Dollard, is too non-experimental on the personality side, and too much a mere 'dictionary' which attempts by analogy to translate psycho-analytic concepts into the terms of learning theory, to generate testable deductions, or to integrate in any genuine manner these two great areas of study. Without in any manner denying the very great importance of the experimental contributions made by all these men to the analysis of anxiety as a learnable drive, we cannot but feel that their intuitive (and contradictory) clinical judgments do not provide a firm basis on the personality side for the construction of a well-based, systematic framework of description, to be integrated with learning theory. This does not mean that their views on the personality side are necessarily mistaken, but merely that they are not based on experiments and observations which are repeatable, non-subjective, and rigorous. It is probable that these writers themselves would not disagree with this judgment, although they would presumably be willing to give more credence to psychoanalytic speculations than would the present writer.

As regards Spence and his colleagues, we have argued that the theoretical inventiveness and experimental ingenuity shown by these men (and women!) have made a very considerable contribution to our knowledge of personality, and of the interaction between anxiety and performance. We believe that we have shown Spence to have been mistaken in his theoretical position regarding the importance of irrelevant drive and its influence on the rate of conditioning; an alternative hypothesis to his will be presented in the next chapter. We believe that we have successfully broadened Spence's theoretical account of the influence of relevant drive (anxiety) on complex learning and performance by relating it to the Yerkes-Dodson law and by including in our formulation not only the deduction relating drive to $_sH_R$, but also the deduction relating drive to $_sE_R$, thus treating the Spence-Farber and the Mandler-Sarason theories as parts of the general Yerkes-Dodson law. Lastly, we believe that we have clarified the dimensional status of 'anxiety', as used by Spence, and related his findings to the dimensions of emotionality (neuroticism) and of extraversion-introversion.

Chapter Four

PERSONALITY AND LEARNING
THEORY: CONSTRUCTIVE

ERFORMANCE in Hull's theory, it will be remembered, is a function of drive and habit. Differences in the rate of conditioning, therefore, may be due either to difference in drive or to difference in the rate of growth of habit $(_sH_R)$. Spence and Taylor, as we have seen, favour the hypothesis that drive (D) is the variable involved. This, however, is a somewhat arbitrary choice and not a rigorous deduction from Hullian theory.

It is interesting to note that Taylor was quite aware of the alternative possibilities, as is shown by this quotation from her discussion of some of her results: 'The consistent superiority of the anxious group in all measures of conditioning and extinction strongly indicates that there is a marked difference in the rate with which the strength of the CR is developed under the two conditions of drive (anxiety) level. This might be interpreted to mean that anxious Ss have a more rapid conditioning rate, or, in Hull's terms, develop habit strength $(_sH_R)$. While this is a possibility, it should be noted that in Hull's theoretical formulation of the assumed relations between response strength, excitatory potential $(_sE_R)$, habit and drive strength, $R = f(_sE_R) = f(H \times D)$, the slope of the rise of the $_sE_R$ value, and hence the response measure, is a direct function of *both* H and D values.'

It will be noted in this quotation that the predilection for differences in D, as opposed to differences in H, as accounting for the more rapid conditioning rate of anxious subjects, is not justified or deduced; Taylor merely argues that 'it is theoretically *possible* for the habit growth curves for two groups of Ss to be identical and yet have both the $_sE_R$ and response curves increase at two quite different rates in the two groups because of different D values' (italics not in original).

This arbitrary choice, as we have seen in the last chapter, was mistaken, and we must now turn to an investigation of the alternative possibility relating differences in rate of conditioning to differences in the rate of habit formation, i.e. to difference in the growth of excitatory potential and possibly also to differences in the growth of inhibitory potential. In doing so we are returning in some measure to a point of view adumbrated, although somewhat obscurely, by Pavlov. Pavlov's theory of personality is rather complicated and by no means consistent; however, in view of its historical importance some discussion of it appears necessary. Its most explicit statement can be found in an article, 'General Types of Animal and Human Higher Nervous Activity', published in 1935; better known perhaps is his chapter on 'The experimental results obtained with animals in their application to men' in his book *Conditioned Reflexes*. As might be expected, Pavlov places importance on observations made on dogs, and attempts to deduce from these the major dimensions of human behaviour. He appears to have postulated three main dimensions: 'In the first place, the *strength* of the basic nervous processes—excitatory and inhibitory—which always constitute the sum total of nervous activity; in the second place, the *equilibrium* of these processes; and, finally, in the third place, their *mobility*.' These he believes to exist in various degrees, but 'leaving aside the gradation and considering only the extreme cases, only the limits of fluctuation, viz. strength and weakness, equality and inequality, lability and inertness in both processes, we obtain eight combinations, eight different complexes of basic properties of the nervous system. If we also take into account that in the absence of equilibrium the predominance may, generally speaking, be on the side now of the excitatory, now of the inhibitory process, and that in the case of mobility, inertness, or lability, may also be a property now of one, now of the other process, then the number of possible combinations increases to twenty-four.' He goes on to emphasize that 'if we also take into consideration even the rough gradations of the three basic properties, we shall thereby again greatly augment the number of possible combinations'. He does not, however, believe that such a degree of complexity is necessary because, as he says, 'It seems to me that this problem was solved —of course, only in general outline—by the Greek genius in his system of the so-called temperaments, where the basic components of the behaviour of human beings and higher animals were exactly emphasized and advanced' (Pavlov, 1955).

Pavlov gives a discussion of the relationships between his three dimensions and the fourfold Greek typology. The main results of this are summed up in the following quotation: 'It is now possible clearly to see how the Greek genius, personified (individually or collectively) by Hippocrates, succeeded in discerning the fundamental features in the multitudinous variations of human behaviour. The singling out of melancholics from the mass of people signified the division of the entire mass of human beings in two groups—the strong and the weak, since the complexity of life must, naturally, tell with particular force on individuals with weak nervous processes and darken their existence. Thus, the paramount *principle of strength* was clearly stressed. In the group of strong individuals the choleric is distinguished by his impetuousness, i.e. inability to repress his temper, to keep it within the proper limits; in other words, he is distinguished by a predominance of the excitatory process over the inhibitory. This, consequently, established the *principle of equilibrium* between opposite processes. Finally, by means of a comparison between phlegmatic and sanguine types the *principle of the mobility* of the nerous processes was established.'

There seems to be little doubt that Pavlov was indeed thinking of human types as homogeneous, non-continuous groups; this is made clear in another quotation: 'Thus, I repeat, the possible variations of the basic properties of the nervous system, as well as the possible combinations of these variations, determine the types of nervous system; as calculated, their number amounts at least to twenty-four. But life shows that the actual number is considerably smaller: we distinguish four types which are particularly distinct and strongly pronounced, and, what is most important, differ in their adaptability to the external environment and their resistibility to morbific agents.' His system, therefore, will not be easily acceptable to modern workers on personality, who stress the dimensional approach and the existence of continuity, and disbelieve in the existence of qualitative, separate types.

Pavlov's personality theories in the normal field may have

suffered from the execrable translations through which alone most English-speaking readers will have been able to become acquainted with them. Even allowing for this, the writer does not, on the whole, find these theories very helpful. It is when we turn to Pavlov's theories of *abnormal* behaviour that we receive some hints which may be worth following up. Thus, it appears that Pavlov thought of psychiatric disorders as being caused by a weak central nervous system which produces strong inhibition in order to protect itself from over-stimulation. While the concepts of a 'strong' or 'weak' nervous system seem to offer little in the way of operational definition, the hypothesis of protective inhibition is amenable to experimental investigation. As an example, we may quote a study carried out by Venables and Tizard (1956), working with reaction times to four different intensities of light: A = 0·26 W., B = 0·52 W., C = 1·33 W., D = 2·25 W. These workers deduced that the higher values of stimulus intensity would produce the effect of an *increase* in reaction time in schizophrenic patients, in contrast to the well-established finding with normal subjects of a non-linear *decrease* in reaction time. Such a prediction would follow from the Pavlovian hypothesis on the assumption that high stimulus levels produce inhibition in the nervous system of schizophrenics as a protection against over-stimulation; this inhibition would in turn cause an increase in reaction time. (Cf. Plate 20 for picture of apparatus used.)

Subjects were asked to release a Morse key as quickly as possible after the onset of a stimulus light which was presented once every 8 sec. A buzzer was sounded 3 sec. before the light appeared, as a warning signal, the timing of buzzer and light being carried out electrically. Twenty presentations of each light intensity were made, all the effects being controlled by the use of a balanced Latin Square design. Three minutes' rest was allowed between each set of twenty presentations. Six groups of four non-paranoid chronic schizophrenic subjects were used, each group completing a Latin Square design; two groups of 4 nurses were used as normal controls. In working out the results only responses in the middle of the range (6 to 15) were used, to avoid possible warming-up effects and 'spurts'.

The main findings are shown graphically in Fig. 23. In each of the six patient groups there is a *decrease* in reaction time from intensity A to intensity B ($p = ·001$), followed by an *increase* in reaction time with intensity C ($p = \cdot$o1), and a slight subsequent decrease with D (which is not significant). In the normal group, on the other hand, there is an insignificant decrease in the reaction time from A to B, no increase in reaction time from B to C, and an insignificant increase with D.

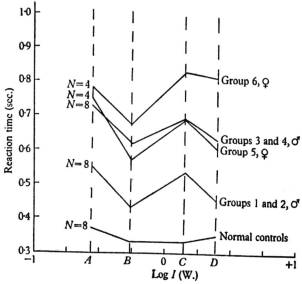

FIG. 23. Reaction time as a function of intensity of signal for normal and schizophrenic subjects.

The increase in reaction time with higher stimulus intensity, which was found in 20 out of 24 schizophrenic subjects, is surprisingly regular and very different from the reactions of the normal group. As Venables and Tizard point out, this effect is similar to the 'paradoxical effect' found in conditioned reflex studies and, as far as it goes, seems to bear out Pavlov's contention. Much further work would, of course, be required before any definite conclusions can be drawn, but it is obvious that in principle the Pavlovian theory does lead to testable predictions, and that in at least one case the somewhat unlikely predictions made from it have been verified. It is not impossible, therefore, that a theory of psychoticism may be built on a modified form of the Pavlov 'protective inhibition' hypothesis. (Cf. a second study by Venables and Tizard (1956) verifying the results of the first.)

In this book, however, we are concerned more with the application of Pavlov's theory to the field of neurosis, and it is here that certain difficulties arise. Pavlov maintains that the disturbances produced in his dogs by the production of 'experimental neuroses', so-called, give rise to two main types of behaviour. 'The type and the degree of pathological disturbance that develops from some definite cause was found in all cases to be determined primarily by the character of the individual nervous system of the animals. Therefore, before describing the different pathological states, it is important to say a few words about the different individual types of nervous system found in our dogs . . . Two definite types, which may be regarded as extremes, stand out with special prominence.'

The first type of animal Pavlov describes is characterized as being lively outside the experimental laboratory, 'extremely vivacious, always sniffing at everything, gazing at everything intently, and reacting quickly to the minutest sounds. Such animals when they get acquainted with men, which they do very quickly and easily, often become annoying with their continuous demonstrativeness. They can never be made to keep quiet either by orders or by mild physical punishment. It was, however, soon found that these very animals when placed in the stand and limited in their movement, and especially when left alone in the experimental room, were the quickest to become drowsy, so that their conditioned reflexes quickly diminished or even disappeared altogether, in spite of frequent reinforcement by food or acid . . . The animals just described must be regarded in the light of the ancient classification as belonging to the pure "sanguine" type. Under quick changes of stimuli they are energetic and highly reactive, but with the slightest monotony of the environment they become dull, drowsy and inactive.

'Our second type of dog is also very definite, and must be placed at the other end of the classical series of temperaments. In every new and slightly unfamiliar set of surroundings such animals are extremely restrained in their movements. They slink along close to the wall in a cringing fashion, and often at the slightest movement or sound from outside—a shout or threatening movement—they immediately cower to the floor. These animals get used to their experimental surroundings and the associated manipulation very slowly, but when they become thoroughly familiar with the new conditions they make invaluable subjects for experimentation . . . It would not be an exaggeration to bring this (type of) animal under the type of "melancholic".

'Both the above types are obvious extremes. In the first the excitatory process predominates in the extreme, and in the second the inhibitory . . . The first needs a continuous and novel succession of stimuli, which may indeed often be absent in the natural surroundings; the other, on the contrary, needs extremely uniform conditions of life and therefore suffers from being unable to react to a sufficient number of stimuli to ensure full use and development of its nervous organization.'

This identification of the 'sanguine' type with extreme predominance of excitatory processes, and of the melancholic type with extreme predominance of the inhibitory processes, does not seem to agree particularly well with the previous quotations from Pavlov's theory, and indeed he himself appears to have recognized that this identification presented some theoretical difficulties. He goes on to argue as follows: 'It has, no doubt, occurred to some that these two types present a contradiction to the theory of the identity of sleep and internal inhibition, in that the type with a predisposition to excitation tends to fall asleep under the conditions of our experiment, while the type who has a predisposition to inhibition remains fully awake.' He then proceeds to argue the case at some length, but the argument appears to be arbitrary and somewhat unconvincing. Indeed, a few pages later he seems to come to a conclusion which is exactly the opposite of that quoted above. In his discussion of experimental neuroses as produced by conditioning experiments, he has this to say: 'It has been seen that the above-mentioned method may lead to different forms of disturbances, depending on the type of nervous system of the animal. In dogs with the more resistant nervous system it leads to predominance of excitation; in dogs with a less resistant nervous system to a predominance to inhibition. So far as can be judged on the basis of casual observation, I believe that these two variations in the pathological disturbances of the cortical activity in animals are comparable to the two forms of neuroses in man—in the pre-Freudian terminology *neurasthenia* and *hysteria*—the first with exaggeration of the excitatory and weakness of the inhibitory process, the second with a predominance of the inhibitory and weakness of the excitatory process.' Here Pavlov would seem to equate the neurasthenic type of neurotic with the lively, sanguine kind of dog described before, by linking both types of behaviour with a predominance of excitatory processes; similarly, he would seem to equate the hysterical type of neurotic with the cowardly, melancholic type of dog, by linking both types of behaviour with a predominance of inhibitory processes. It is very difficult to follow his argument here; if anything, it is the hysteric who is lively and sanguine, and the neurasthenic who is 'cowardly' and melancholic. The writer has spent a considerable amount of time trying to reconcile the contradictions in Pavlov's theory, only a few of which have been quoted. He has come to the conclusion that no such reconciliation is possible and that Pavlov does not, in fact, present us with a proper theory of personality derived from his conditioning experiments, but rather is concerned to point out certain analogies and possible methods of research in the fields of normal and abnormal personality. As such, Pavlov's comments are worthy of the most serious consideration, coming as they do from one of the great masters of psychological observation and experimentation. It would, however, be an error to regard these hints as a fully-fashioned theory from which rigorous deductions of any kind could be made. It is in this spirit that the writer, in formulating his own hypothesis, has made use of Pavlov's work, and it is to this more precise formulation that we must now turn.

In doing so, we receive relatively little help from Hull, although he quite clearly recognized the problem of individual differences (Hull, 1945). His last postulate (Hull, 1951; Postulate XVIII. Hull, 1952; Postulate XVII) is in fact a postulate of individual differences, and reads as follows: 'The "constant" numerical values appearing in equations representing primary molar behavioural laws vary from species to species, from individuals to individuals, and from some physiological states to others in the same individuals at different times, all quite apart from the factor of behavioural oscillation $(_sO_R)$.' This postulate serves as a statement of the problem, and indicates Hull's recognition of its importance; it does not contain any suggestions specific enough to generate experimental proof or disproof. It might appear that this is a somewhat severe judgment, and that surely it might be possible to investigate the 'constant' numerical values mentioned by Hull in a systematic fashion.

Unfortunately, these values, as Koch (1954) has so clearly shown, are numerical only in a purely notional sense; there is no empirical method available at present by means of which we could convert Hull's programmatic developments into actual mathematical measurement. Consequently it would appear that we must have recourse to a somewhat less advanced, and more qualitative, type of approach. Following the lines of the general theory developed in a previous chapter, then, we present the two postulates in terms of which we hope to be able to integrate important areas of personality and learning theory. The first of these two postulates may be called the *Postulate of Individual Differences*; it runs as follows: '*Human beings differ with respect to the speed with which excitation and inhibition are produced, the strength of the excitation and inhibition produced, and the speed with which inhibition is dissipated. These differences are properties of the physical structures involved in making stimulus-response connections.*'

To make our theory complete, we must add another postulate, which may be called the *Typological Postulate*. It runs as follows: '*Individuals in whom excitatory potential is generated slowly and in whom excitatory potentials so generated are relatively weak, are thereby predisposed to develop extraverted patterns of behaviour and to develop hysterical-psychopathic disorders in cases of neurotic breakdown; individuals in whom excitatory potential is generated quickly and in whom excitatory potentials so generated are strong, are thereby predisposed to develop introverted patterns of behaviour and to develop dysthymic disorders in case of neurotic breakdown. Similarly, individuals in whom reactive inhibition is developed quickly, in whom strong reactive inhibitions are generated, and in whom reactive inhibition is dissipated slowly, are thereby predisposed to develop extraverted patterns of behaviour and to develop hysterical-psychopathic disorders in case of neurotic breakdown; conversely, individuals in whom reactive inhibition is developed slowly, in whom weak reactive inhibitions are generated, and in whom reactive inhibition is dissipated quickly, are thereby predisposed to develop introverted patterns of behaviour and to develop dysthymic disorders in case of neurotic breakdown.*'

We now have a small postulate system allegedly accounting for certain major personality variables. We must now attempt to decide, on experimental grounds, the degree to which our system can account for the known facts, and predict previously unknown ones. First of all, let us return to the question of conditioning and personality which we raised in connection with

Spence's hypothesis. The theory just outlined tells us that individuals in whom excitatory potentials are generated quickly and strongly and in whom inhibitory potentials are generated slowly and weakly, will tend to be introverted in personality. It also follows directly from our statement of the laws of excitation and inhibition that such people should form conditioned reflexes quickly and strongly. Conversely, individuals who generate weak excitatory potentials slowly, and who generate strong inhibitory potentials quickly tend to be extraverted in personality; such people, according to the statement of the law of inhibition and excitation should form conditioned reflexes slowly and with difficulty. There is no indication in our system that differences in irrelevant drive should produce any differences in conditionability; consequently our prediction points to a correlation between conditionability and extraversion-introversion, but not to any correlation between neuroticism and conditionability. Thus our prediction of finding introverts to be more conditionable should apply to neurotic introverts (dysthymics) just as much as to normal introverts, and our prediction that extraverts would be difficult to condition should apply to neurotic extraverts (hysterics) just as much as to normal extraverts.

We can now design a crucial experiment to test the predictive accuracy of our theory as compared with Spence's. The Taylor scale, as we have seen, is very largely a measure of neuroticism; consequently hysterics should have high scores on it. (Franks, 1954, reports mean scores of 31·55 for dysthymics, 21·30 for hysterics, and 17·00 for normals. The difference between dysthymics and hysterics is accountable for in terms of the failure of the Taylor scale to be a *pure* measure of neuroticism; as mentioned before, it also has a projection on the introversion axis.) High scores on the scale, according to Spence's theory, mean ease of conditionability, so that Spence would have to predict that hysterics would develop conditioned reflexes speedily and strongly, as compared with normals. According to our hypothesis, as pointed out above, hysterics should be very difficult to condition in view of their extraverted personality. We thus have here a crucial experiment which should enable us to decide between these two theories. Such an experiment was carried out by Franks (1954, 1956), who used eyeblink conditioning on 20 hysterics, 20 normal subjects, and 20 dysthymics. Details of the apparatus used, and the procedures, have already been given in a previous chapter. Results are shown in Fig. 24 for both acquisition and extinction trials. It will be seen that dysthymics show much quicker conditioning than do the other groups, and the hysterics condition less well than the other groups. (The difference between normals and hysterics falls short of full significance statistically. All other differences are significant.) These results go counter to Spence's theory and support the hypothesis outlined above.

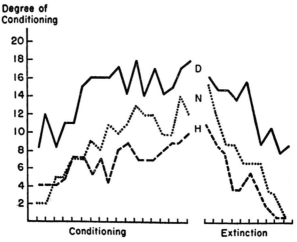

FIG. 24. Course of conditioning and extinction of groups of dysthymic (D), normal (N), and hysteric (H) subjects.

When the hysterics and dysthymics in this experiment were scored in terms of the number of conditioned responses given during the 18 test trials, it was found that only 4 hysterics had a score above 8, while only 2 dysthymics had a score of 8 or below. (Fig. 25 shows the actual distribution.) When similar historgrams were plotted in connection with the PGR response, which had been conditioned simultaneously with the eyeblink, a total misclassification of 30 per cent was obtained. 'When a double criterion is used, however, in which to be classified as hysteric the patient must have 8 or less eyeblink CR's *and* also 3 or less PGR CR's, then the two groups may be separated with no misclassification whatsoever.' It should also be noted that 'when the normals are compared with the neurotics as a combined group, there are no significant differences in the number of CR's produced.'

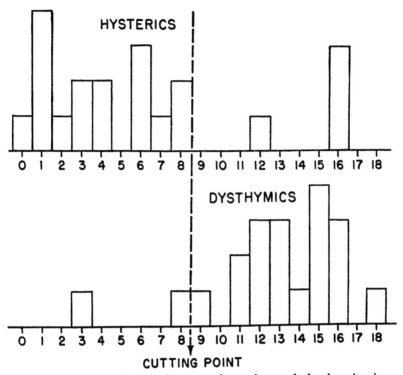

FIG. 25. Differentiation between hysterics and dysthymics in terms of number of conditioned eyeblink responses during standard test.

The subjects of this experiment had been given the following questionnaires:

(1) Guilford's R scale as a measure of extraversion;
(2) Taylor's MAS as a measure of anxiety;
(3) Eysenck's Maudsley Medical Questionnaire as a measure of neuroticism.

It was expected, in terms of our theory, that the MMQ would have zero correlation with conditioning, that the MAT would have a slight positive correlation with conditioning, by virtue of its slight loading on introversion, and that the R scale would have a high negative correlation with conditioning, by virtue of its loading with extraversion. In terms of the Spence-Taylor theory, it would be expected that the MAT would have the highest correlation, followed by the MMQ (which correlates about ·9 with the MAT); the R scale would not be expected to correlate at all with conditioning. The results are given below in Table VII; they are clearly in accordance with our theory, and contradictory to that of Spence and Taylor. (It should be noted that the correlation of conditioning with R is slightly inflated because the R scale was used as a secondary selection device additional to clinical psychiatric judgment; this results in the choice of extraverted and introverted groups slightly more extreme than would have been obtained by reliance on psychiatric selection alone. However, as will be shown in the next experiment, the omission of such selection does not depress the actual correlation between R and conditioning found.)

TABLE VII

Scale:	Eyeblink Conditioning:		P.G.R. Conditioning: Acquisition
	Acquisition	Extinction	
R	− ·48	− ·37	− ·25
MAS	+ ·15	+ ·16	+ ·17
MMQ	+ ·08	+ ·20	+ ·20

Curve-fitting is frequently resorted to in connection with learning curves, and in the hope of obtaining further information from our data an attempt was made to use these techniques and fit a general exponential function to our data. The formula used is $y_i = PF^i + M(1 - F^i)$, where $P = y_0$ is the initial value of y when $i = 0$, M is the asymptotic final value of y as $i \to + \infty$, and F is a constant related to the rate of rise. The first difference of y_i is $\triangle y_i = (1 - F)(M - y_i)$, so that the increment $\triangle y_i$ is a constant fraction of the unachieved remainder $(M - y_i)$, the fraction being $(1 - F)$. If $\tau_{\frac{1}{2}}$ is the value of i at which y_i has increased by one half of its maximum possible increase, then $\tau_{\frac{1}{2}} = - \log 2 / \log F$. For values of i from 1 to 18 there are values of p_i, namely the proportion of subjects responding, for each of the three groups (normals, hysterics, dysthymics). The curves were fitted to these data assuming $P = p_0 = 0$, so that $p_i = M(1 - F^i)$; the fitted curves are a least-squares fit, and are shown in Fig. 26. (The assumption that the probability of evocation of the conditioned response at trial $i = 0$ is $p = 0$ is more than an assumption in view of the unreinforced trials preceding the experiment, each one of which might be regarded as representing p_0.) By converting the p_i values through the arcsin transformation $q_i = 2 \arcsin \sqrt{p_i}$,

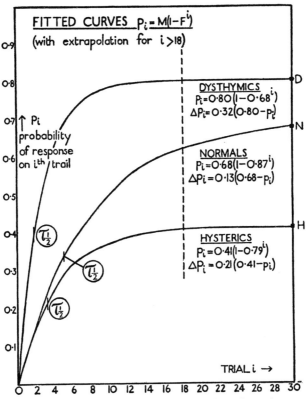

FIG. 26. Fitted curves for conditioning data shown in Fig. 24, using formulae and methods discussed in text. (Values for $i > 18$ are extrapolated.)

the sampling variance of which is $1/n$ where the size of the sample is n, the goodness of fit of our curves may be roughly tested. The values of q_i given by the fitted curve are shown in Fig. 27 a, b, c, together with a band on either side of $\pm \sqrt{1/n}$; it will be observed that nearly all the similarly transformed observed values fall within this band. (The fit is least satisfactory for the hysterics.)

Our interest centres most on the asymptotic maximum values and the 'half-life' values $\tau_{\frac{1}{2}}$. The maxima fall in the predicted order: Dysthymics ·80, Normals ·68, and Hysterics ·41, thus supporting the conclusions from the raw data regarding the respective 'conditionability' of these groups. The 'half-life' values, however, contrast the neurotics with the normal groups; the values for Normals = 5·0, for Dysthymics = 1·8, and for Hysterics = 2·9. The interpretation of these figures is not at all obvious, but if future research should show these findings to be repeatable, then we might have a possible measure of neuroticism or drive in τ, in the sense that neurotics tend to approach their asymptote values more quickly than normals. In advance of such duplication, psychological speculation about the possible causes of this difference does not seem called for.

Franks (1957) followed up his first experiment with another one in which 55 normal paid undergraduate male volunteers acted as subjects. The same experimental set-up was used, but the Maudsley Personality Inventory (Eysenck, 1957) was substituted for the R scale and the MMQ in order to obtain an estimate of the subjects' extraversion and neuroticism. The correlation between conditioning and extraversion was − ·46 (acquisition) and − ·34 (extinction); that between conditioning and neuroticism ·04 and ·15 respectively. Using a one-tail test of significance, it was found that the two correlations between conditioning and extraversion were highly significant ($p <$ ·01), while the two correlations between conditioning and neuroticism were insignificant. These results strongly suggest that in normal subjects also conditionability is related to introversion, and not to neuroticism—emotionality—anxiety.

For the sake of comparison, a diagram is given showing the rate of conditioning for the 15 most extraverted and the 15 most introverted subjects in this group (i.e. those roughly one S.D. above and below the mean). The differences are striking (Fig. 28). A similar diagram was prepared for the 15 most neurotic or emotional subjects and the 15 least neurotic or emotional subjects. No separation of any kind was found, in spite of the fact that the neuroticism scale used correlates very highly with the Taylor Anxiety Scale. We may conclude from these two studies that questionnaire scores of extraversion-introversion account for about 25 per cent of the total variance of the eye-blink conditioning rate of acquisition, while questionnaire

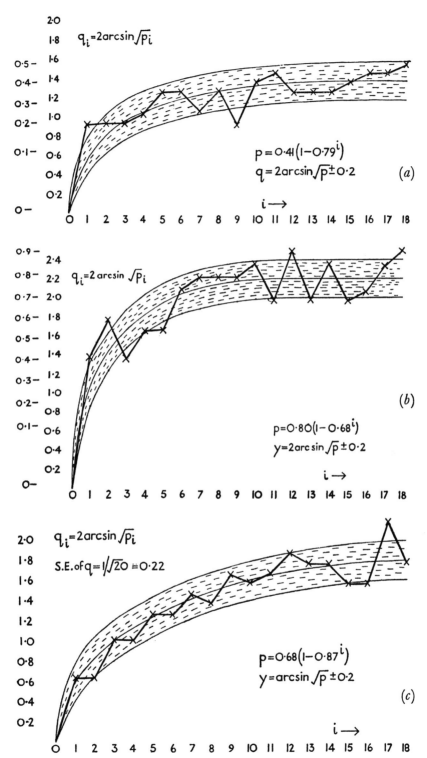

FIG. 27. Curves showing goodness of fit for the formula used to derive the curves shown in Fig. 26.

scores of neuroticism account for none of the variance. According to Taylor, the MAS scores account for 6 per cent of the variance, an amount which is not only significantly lower than the 25 per cent contributed by introversion, but also well in line with the projection of MAS scores on the introversion-extraversion factor. These results thus not only support our hypothesis as against the Spence-Taylor one, but they also account for all the findings reported by the Iowa group, in more inclusive terms.

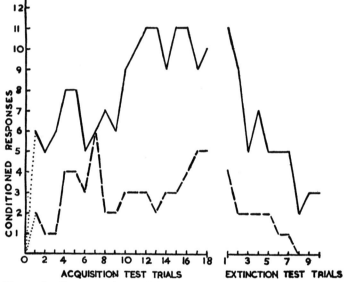

FIG. 28. Course of conditioning and extinction in group of normal introverts (——) and extraverts (----).

So far our studies have dealt with normal extraverts and with hysteric neurotics; it will be remembered, however, that in terms of their test behaviour psychopaths should be classed with these groups, and that consequently we would expect them also to have low conditioning scores. Only one study has been reported in the literature dealing with this problem (Lykken, 1957), and as this experiment was conceived in rather a different framework from that presented here, the reader is recommended to read the original report for a detailed statement of Lykken's own hypotheses; we shall only be concerned with predictions deriving from our general theory. Lykken makes a useful differentiation between *neurotic* and *primary* psychopathy, or *sociopathy* as he prefers to denote this behaviour pattern; in terms of our theory, the former would denote extreme extraversion with high neuroticism, the latter extreme extraversion with average or low neuroticism. As far as lack of conditionability and general behaviour are concerned, both groups should be similar with respect to extraverted traits and symptoms, and dissimilar with respect to neurotic traits and symptoms. It might be useful to denote the neurotic extravert with strong asocial tendencies a psychopath, as we have done hitherto, and the non-neurotic extravert with strong asocial tendencies a sociopath. This usage, which is different from Lykken's, we shall adhere to in this book.

Lykken selected three groups of subjects, corresponding in our terms to a psychopathic group, a sociopathic group, and a normal group, and subjected all his subjects to a lengthy series of experimental tests, including one of PGR conditioning. Our prediction would be that both psychopaths and sociopaths would be more difficult to condition than would the normal group, and indeed this is the result reported by Lykken, at an acceptable level of statistical significance. The actual scores for the three groups may be of some interest; they were: sociopaths, 478; psychopaths, 483; normals, 551. It is regretted that no dysthymics were included in this study; their scores would be confidently expected to be in excess of those of the normal group. One other feature in Lykken results is of particular interest. On the Taylor MAS, the sociopaths scored at the same level as the normals, while the psychopaths had very much higher scores ($p = \cdot 01$). In spite of their high 'anxiety' scores, then, the psychopathic group did not give the high rate of conditioning that would be expected on the basis of the Spence-Taylor hypothesis. Thus these results agree well with those of Franks, and support the theory here advocated. Lykken did not administer an extraversion scale, but he did make use of the MMPI Pd (psychopathy) scale, which as shown by Franks *et al.* (1957) is to some extent a measure of extraversion. As expected, both psychopaths and sociopaths have significantly higher scores on this scale than do normals; there are no differences between psychopaths and sociopaths.

In this theorizing, Lykken introduces an interesting distinction. He would appear to suggest that while sociopaths present genuine cases of low conditionability, psychopaths, 'having quite normal anxiety conditionability, may show deficient reactivity, provided something interferes with the development of emotional set and verbal mediation, which in the normal S are acting to supplement the new conditioning to produce generally higher GSR reactivity curves. Suppose, for example, an S fails for some reason to perceive any threat whatever in the experimental situation and similarly fails to consciously recognize the contingency between CS and shock. Such failure must be regarded as abnormal, and one thinks, of course, of the phenomenon of repression (or dissociation?)' In other words, Lykken seems to think of the failure of psychopaths to condition readily as being due to the action of certain psychoanalytic defence mechanism. It is difficult to accept such a view. Repression as a mechanism is itself in need of an explanation—an attempt at such an explanation in terms of inhibition theory will be made later—and can hardly be invoked to act as an explanatory mechanism. It belongs to quite a different universe of discourse to that of conditioning, and cannot be introduced as a kind of *deus ex machina* to explain the results of conditioning experiments. In any case, no such additional hypothesis appears necessary, as the results reported fit in very well with the theory here adopted.

While all these results, then, support our position, it should be noted that many questions are left to be answered. It is well known that correlations between different types of conditioning, or even between different indices for the measurement of the same type of conditioning, do not correlate together very highly. It is possible that the low correlations found in the literature are due to the use of very small and often homogeneous samples of subjects; it is also possible that they may be due to the low reliability of the measures used. This field is a very complex one and technical and statistical difficulties abound. However, when the proper indices are taken for each conditioning variable, when properly selected samples are tested in sufficient number, and when the technical conduct of the investigation is unexceptionable, then it would follow from our postulate system that a general factor of conditionability should become apparent. It should also follow that personality measures of introversion should correlate more highly with this factor than with any single constituent test. It is possible, of course, that in addition to such a general factor, group factors may be discovered contrasting, say nocive, with nutrient types of conditioning (cf. a paper by Bindra *et al.* (1955) in this connection). A proper programme of research in this area, geared to the study of individual differences in the manner outlined, appears to be essential if these questions are to be answered. Another problem which is posed by our results relates to the dual nature of our theory and consequently to the lack of specificity of our experimental results. A high rate of conditioning could be produced *either* by the development of strong excitatory potential or the failure to develop strong inhibitory potential, or both. (Inhibitory potential is expected to be generated during the unreinforced trials interspersed with the reinforced trials in order to measure the strength of the conditioned response.) General theoretical considerations make it appear unlikely that in the present experiment inhibitory potentials would assume a very prominent place, but that is merely a surmise. Clearly more direct ways of isolating excitatory and inhibitory potential are required, and possible ways of dealing with this problem will be indicated later on in this chapter.

Several possibilities for the independent measurement of inhibitory potential are furnished us in terms of the general theoretical system discussed in Chapter Eleven. The only one for which sufficient experimental evidence exists at present relates to the so-called reminiscence phenomenon already described. It will be recalled that according to the theory massed practice produces inhibition which is not given time to dissipate, and which accordingly depresses performance. If, now, a rest pause is introduced, this should enable inhibition to dissipate, while leaving $_sH_R$ unaffected; performance after the rest pause should therefore now be superior to performance before the rest pause. The amount of increase in performance (reminiscence) would be a direct measure of the inhibition generated during the massed practice. Our theory predicts that extraverts should generate more inhibition during the practice period, and it would seem to follow that they should show larger reminiscence effects. This theory was formally advanced by the writer (Eysenck, 1956) in connection with an experimental study making use of the pursuit rotor described on a previous page. Five minutes of massed practice were followed by 10 minutes of rest, a further 5 minutes of massed practice, another 10-minute rest, and a final 5 minutes of massed practice. The improvement from the end of one practice period to the beginning of the next was taken as the reminiscence score. (The theoretical justification for this choice of score has been discussed elsewhere, together with an experimental exploration of certain problems of measurement arising in this type of test. Eysenck, 1956.)

Using the Maudsley Personality Inventory (Eysenck, 1957) as a measure of personality, it was found that, very much in line with prediction, extraversion correlated significantly with reminiscence scores after the first interval; after the second interval the correlation was still positive but no longer significant. This was explained in terms of the interference of conditioned inhibition, which exerted a much stronger influence at the later stages of practice than at the earlier stages. Experimental proof for this suggestion was independently given (Eysenck, 1956). Admittedly the correlation is not high ($r = \cdot 29$) but this appears largely due to the lack of reliability of the reminiscence score. (The correlations between first and second reminiscence score were only $\cdot 44$.) The fact that in spite of the unreliability of the score significant results are obtained suggests that improvements in the technique would result in considerably higher correlations. (Correlations were also found between reminiscence and neuroticism, at a highly significant level. An explanation of these correlations has been given elsewhere (Eysenck, 1956) but would not be relevant at this point, as our main concern is with the extraversion variable and its relation to inhibition.)

A single experiment, even though the results be significant, is less convincing than an independent duplication. Consequently, much importance attaches to the work of E. Treadwell (1956), who tested our general theory along somewhat different lines. Instead of the pursuit rotor, she used a metal drum with a track which had to be followed by the subject with a metal stylus; the drum was driven by an electric motor, and errors in following the winding path were automatically recorded by the stylus touching the raised sides of the track. Instead of the R scale or the M.M.I. she used an extraversion scale from the Minnesota Multiphasic Personality Inventory. And instead of a correlational design she made use of analysis of variance, as this method was better adapted to her set of hypotheses. From the general theory she deduced the following three hypotheses:

H_1: Extraverts will show more reminiscence than introverts after any given period of pre-rest learning, and after any given rest interval.

H_2: Extraverts will show maximum reminiscence after a *shorter* period of pre-rest learning than introverts.

H_3: Introverts will show maximum reminiscence after a *shorter* post-learning rest interval than extraverts.

It will be seen that these hypotheses can be tested in an experimental design involving a group of extraverts and a group of introverts, a long and a short rest period (10 minutes *vs.* 5 minutes) and a long and a short practice period (459 seconds *vs.* 108 seconds). All the possible eight combinations (2 × 2 × 2) were investigated, making use of the most extraverted 20 subjects and the most introverted 20 subjects out of a group of 107 who had been administered the questionnaire. Reminiscence scores were determined by subtracting the two last pre-rest trials from the first two post-rest trials. The results are shown in Table VIII. They give support to all three hypotheses, but in particular they show at a statistically significant level that extraverts (293·5) have higher reminiscence scores than introverts (210.0). Thus these results, obtained under quite different circumstances, agree with our own work in supporting the view that inhibition is stronger in extraverts than in introverts.

TABLE VIII

Source of Variance:	Sum of Squares:	d.f.:	F. Ratio:
Questionnaire Score			
(I *vs.* E)	174·306	1	4·85*
Rest (L *vs.* S)	·156	1	—
Practice (L *vs.* S)	432·306	1	11·38†
Interaction Q × R	127·806	1	4·26*
„ Q × P	35·156	1	—
„ P × R	23·256	1	—
„ P × Q × R	107·258	1	3·577
Within groups	1216·700	32	
Total:	2116·944	39	

Significance Levels: * $F_{.05}$ = 4·15.
† $F_{.01}$ = 7·50.

After reviewing work on *conditioning* and *reminiscence*, we must now turn to studies of the *work decrement*. In saying that mental work decrement is due to accumulating inhibition, as we have done in Chapter Two, we have implied that when this hypothesis is taken in conjunction with our typological postulate, it would follow that extraverts would show greater work decrement than introverts. Some direct evidence on this point has come from the work of the Cambridge Applied Psychology Research Unit, where Mackworth and his colleagues have done a considerable amount of experimentation on continuous perceptual work ('vigilance'—Mackworth, 1948; 'human watch-keeping'—Broadbent, 1953). Under conditions of continuous watch-keeping, errors of omission arise in spotting stimulus changes which may with advantage be conceptualized as inhibition phenomena. Under these conditions, we would expect to find marked differences between extraverts and introverts. Such differences do in fact appear to exist. Broadbent (1956) has reported that 'individual differences in human beings performing inspection watch-keeping tasks are large. Significant correlations have been found . . . between "fatigue" decrements in a number of such tasks and tests normally found to distinguish hysterics from dysthymics. There is thus some reason for holding that extraverts deteriorate more seriously in prolonged work; we may say, they are more liable to "inhibition".' The personality tests used by Broadbent included the Guilford R scale and measures of 'level of aspiration'; the watch-keeping tasks used included a choice serial reaction task, mental arithmetic, and the 20-dials and 20-lights tests, in which random changes on one of twenty presentation panels had to be signalled. (Correlations on small groups of subjects averaged between ·3 and ·5 in a number of studies. A description of the tests used can be found in Broadbent (1950, 1951). Broadbent's own theory of 'vigilance' phenomena is somewhat different from that here adopted, and can be consulted in his 1953 paper. The two theories are not necessarily incompatible.)

Another application of the concept of inhibition to the work decrement can be found in a study by Claridge (1956). Working with imbeciles, this writer used a task originally devised by Gordon (1953), consisting of a frame covered with a sheet of perforated zinc containing 82 holes to the square inch. A column down the shorter side of the board consisted of exactly 60 holes, and subjects worked to insert small escutcheon pins into the holes, working vertically down a column and completing it before starting the next. Each subject was given a small tray, containing a large supply of pins, which was placed by the side of the board. Subjects worked variously for 30-minute and 60-minute periods under different conditions of motivation. (Cf. Plate 23.)

In view of the large individual differences in performance and work decrement, Claridge constructed a rating scale which could be used as a measure of temperament for imbeciles. This scale, which was very carefully constructed and validated by him, is given below. He called it the 'excitability' rating scale, denoting by 'excitable' the aggressive, active, 'hysterical', sociable person with high verbal activity and considerable inter-personal response, intractable, unpredictable and variable in behaviour. The close similarity of the items on this scale to standard questionnaires of extraversion makes it reasonable to identify Claridge's 'excitability' with extraversion and to predict that on the task used, negative correlations would be found between extraversion-excitability and improvement during the course of the experiment.

EXCITABILITY RATING SCALE[1]

Weighted
Score

Item I. Emotionality level

0	A	Is a placid patient who rarely gives recognizable signs of emotion.
9	B	Is normally a cheerful patient, who has few extreme changes in mood.
22	C	Is an excitable patient who is easily pleased or cast down.
25	D	Is 'hysterical' and liable to frequent outbursts of temper or sullenness at minor things.

Item II. Aggressive behaviour

0	A	Always remains passive in encounters with other patients.
9	B	Can be roused, but usually only under extreme circumstances.
17	C	Sometimes becomes aggressive, but usually only in quarrels, when upset by others.
26	D	Sometimes has outbursts of violence against other patients for no apparent reason.

Item III. Activity level

| 0 | A | Would sit all day if left alone. |

[1] Rater is asked to choose the statement, A, B, C, D (E), from each item which most closely describes ratee. Subject's excitability score is the total of the weighted scores for one statement chosen from each of the nine items.

Weighted
Score

1	B	Is slow, but gets things done with occasional prodding.
15	C	Is active and gets things done at a reasonable speed.
17	D	Is restless and extremely quick in movement.
29	E	Is so jerky and overactive that this interferes with what he/she is doing.

Item IV. Variability of work activity

0	A	Will continue repeating the same task until moved on to another.
14	B	Seems to want to complete a task before starting on the next.
16	C	Often starts a new job before he/she has finished the previous one.
24	D	Extremely distractable, so that the job is never finished.

Item V. Verbal activity

0	A	Speaks only occasionally or when spoken to.
11	B	Speaks spontaneously and will carry on short conversations.
19	C	Will talk at some length whenever there is an opportunity.
24	D	Talks incessantly and often without meaning.

Item VI. Sociability

0	A	Is completely solitary and almost always sits in a corner away from the other patients.
5	B	Is usually seen with only one or two special friends, but tends not to mix with the other patients in the ward.
9	C	Has a number of friends and mixes with most of the other patients in the ward.
25	D	Is frequently seen with someone different and is into everything that goes on.

Item VII. Inter-personal response

0	A	Is completely unmoved by visitors to the ward and will not answer when they speak to him/her.
6	B	Will show some interest in visitors but will answer only briefly when spoken to.
20	C	Will wave to visitors when they enter the ward and answer freely when spoken to.
31	D	Will rush excitedly towards visitors and often engage them in conversation.

Item VIII. Amenability

0	A	Always obeys passively and without comment if asked to do something.
9	B	Usually does most things he/she is asked to do with apparent willingness.
17	C	Seems to like to do things to please people and sometimes offers spontaneously.
25	D	Tends to be intractable, often grumbling and sometimes refusing outright to do things when asked.

Weighted
Score

Item IX. Predictability

0 A Remains steadily the same for long periods, so that it is always easy to tell how he/she will respond to the approaches of others.

14 B Usually responds as expected to the approaches of others, since there is little variation in his/her response.

18 C Has the usual periodic ups and downs, but it is relatively easy, knowing his/her mood, to guess how he/she will react.

26 D Only when you know him/her well can you tell what the response will be to other people.

30 E Varies very rapidly in response to others, so that it is impossible to tell whether he/she will be hostile or friendly when approached.

There were no significant differences between extraverts and introverts on the initial trials. On a small group of 18, the correlation between excitability score and absolute improvement for the first 10 trials had a value of $-\cdot56$ which closely approached the $\cdot01$ level of significance. These trials were 60-minute trials, but similar, though slightly lower, correlations were found on another group ($N = 20$) with 30-minute trials ($r = -\cdot44$). A last correlation was obtained for 48 subjects all of whom had worked for 10 trials, and for whom the observed value of the correlation turned out to be $-0\cdot41$, which was significant at the $\cdot01$ level of confidence. These results bear out our prediction of greater inhibition effects in extraverts, as long as the assumption can be justified that 'excitability' bears some relationship to extraversion.

Claridge furnishes some evidence that the negative correlations observed between improvement and extroversion vanish when motivation is increased. Unfortunately, the results are non-significant and the experiment was carried out on too small a group to make it possible to be certain of the repeatability of the observation. This interaction between drive and decrement is an interesting one and should be verified, if possible, in future experiments. As we shall see presently in connection with another experiment, Claridge's findings relating to this interaction are not untypical, and are well in line with our theory.

Deductions of the kind just considered are traditionally made with respect to routine manual or cognitive tasks. Yet, as the writer has pointed out elsewhere (Eysenck, 1955), the type of work represented by a lengthy intelligence test, in which similar problems are presented one after the other to the candidate without any rest pauses in between, is equally subject to the law of inhibition. Changes in rate of work, involuntary rest pauses, changes in total drive with increase of D_—these predicted effects have not been observed because they have not been looked for. The non-analytic methods adopted by psychrometricians, who only analyse total scores and neglect the many different ways in which such total scores can be built up, have been criticized by Furneaux (1955), who has substituted much more rigorous methods in the construction of his Nufferno tests; it is appropriate that the data to test our hypothesis should come from an experiment carried out and analysed by him.

The test used consisted of sixteen easy letter-series problems, preceded by two problems which were not scored, and followed by an insoluble problem, also not scored. The problems are so easy that in the population of university students tested errors do not occur; consequently, the score used is the time taken over each problem. The problems are roughly equal in difficulty, as determined by prior research. Under these conditions we would expect inhibition to affect the speed of work, and we would expect it to do so differentially for extraverts and introverts. No more precise prediction can be made as the test which is being analysed was preceded by other tests of intelligence, thus making the situation too complex to allow of precise prediction.

Subjects were given the Guilford scales, and 12 markedly extraverted and 15 markedly introverted subjects chosen for a comparison of their scores. The most reliable type of score was found to be the rate of work for a given item, divided by the average rate of work for the whole test; these scores are plotted in Fig. 29. The difference between the groups was found to be statistically significant, thus lending support to both our points —inhibition affects the rate of work, and it does so differentially for extraverts and introverts. Furneaux took one further step. Using a new sample of 130 students, he plotted each subject's scores and gave him a new score (pattern score) according to the degree to which his pattern of scores approached the extraverted or the introverted pattern in Fig. 29. These pattern scores would be expected to correlate with extraversion-introversion scores on the questionnaire, and indeed a very significant correlation of ·35 is reported by Furneaux, thus cross-validating the differential patterns found.

These results on the whole favour the hypothesis, but it is much too early to say very much about them. The experiment was not specifically designed to test our hypothesis, but use was made of data accumulated in the course of a rather different experiment; consequently, no very specific predictions could be made. The analysis has been included here largely because, as far as they go, the results suggest that this approach to the more detailed study of intellectual performances is a fruitful one, and

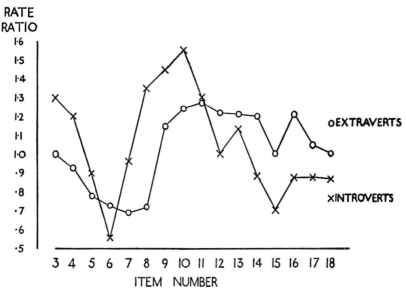

FIG. 29. Rate ratios (rate of work while attempting item/ average rate during whole test) of extraverts and introverts for 16 easy items of Nufferno Intelligence Test, Form AA (Unstressed).

because this approach has been so badly neglected by psychometrists. The writer has no quarrel with statistical methods of analysis, such as those routinely applied to intelligence tests; what he would criticize is the neglect of psychometrists to make use of psychological theories in their analyses even when, as in the case of inhibition, there is ample evidence to suggest that these factors are likely to exert a powerful influence on test scores. Here, it would appear, is a wide-open field for fruitful and practically as well as theoretically important research to be carried out.

THE DYNAMICS OF ANXIETY AND HYSTERIA

A somewhat different type of deduction is represented in the work of Cain (1942). We have argued that feelings of monotony and boredom are the mental equivalent of temporal inhibition. Assuming this relationship to be as stated, we would expect a correlation between extraversion and susceptibility to monotony (cf. also Wyatt & Langdon, 1937). Cain studied some 70 female workers engaged in repetitive semi-skilled work, and found that 'the monotony-susceptible worker tends to be less content with her life in general than the worker who is non-susceptible. The monotony-susceptible also tends to be more poorly adjusted in her relationships to family and the home. The non-susceptible liked better the more routine kinds of housework and preferred the quieter forms of recreation. She also tended to prefer regular habits of daily activity outside work.' While this study was not carried out with the intention of providing evidence relating to our hypothesis, the description of the worker who is not susceptible to monotony as one who 'liked better the more routine kinds of housework and preferred the quieter forms of recreation', and as one who preferred 'regular habits of daily activity outside work' fits in well with the theory that this type of worker would be characterized by introverted traits. There is much material along these lines in research reports from the industrial field, but unfortunately none of these appear to be designed to test a theory such as that here presented, and consequently most of this work is only tangential, and cannot be regarded as providing acceptable proof for our contention. It is to be hoped that studies designed with this hypothesis specifically in view will soon provide more definitive evidence in connection with this problem which appears of some practical importance in vocational guidance and in occupational selection.

While the evidence is rather meagre with respect to the three deductions just discussed, there is fortunately a considerable amount of experimental support for another deduction which also relates to the personality differences to be expected from continuous work. In discussing this prediction, it must be borne in mind that the manifestation of temporal inhibition which is to be looked for in any particular experiment depends very much on the exact specification of the task in question. Inhibition may show itself as a slowing-down in speed when accuracy is controlled, or a loss in accuracy when speed is controlled; it may show itself as a change in both speed and accuracy when neither is controlled. What would we expect to happen under conditions where subjects are required to make accurate and well-controlled movements in order to return changing dial-settings to zero position, or, more generally, where their task consists in a quick and precise response to a variety of constantly changing visual stimuli? The answer dictated by our general theoretical position surely must be that the neural structures mediating the stimulus-response connections develop temporal inhibition and periodically produce involuntary rest-pauses, and that this combination of inhibition and I.R.P.s would have the effect of producing a slowing down of reactions, i.e. a general inertia. If the experimental situation is such that failure to make prompt and accurate responses aggravates the faults in the stimulus-complex which the subject has to rectify, then inertness of response would allow larger errors or faults to develop; these in turn would require large and more complex movements for their correction. Conversely, a failure of inhibition to develop would lead to immediate correcting responses to the changing stimulus situation, thus preventing any large errors; in an exaggerated form, this type of behaviour could easily lead to over-activity, i.e. to a tendency to react too quickly to possibly chance disturbances, and to over-correct relatively slight deviations.

We are thus led to postulate two extreme types of reaction, dependent on the presence or absence of strong inhibitory potential. The strongly inhibitory type (extravert; hysteric) should on this hypothesis be subject to sluggish, inert response behaviour; the weakly inhibitory type (introvert; dysthymic) should be subject to over-active, over-responsive behaviour. Historically, Bleuler (1906) appears to have been one of the first to note the differentiation between the type of person in whom there is a quick and intensive reaction to emotional impressions and the type of person in whom the effect is suppressed, leading to displacements and conversions. Nunberg (1918), one of Jung's associates, produced experimental evidence for the existence of this continuum in his work on motor movement in response to word association; he showed that some subjects make excessive, others decreased motor movements under affect. Berrien (1939) also found evidence of two extreme types of reaction to emotion-provoking stimuli which he labelled 'excitatory' and 'inhibitory' respectively. It is the work of Davis (1946, 1948,

1949), however, which is of particular relevance here, as he appears to have been the first to relate over-active and inert types of behaviour to personality differences.

Davis was concerned with the causes of pilot error, and carried out a series of experiments in a simulated cockpit; this was similar to the well-known Link trainer except that it did not itself move. Instruments of the panel respond realistically to movements on the controls; the effects of these control movements were less complex than those of an aircraft, but the test was apparently accepted by the subjects as an exercise in instrument flying. This exercise consisted of a series of four manœuvres, together occupying ten minutes, repeated between intervals of straight and level flying. Only the periods of manœuvre were scored; instructions and recording were so arranged that a perfect performance was recorded as a straight line, and deviation indicating an error. Other detailed records of performance were also made.

Two types of error were observed; *errors of over-action* and *errors of inertia*. Subjects exhibiting over-activity 'obtained large scores on control movements. Their errors in instrument reading were small and of short duration. . . . Responses to instrument deviations were excessive, the extent and gradient of the movements being greatly increased and over-correcting frequent, with the result that secondary responses were required. Numerous restless movements were observed. . . . Subjects felt excited and under strain, tense and irritable and sometimes frankly anxious. They felt that correction was urgent and made it impatiently. . . . Although . . . subjects were dissatisfied with their performance, they were not discouraged, but keen to improve and continued to try to do the test well. . . . Several pilots reported preoccupation with the test for some time after it was finished. Some returned later in the day and asked for a further opportunity of doing the test.'

Subjects exhibiting the inertia reaction made 'errors which were large and of long duration, whereas activity, represented by scores of control movements, was relatively little. . . . The individual responses were less hurried and less disturbed by restless movements than were those of the pilots showing the over-activity reaction, but they were often more extensive than at the beginning of the test, due probably to the large size of the instrument deviations and the tendency to make responses proportionate to the size of the deviations. . . . Subjects reported that their interest had flagged and that their concentration had failed. A feeling of strain had now given way to one of mild boredom, tedium or tiredness. . . . In contrast to the restless striving of the over-active class, the pilots in the inert class gave the impression that they had lowered their standards of performance to a level well within their powers. . . . Subjects' judgment of the degree of accuracy to which they had attained was usually faulty, and they were unaware of the degree to which they had failed to correct deviations of the instruments. . . . There was . . . an emotional indifference as far as the test itself was concerned.'

These results are closely in accord with Nunberg's observation in his original work. They also link up well with experimental work on the extravert-introvert dimension reported elsewhere (Eysenck, 1947) showing that introverts (like the over-active response type) tend to show anxiety, to be irritable, to have a high level of aspiration, and to be dissatisfied with their performance. Extraverts (like the inert response type) tended to show emotional indifference, to have low levels of aspiration adjusted to actual performance, and to be satisfied with their performance, however poor. So far, then, our predictions appear to be borne out. More direct proof, however, appears desirable of the two main hypotheses deducible from our theory:

(1) Pilots who are neurotic should show a larger proportion of abnormal (over-active or inert) reactions than pilots who are not diagnosed as neurotic, and

(2) pilots who are diagnosed as suffering from dysthymic disorders show the introverted, over-active behaviour pattern, while pilots suffering from hysterica disorders should show the extraverted, inert behaviour pattern.

Both these hypotheses were tested by Davis on 355 normal and 39 neurotic pilots. Taking the comparison between normal and neurotic pilots first, it will be seen from Table IX that both predictions are verified: 75 per cent of the normals show normal reactions, but only 33 per cent of the neurotics do so. Seven per cent of anxiety states show inert reactions, while 75 per cent of hysterics do so. These conclusions are statistically significant. Repetition of the experiment, using a modified and much simpler type of apparatus, gave results which show again, at

TABLE IX

Test Results of Normal and Neurotic Pilots

	Reactions						Total N
	Normal		Over-active		Inert		
	No.	%	No.	%	No.	%	
Normal Pilots	268	75	59	17	28	8	355
Neurotic Pilots	13	33	11	28	15	38	39
Acute Anxiety State	6	43	7	50	1	7	14
Hysteria	1	12·5	1	12·5	6	75	8
Other	6	35	3	18	8	47	17

an acceptable level of statistical significance, that the acutely anxious (introvert) type of patient tends to make more extensive responses than did the normal subject, while the hysteric (extravert) patient tends to make less extensive ones. (This apparatus is illustrated in Plate 13 in Eysenck, 1952.) The task consists of aligning a central pointer with a line at the right or at the left, according to the brightness of two lights flashed on at both sides. Movement of the pointer is mediated through an integrating disc, and is produced by turning the handwheel. Provision is made for automatic recording of movements, time sequences, etc. (Cf. Davis, 1948.) Scores for 'extent of responses' are given below in Table X. Dysthymics clearly give more extensive, hysterics less extensive response.

TABLE X

	Distribution of Cases (Extent scores—arbitrary units)						Total
	3	4	5	6	7	8	
Healthy pilots	1	3	21	29	14	1	69
'Acutely anxious' patients	1	1	2	3	6	2	15
'Hysterical' patients	4	5	2	1	0	0	12

The hypothesis of a normal-neurotic continuum would also require that within the normal group there should appear a correlation between neurotic predisposition and percentage of abnormal responses. The percentage of abnormal responses made by the 355 normal pilots is given in Table XI after they had been divided into three groups according to psychiatrically assessed degree of neurotic predisposition; it will be seen that there is an increase in abnormal responses from 16 per cent in the group showing the least predisposition, through 27 per cent to 46 per cent in the group showing the greatest amount of predisposition. Thus this third hypothesis is also confirmed by Davis's results at a reasonable level of statistical significance. We may take it as established, therefore, that under emotional stress there is a disorganization of motor processes, a disorganization which is closely correlated with neuroticism or lack of emotional stability. We may also take it as established that the direction taken by this disorganization—inertia or overactivity—is related to extraversion-introversion, as postulated by our theory.

TABLE XI

Association of Neuroticism and Test Scores

Predisposition to Neurosis	Normal	Over-active	Inert	Percentage Abnormal
Nil	130	13	12	16
Slight	113	32	9	27
Moderate	25	14	7	46

This interesting work has been extended recently by Venables (1953, 1955) in an experiment which was conducted as part of a larger investigation into the effects of psychological handicap. It occupied approximately 8 minutes of a session lasting $1\frac{1}{2}$ hours; during this session the subjects completed a battery of intelligence and personality tests. A normal sample was tested consisting of 210 male trainees for the job of bus conductor. Data were available for each subject to make it possible to allocate factor scores on intelligence, neuroticism, and extroversion to him; these scores were derived from the analysis of results on 15 psychometric tests. Also tested were male neurotics of similar age: 11 hysterics and 11 dysthymics were allocated to the experimental group from a population of patients interviewed at a psychiatric hospital. To enable results from these two samples to be compared, two groups of 11 subjects each from the normal sample were chosen on the basis of high scores on the neuroticism factor and extreme scores on the introversion-extraversion factor; these groups, chosen to have characteristics which were similar to those of the two neurotic groups, may be called quasi-anxious (QA) and quasi-hysteric (QH).

The apparatus used by Venables is shown in Fig. 30. It is described by him as follows: 'From the subjects' viewpoint the apparatus consisted of a milk-white screen $8\frac{3}{4} \times 5\frac{1}{2}$ in., set in a brass frame, at an angle of 45° from the base. On either side of the centre line of the frame and at $2\frac{3}{8}$ in. from it were two marks over which the stimulus lights appeared. In the horizontal shelf in front of the display screen was a slot $8\frac{1}{2}$ in. long through which

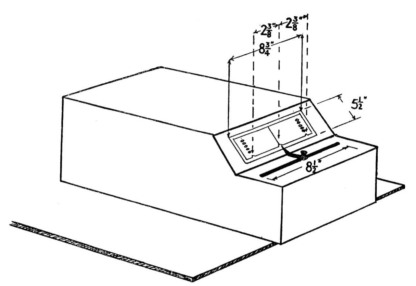

FIG. 30. Apparatus used by Venables in experiment on motor response to stress.

a knob protruded. A pointer attached to the knob indicated its position against the marks on the display panel. Five stimulus lights were set vertically behind the display panel above each lateral mark. Their position was not visible until alight. Reading from the bottom the stimuli were (1) white, (2) green, (3) red, (4) showing the word YES, (5) showing the word NO.

The subject was given the instructions, 'When you hear this click' (a signal indicating that new stimulus was being presented), 'move the pointer from the mark in the centre to the mark under the white light, if it is on its own, or has green or YES over it. However, if it has red or NO over it move it to the mark on the opposite side. After this, move the pointer as quickly as possible to the centre mark.'

The pointer was attached to a lever controlling a pen which recorded the subject's movement on a moving paper. The stimuli were automatically presented in predetermined sequence *via* the contacts of three uniselectors. The presentation of stimuli was divided into three consecutive periods of 50 displays each. In the first easy period A, white lights only were used at a 2 sec. periodicity; this was followed by a difficult period B, using all the lights at 1·5 sec. per display, and a final easy period

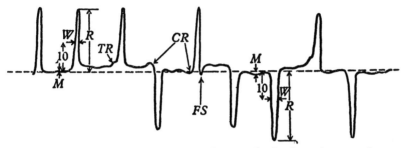

FIG. 31. Artificial example showing method of scoring psycho-motor task records.

C, identical with A. The whole task thus took 275 sec. to complete. The order of presentation of lights was such that each direction of movement to each type of display was balanced. Every fifth response in the difficult period B was to a simple white light stimulus. This scheme was adopted as it was required to measure characteristics of response which were not themselves reactions to difficult stimuli, but were set in an environment of difficult stimuli. By this means it was hoped to measure not the immediate effect of distraction, but the effect on response to a standard stimulus of the emotional condition produced by having to respond to more complex stimuli.

As regards procedure, the subject was seated in front of the apparatus, which was placed on a low table so that his forearm was parallel to the ground; he was asked to use his preferred hand. The task was explained to the subject, who was allowed to practise at his own speed whilst 50 displays were presented. It was then explained that his responses would be recorded and that he should expect a period of white lights only at a slow speed, a period using all the lights at a slightly faster speed, and finally white lights only again at a slow speed, there being no break between the periods.

The scoring on the records was as shown in Fig. 31, which illustrates the definition of the following concepts:

R = Maximum extent of response.

W = Width of response measured at a fixed distance (10 arbitrary units) from the centre line.

M = The deviation from the centre line of the point of return after each response.

Ten responses were measured in each period A, B and C, and means and standard deviations were calculated for each variable. The means were designated $\bar{R}$, $\bar{W}$ and $\bar{M}$, and the standard deviations, giving measures of variability within each period, were denoted by S_R, S_W and S_M.

In addition to this measurement, selected secondary features of all the responses in each period were counted. These were:

FS = False starts, where the subject started initially in the wrong direction.

TR = Trailing returns, where the subject did not make a simple direct return movement to the centre line after a response.

CR = Corrected returns, where the return movement overshot the centre mark and had to be corrected.

The best measure for the over-active–inert continuum was found to be the amount of response per unit time, measured by R/W. This score was found to have a split-half reliability of ·970 in period A. Five types of measure altogether were analysed for each subject, namely, his score in period A, his score in period B, his score in period C, change in score between periods A and B, and change in score between periods B and C. Some of the results are given in Fig. 32. They are summed up by Venables as follows:

'If we examine the results from either the whole of sample 1 or the subgroups drawn from it, it is seen that extravert and quasi-hysteric subjects show a significant tendency to change their performance in the inert direction under increased difficulty. The reverse tendency is shown in introvert, quasi-anxious, and anxious subjects. The hospitalized, hysteric patient presents an initially inert type of response. Commencing performance on this level, he does not change his performance in the inert direction under increased difficulty, but maintains a performance which is substantially similar to his starting performance.

'With decrease in task difficulty there is in all cases a significant tendency for the extravert or hysteric subject to per-

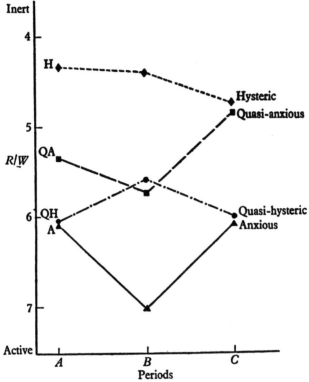

FIG. 32. Changes in activity of response (R/W) between periods A, B, and C in four groups.

form more actively whilst the introverted or anxious patient subject shows a decrease in activity.

'On examination of the measures which make up the index R/W it is seen that response length tends to shorten in the difficult period and lengthen subsequently, although to different extents, in different groups of subjects. On decrease of difficulty there is a general lengthening of response in all groups.

It is the measure W, the time for which the response lasts, that seems to be responsible to a greater extent for differential behaviour between the groups. In both dysthymic groups there is a speed up of response under difficult followed by a slowing down with decrease in difficulty. In the hysteric patient group performance is slow initially whilst in the extraverted group drawn from sample 1 there is a slowing down on increase of difficulty. In both of these groups there is a speed up on decrease of difficulty.'

Individual differences on the inert-active continual, as measured by R/W, are related exclusively to extraversion-introversion; correlation of task variables with intelligence and neuroticism show that they are, in general, independent of these factors as well as of age. The results on the neurotic groups bear out those reported by Davis. It is found that in all three periods hysterics are inert and dysthymics overactive. In the normal group and particularly in the quasi-anxious and quasi-hysteric groups, it appears that such differences are brought out only with an increase in stress. As stress increases from period A to period B, the quasi-hysteric group gets more inert, the quasi-anxious group more overactive, while on the removal of stress, i.e. in period C, both groups move in the opposite direction. These results should be seen in the context of our discussion of the Yerkes-Dobson law where it is pointed out that objective differences in stress, as defined by the total stimulation configuration, must be supplemented by a consideration of individual differences in reactivity or emotionality. For the two neurotic groups, therefore, who according to our theory are especially high on emotionality, the period A task must be assumed to have been highly stressful to bring out the overactivity-inertness reactions, which in the quasi-hysteric and quasi-anxious groups (who according to our theory are somewhat less emotional) require the added stress produced in period B. These findings then are well in agreement with a theory postulating a multiplicative function as describing with some accuracy the relation between drive on the one hand and excitation and inhibition on the other.

Also in agreement with this conclusion is another study by Venables (1956) in which he studied car driving performance in relation to personality. He showed that there was a significant tendency for inconsistency of performance to be associated with

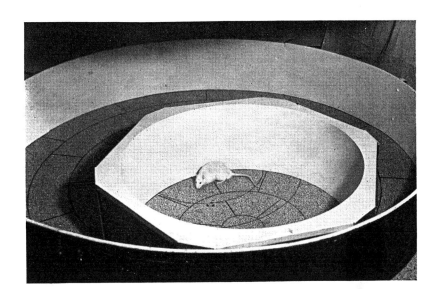

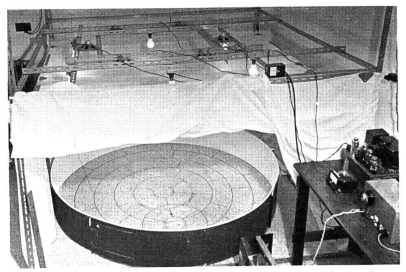

13*a*. Open field test: rat in enclosure showing alternative sizes of test-field.

13*b*. Open field test: superstructure for changing stress of test by changes in noise level and illumination.

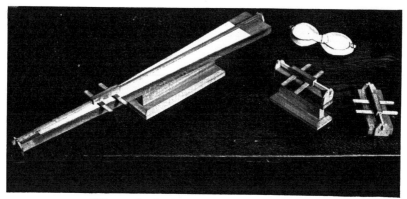

14. Kinaesthetic figural after-effect apparatus.

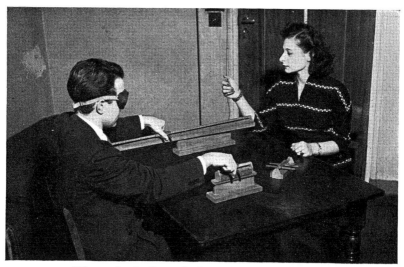

15. Kinaesthetic figural after-effect: test in progress.

neuroticism and also with extraversion. This result was in line with expectation in view of the relation of extraversion to the tendency towards inert performance. 'This inertia would, it is thought, produce lax control of the car which would show as inconsistent behaviour between occasions.' Though the numbers used are not large, the results are statistically significant and would certainly deserve following up in a more extended study.

Before leaving a discussion of motor phenomena related to our theory, we may perhaps quote some work connected with brain damage. We have previously noted the fact that brain damage tends to produce extraverted behaviour patterns; we may now state a more fundamental postulate in the following form: *brain damage leads to an increase in inhibitory potential, both temporal and spatial.*[1] Most of the evidence for this postulate is to be found in the perceptual field, and will be discussed in the next chapter; here we will draw attention to three sets of phenomena only. The first of these is concerned with conditioning; it follows from our theory, taken in conjunction with our postulate, that brain damage should lead to a decline in the

---

[1] This postulate should be read in the context of our discussion in the first chapter of the work of Petrie and LeBeau. It is intended to have two implications, one of which is *quantitative*, the other *qualitative*. The quantitative corollary simply states that: *The growth of inhibitory potential is proportional to the percentage of brain tissue destroyed*; this form of statement clearly relates to Lashley's classical work on rats (1929) and his conclusion regarding cognitive loss after brain surgery. The evidence is by now fairly definite that this corollary is too broad and general to cover all the facts, and that a second corollary is needed. This refers to the particular location and/or type of tissue destroyed, and reads as follows: *Growth of inhibitory potential is related to the precise location of the injury to the cortex*, being particularly marked, for instance, after destruction of parts of areas 9 and/or 10. The admission of both general and localized effects seems necessitated by the experimental evidence (Tizard, 1956; Meyer, 1957); it is realized of course that both the postulate and the corollaries must be stated much more precisely before they can be considered to be particularly useful. Such a statement is at present impossible, and the postulate is given here because it suggests profitable methods of investigation rather than as a final, definitive summing-up of research. It should be noted that the brain-damage postulate was originally put forward by Shapiro (1956), whose work will be discussed in the next chapter: 'Brain damage results in the increase in the strength of inhibitory effects in some, at least, of the remaining parts of the brain.'

Our general conclusion is similar to that reported by Teuber and Weinstein (1956) as a result of their studies of the impairment of brain-injured persons to discover hidden figures in the Gottschaldt test; they maintain that cerebral lesions in man have twofold effects, *specific* and *general*. It may be noted that the experimental findings of these writers are in good accord with an inhibition theory, and in fact a prediction to this effect was made by M. Shapiro in discussion with the writer several years ago, specifying the particular test used by Teuber and Weinstein.

rate of conditioning. Gantt (1950) and Reese *et al.* (1953) have provided some evidence to indicate that this deduction finds some support in experimental fact. The other deduction is a little more indirect. Lepley (1934) and Hull (1943) have elaborated the inhibition theory here adopted to include the well-known bowing effect observable in serial nonsense syllable learning. Following them we may take the amount of bowing observed as a measure of the degree of inhibition shown by a given subject. It follows that extraverts should show a greater degree of bowing than introverts, and equally that brain-damaged subjects should behave on this test very much like extraverts. No formal experiment appears to have been done in this connection, but Malmo and Amsel (1948) have published some incidental observations on four brain-damaged patients, showing a considerably increased degree of bowing in their learning curves. These curves are reproduced in Fig. 33. A repetition of this experiment would appear necessary before the results could be claimed as supporting our theory very strongly, in view of the small number of cases used.

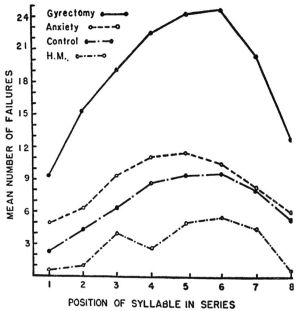

FIG. 33. Serial position effect in nonsense syllable learning, showing extreme bowing after brain injury.

Our third example comes from the field of work decrement studies. It would seem to follow from our theory of brain-injury as productive of inhibitory potential that continuous work should produce more inhibition in brain-damaged than in normal or functionally disturbed control subjects, such as schizophrenics. The only study along these lines which has come to our attention is one carried out recently by Rosvold *et al.* (1956). The authors of this large-scale and particularly well-controlled experiment do in fact report the predicted effects at acceptable levels of statistical significance, and we may conclude, therefore, that the experimental data do not contradict our deduction.

It will be seen that out of the many hundreds of deductions which learning theory, taken in conjunction with our typological postulate, could mediate, only a very small number has in fact been tested. The fact that the results have been promising does not necessarily carry any implication that similar success would attend attempts to verify other deductions. There appears to be in prospect a very large experimental programme to be carried out before any kind of definitive judgment can be formulated about the value of the theory here advocated.

Chapter Five

PERSONALITY AND PERCEPTUAL PROCESSES

PERCEPTUAL processes are probably connected with personality structure just as intimately as are learning and conditioning. Yet here also there has been a remarkable dearth of properly conceived and theoretically based experimentation. An irresponsibly high percentage of the total work in this field appears to have gone into the development of so-called 'projective' tests. Nothing more will be said here about the Rorschach and other similar tests; the critical reader who is familiar with its almost complete lack of reliability and validity, or who has followed the fate of such concepts as 'colour shock' at the hands of the experimentalist, will not require a detailed substantiation of the view outlined above (Eysenck, 1957).

Leaving out then the so-called projective devices from our account, we are still faced with a vast literature devoted to the exploration of objective differences between normal and various neurotic and psychotic groups. This whole field has been surveyed quite recently by Granger (1953), and a large battery of tests has been applied to normal, neurotic and psychotic subjects by Eysenck, Granger and Brengelmann (1957). The results of all this work show that very marked differences can be observed between these groups, and that objective measures of the kind considered can be of great value in both diagnosis and prognosis. However, from our present point of view, these results have one undesirable feature: there is no theoretical framework to bind them together, and consequently from the point of view of scientific advance, they must be regarded as accidental findings—data in search of a theory, as it were. That would seem to rule them out of consideration from our present

148

point of view, and we must turn rather to a much more limited set of experiments which, however, have the advantage of being derived from a clearly formulated theory and of linking up with the data reported in our last section.

It will be remembered that we postulated two varieties of inhibition: temporal or reactive inhibition and spatial or induced inhibition. It will also be remembered that the locus of inhibition was assumed to be central, as Pavlov thought, rather than peripheral, as was Hull's view. If these assumptions are correct, and if these processes of inhibition are of fundamental importance in cortical behaviour, then we would expect to encounter them also in the perceptual field. Our task therefore would be a twofold one: first to find perceptual analogues of temporal and spatial inhibition, and second, to show that on such perceptual measures of inhibition predicted differences between extraverts and introverts, or between brain-damaged and non-brain-damaged subjects, occur in the expected direction. As we shall show presently, both these expectations are, in fact, fulfilled. We will first turn to temporal inhibition or 'satiation'.

The general postulate of reactive inhibition states in effect, as pointed out by Hull, that 'all responses leave behind in the physical structures involved in the evocation, a state or substance which acts directly to inhibit the evocation of the activity in question. The hypothetical inhibitory condition or substance is observable only through its effect upon positive reaction potentials. This negative action is called *reactive inhibition*. An increment of reactive inhibition ($\triangle$ I_R) is assumed to be generated by every repetition of the response (R), whether reinforced or not, and these increments are assumed to accumulate except as they spontaneously disintegrate with the passage of time.' Now, from the behaviourist point of view perception is in fact a stimulus-response connection (cf. Garner *et al.*, 1956, for a thorough discussion of this point of view), so that this general principle should apply with equal force to the so-called perceptual phenomena. It may be surmised that here, as in the learning field, special conditions will have to be created to make the phenomenon amenable to observation and measurement. Just as in the field of learning theory reminiscence phenomena are only obtained under highly specialized laboratory conditions of massed practice, so inhibition phenomena in perception are also likely to require highly specialized laboratory conditions for their observation. Fortunately there has, in recent years, been a considerable degree of interest in the investigation of such phenomena, and Kohler (1940, 1944) has given them the general name of *satiation phenomena*, or figural after-effects.

Köhler's own formulation of the general hypothesis underlying his work postulates that 'a specific figure process occurs whenever a figure appears in the visual field. And this process tends to block its own way if the figure remains for some time in the same location. . . . Continued presence of *any* figure in a given location must change conditions for subsequent figure processes in the same region of the field.' This statement of the satiation hypothesis in perception is formally identical with Hull's statement of the reactive inhibition hypothesis in learning, and both are, in fact, deducible from Spearman's (1927) general law of fatigue, which was postulated many years before Hull or Köhler constructed their respective postulate systems: 'The occurrence of any cognitive event produces a tendency opposed to its occurrence afterwards.'

Some of the similarities between learning and perception phenomena were noted by Köhler and Fishback (1950), in particular the favourable influence of rest intervals and the phenomenon of reminiscence, and they suggested that the processes responsible for these phenomena in learning, and neural satiation in perception, might be similar. Eysenck (1955) formally proposed the general 'identity' hypothesis outlined above, discussed methodological problems in the way of proving theories of this kind, and furnished an experimental demonstration of the identity of underlying processes, which will be discussed presently. Duncan (1956) has reviewed the formal points of similarity between reactive inhibition and satiation, and a brief summary of these points may serve as a good introduction to the experimental part of this section.

(1) *Source*. Both inhibition and satiation develop as a consequence of afferent stimulation, or, as we would prefer to put it, both are a consequence of the repeated passage of neural currents from the stimulus to the response side. (2) *Locus*. Both inhibition and satiation are central; this point has been demonstrated by Köhler and Wallach (1944) in connection with figural after-effects, and has been argued by us with respect to inhibition on a previous page. (3) *Effects*. Both inhibition and

satiation distort behaviour in the direction of departing from some criterion or standard. (4) *Rate of growth.* Duncan reviews the evidence and concludes that 'it can probably be concluded that with continuous stimulation the effects of both processes will be manifest after periods of stimulation as brief as 5–10 sec.' (5) *Maximum effect.* 'With continued stimulation there is a point reached beyond which the distortions produced by either satiation or reactive inhibition do not further increase.' (6) *Rate of decay.* 'Both satiation and reactive inhibition dissipate over rest, and the rates of decay for both are quite rapid at first.' Summarizing, Duncan wrote: 'It appeared that the two processes are quite similar on most, perhaps all, characteristics. Although more research is needed on some points, present evidence suggests that reactive inhibition and neural satiation may refer to the same process.'

It is one thing to suggest that two processes are identical, but quite another to furnish proof of this identity. Logically, there are three types of 'proof', i.e. three types of deduction from the hypothesis that two processes, which we may call A and B, are in fact identical. (This argument is quite general, and while it applies to the two processes under review, it is by no means restricted to them. For this reason we shall talk about A and B, rather than about inhibition and satiation, so that the argument may retain its air of generality.) The first proof may be called the *neuro-physiological proof*, and it depends on the discovery in the microscopic realm of neurological substrata for the molar phenomena we call A and B. If these substrata are identical, then we may rest satisfied that the molar phenomena mediated by them are identical. While this method of proof will probably appeal to readers as the most satisfactory, and while quite probably neurophysiology will advance sufficiently one day to make possible the identification of molar and molecular phenomena, it is not possible at present to pretend that this stage has been reached, or even that it has been approached sufficiently closely to make us at all confident that success will be reached in our lifetime. However desirable, therefore, this method does not seem readily applicable.

The second type of proof may be called the *functional proof*, because it is based on similarities of functioning, rather than on similarities of structure underlying function. The arguments advanced by Duncan are typical of this method of argument; it is demonstrated that two phenomena obey similar laws, and consequently the similarity of the processes is asserted. This is the traditional argument in psychology, and its cogency can hardly be denied. Its weaknesses are twofold. In the first place the numerical results from the experimental study of the processes in question are not usually precise enough to make the proof very rigorous, and in the second place the presence of different types of extraneous and interfering variables may produce differences in the observations although the underlying processes are identical, just as easily as they may counteract differences in the underlying processes and thus give rise to (spurious) similarities in the observations. Cautious experimentalists are of course well aware of these sources of error and try to reduce their import, but in our present state of ignorance proof of the functional type is not always as impressive and convincing as one might wish.

The third type of proof may be called the *differential proof*, because it is based on the existence of individual differences which are relevant to the processes to be compared. This proof rests on a postulate which we may call the correlational postulate, and which is fundamental to factor analysis, correlational analysis, and all the statistical methods of the analysis of interdependence (Kendall, 1950; Eysenck, 1953). It may be stated as follows: *If two processes are mediated by one and the same source variable, and if the strength of this source variable differs from one person to another, either innately or for other reasons, then the two processes will be found to covary (correlate) in the population, when all other influences relevant to the manifestation of the two processes have been eliminated or held constant, either statistically or experimentally.* In practice, this means that we may search for proof of the identity of processes A and B in the correlations between reliable and valid measures of these processes under appropriate experimental conditions. In terms of our specific problem, if inhibition and satiation are at bottom identical ('mediated by one and the same source variable'), and if there are individual differences in the rate of growth, the maximum strength, and the rate of dissipation of these processes, then reliable and valid measures of inhibition and satiation should correlate positively, provided that sources of interference and contamination are properly controlled.

This method of correlation may be called the direct form of

the differential proof; it lies at the bottom of the factor analytic method. If visual and kinaesthetic figural after-effects are both produced by the same hypothetical process of 'satiation', and if there are individual differences in satiation, then measures of visual and kinaesthetic figural after-effects ought to intercorrelate, i.e. people with high rates of satiation should have strong after-effects of both types, and people with low rates of satiation should have weak after-effects. Wertheimer (1955) has shown that this prediction is indeed borne out in fact. Similarly, and for the same reasons, if inhibition and satiation are both due to some common central process, then measures of satiation and inhibition should be correlated with each other. Livson and Krech's (1955) demonstration of such a correlation between retroactive inhibition in nonsense syllable learning and the magnitude of the kinaesthetic figural after-effect may be quoted as an example relating to this deduction.

However, the direct form of this proof is not the only one, and it may not always be the most efficient or the most practical. We may make use of the typological postulate advanced in a previous chapter, and formulate an indirect form of the differential proof. This form makes use of the fact that we have available a theory which tells us what kind of people are likely to have high satiation and inhibition scores (extraverts, hysterics, brain-damaged), and what kind of people are likely to have low scores (introverts, dysthymics). Instead of correlating large numbers of tests of satiation, inhibition, and so forth with each other, which is a very time-consuming, difficult, and expensive procedure, needing considerable resources, this method uses personality measures or psychiatric diagnoses as intermediary of connecting variables. Thus instead of correlating a measure of satiation, say, and a measure of reminiscence, this method would mediate the proof by showing that (1) satiation correlates with extraversion (Eysenck, 1955), and (2) reminiscence correlates with extraversion (Eysenck, 1956). The groups on which the tests are done need not be the same, and indeed the experiments need not be done by the same person nor in the same laboratory. Thus the indirect form obviates the necessity implicit in the direct form of the proof of concentrating all the work in one single, huge, centralized project, and makes possible the easy comparability of different pieces of work carried out in different laboratories by different investigators,

While theoretically the direct method is perhaps slightly prefer-able, practical reasons will make many research workers prefer the second method.

The difficulties of the differential proof will be as evident as its advantages. Experimental methods of investigation, such as those elaborated for the study of satiation and inhibition, are not usually well adapted to the exigencies of psychometric pro-cedures; they usually have low reliabilities, and may necessitate much work before a suitable method of scoring is discovered. (Cf. H. J. Eysenck, 1956, for the scoring of reminiscence tests, and S. B. G. Eysenck, 1957, for scoring the P.G.R.) The neces-sity to partial out disturbing influences, or eliminate them experimentally, presupposes more definite knowledge than we usually have; to keep constant sex, age and intelligence is usually as much as can be done. Occasionally other variables are of obvious importance, to such an extent that they may make it impossible to interpret the results of experiments where they have not been adequately controlled. Thus the results reported by Nicholls (1955) on visual satiation effects in neurotics are impossible to interpret because of the failure of neurotics to obey instructions to fixate the inspection figure. We suspect that much of the work of visual satiation, speed of reversal of ambiguous figures, after-effects of rotating spirals, and dark vision is vitiated by failure to control this very simple and obvious variable. More will be said about this point later on.

The differential method, thus, is beset with difficulties no less than is the functional method, and indeed the difficulties in both are similar, and spring from our relative ignorance of the factors which determine the phenomena we are studying. What is suggested here is that the differential method is a useful and valuable adjunct to the functional method, so that when both methods agree in the answer which they give to our experi-mental probing, we may feel somewhat more certain that this answer is indeed the correct one. However, in the absence of the neuro-physiological proof complete certainty is not likely to be felt by anyone familiar with the difficulties of work in this field.

Applications of the indirect form of the differential method to motor phenomena, such as conditioning, reminiscence, work decrement and others, have been discussed in previous chapters;

we must now turn to its application to the phenomena of satiation. The main experiment here is one reported by the writer (Eysenck, 1955), using the kinaesthetic figural after-effect.

The apparatus used in this experiment is an adaptation of that described by Köhler and Dinnerstein (1947); the exact form of apparatus and procedure was taken from Klein and Krech (1952), who used it in their work on cortical conductivity in the brain injured. As a full description and rationale are given by these authors, our own will be brief. Plates 14 and 15 show the apparatus set out on a table and the test in progress, and may serve to facilitate comprehension.

The apparatus consists of a comparison scale (marked 'A' in the photograph), a test object (marked 'B'), and a stimulus object (marked 'C'). Movable riders are affixed to all three objects in such a way that the position of thumb and forefinger is fixed as the subject moves these two fingers up and down along the sides of the object. All objects are made of unpainted, smoothed hardwood. The apparatus is so arranged as to present the comparison scale to the left of the seated subject and either the test or stimulus object to his right.

The subject is blindfolded before he has an opportunity of viewing any part of the equipment. Having taken his seat in front of the apparatus, he is given an explanation of his task as well as a demonstration. Then the experiment proper commences. Putting thumb and forefinger of his right hand into the rider of the test object, and thumb and forefinger of his left hand into the rider of the comparison scale, S is required to adjust the position of the rider on the comparison scale until the distance between the fingers of his left hand feels equal to the distance between the fingers of his right hand. This is the point of subjective equality, and all changes are measured from this point as the baseline. Four separate determinations are carried out, and the results averaged, to make this baseline more reliable.

The next step in the experiment consists in providing the subject with varying periods of constant tactile stimulation. For this purpose he is instructed to put his fingers into the rider on the stimulus object, which is slightly broader than the test object ($2\frac{1}{2}$ in. as compared with $1\frac{1}{2}$ in.), and to rub the sides of the stimulus object at an even rate for periods of 30 sec., 60 sec.,

90 sec., and 120 sec. respectively. Four determinations of subjective equality are made after each period of rubbing in order to obtain more reliable measures. In this way the effect of rubbing the stimulus object on the perception of the test object is ascertained. Finally, after a five-minute rest period and again after another ten-minute rest, the subjective width of the test object is again ascertained in order to establish the perseverative effects of the stimulation periods. These two sets of judgments are again obtained four times each in order to increase reliability.

The predicted after-effect consequent upon the rubbing of a stimulus object *broader* than the test object is an apparent *shrinking* of the test object, which should manifest itself in terms of a decrement in the width on the comparison scale judged equal to the text object. For each subject this decrement is expressed in terms of his own original baseline, so that individual differences in perceived equality are taken into account in the score, which thus is essentially a percentage decrement score, i.e. an estimate of the shrinkage that has occurred as a percentage of the original width of the object as perceived by each subject.

The following scores were obtained: (1) average percentage decrement after 30 sec.; (2) average percentage decrement after 60 sec.; (3) average percentage decrement after 90 sec.; (4) average percentage decrement after 120 sec. In addition to these post-stimulation after-effects, the following recovery period scores were obtained: (*a*) average percentage decrement after 5-min. rest; (*b*) average percentage decrement after (10 min. + 5 min. =) 15 min. rest.

The subjects in this investigation were selected on the basis of a combination of psychiatric criteria (diagnosis of 'hysteria' or 'anxiety') and questionnaire score (Guilford R scale); all subjects were male, equated for age and intelligence. There were 14 extraverted and 14 introverted neurotic patients in the experiment altogether. Reasonable reliability was demonstrated for the scores used, the Hoyt (1941) formula being employed. The main results are shown in Fig. 34; it will be clear that satiation effects arise more quickly in the extraverted group, attain greater strength, and dissipate more slowly. An overall test of significance (Hotelling's T test, 1931) invalidated the null hypothesis between the ·01 and the ·05 levels of significance.

Correlations between R-scale scores and extent of figural after-effect were in the neighbourhood of ·3 for the different periods of stimulation, decreasing in size with increasing length of stimulation. (For 30 sec. stimulation, $r = ·374$; for 120 sec. stimulation, $r = ·218$.)

These correlations were run on 35 subjects altogether, namely, the 28 patients included in the main experiment and 7 patients who had been excluded because their R scores disagreed with their diagnosis. It is interesting to note that in each case where

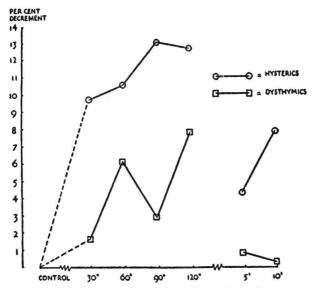

FIG. 34. Amount of figural after-effect shown as percentage decrement after four different periods of stimulation and two different periods of rest.

a patient had been diagnosed hysteric but had an R score which put him on the introverted side, relatively small figural after-effects were found. In each case where a patient was diagnosed dysthymic but had an R score which put him on the extraverted side, relatively large after-effects were found. In other words, when diagnosis and questionnaire disagreed, the experimental test agrees much more closely with the questionnaire than with the psychiatric diagnosis. In view of the widespread habit of heaping contumely upon questionnaires, this fact may deserve stressing.

A repetition of this experiment was carried out by Nicholls (1955), who also included in his study a variety of visual and other types of satiation measures. Unfortunately he did not find it possible, as mentioned already, to induce neurotic patients to fixate the inspection figure properly for the requisite period of time, so that the major sections of his data are impossible to interpret. (It was for this reason that the writer originally decided on a kinaesthetic test as the preferred measure of satiation.) However, this criticism does not apply to Nicholls's use of

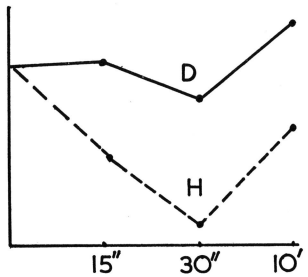

FIG. 35. Amount of figural after-effect shown by dysthymics (D) and hysterics (H) after two periods of stimulation and one period of rest.

the same instrument employed by the writer in the experiment just described, and consequently his results, obtained from 27 hysterics and 26 dysthymics, may be of interest. Using two stimulation periods of 15 sec. and 30 sec. respectively, and a recovery period of 10 min., he found results which tended to support those of the previous study, at confidence levels between 5 and 1 per cent for the different measures taken. Fig. 35 shows the absolute decrement after stimulation for the two groups expressed as deviations from their respective pre-stimulation level. A greater effect of the stimulation period on the hysterics as compared with the dysthymics is obvious here also.

Nicholls's data showed some rather marked differences between the initial (pre-inspection period) scores of hysterics and dysthymics which throw some doubt on the admissibility of the type of score used. No such difficulties were encountered by Bartholomew in an unpublished study, using the same measuring instrument on 64 male criminals, together with the Maudsley Personality Inventory. He obtained correlations between extraversion and the figural after-effect (15 sec. stimulation) of ·4057, and between extraversion and return to rest of ·3532, both being fully significant statistically and in the predicted direction. On the whole, therefore, the evidence is rather favourable as far as this particular deduction is concerned.

We have so far concentrated on hysterics and dysthymics as the groups mediating our predictions; there is also some work, however, relevant to brain-damage as the mediating variable. Reference here is to the study of Klein and Krech (1952), who compared, on the kinaesthetic figural after-effect apparatus already described, 12 brain injured and 16 control subjects. The results are summarized as follows by Klein and Krech. 'Consistent trends were: (a) frequency and intensity of satiation effects were significantly greater in the brain-injured; (b) the brain-injured reached maximal satiation more quickly; (c) the satiated state persisted longer in the brain-injured, recovery being less pronounced and slower . . .; (d) correlations of satiation indices with neurological ratings ranged from + ·63 to + ·92, clearly suggesting a relation between extent of clinically observed disturbance and figural after-effect measures.' These results are clearly much in line with our hypothesis and they serve to support it.

More recently, Jaffe (1954) attempted to duplicate the Klein and Krech study; he was unable to discover any statistically significant differences between his brain-injured and his controls. Wertheimer (1956) has summed up the position thus: 'Clearly further research is needed concerning figural aftereffects in people with brain injury; until it is done, the only ways to account for these differences in results seem to be in terms of locus or extent of cortical damage in the subjects used by Jaffe as compared with those used by Klein and Krech; perhaps, also, the low statistical criterion used by Klein and Krech may have led them to reject the null hypothesis erroneously.' Until this controversy is clarified by further research, therefore, it must be doubtful whether we can legitimately use the results quoted as support of our hypothesis.[1]

One further finding may be mentioned. Sheldon (1940, 1942), as is well known, posits the existence of introverted personality traits in individuals of asthenic, leptomorph, or ectomorph body build, while he posits the existence of extraverted personality traits in individuals of pyknic, eurymorph, or mesomorph body build (cf. Eysenck, 1953, for a discussion of the evidence). Rees and Eysenck (1945) have demonstrated independently that hysterics tend to be eurymorph in body build, while dysthymics tend to be leptomorph. We would expect, therefore, that a slight positive correlation would exist between strength of figural after-effects and mesomorph body build, and a slight negative correlation between strength of figural after-effects and ectomorphic body build. Such correlations, significant and in the predicted direction, have indeed been demonstrated by Wertheimer (1955). While his sample was small and not well chosen from the point of view of this demonstration (which was only incidental to his major purpose), nevertheless as far as they go his figures support our hypothesis.

Before leaving the subject of figural after-effects, a word may perhaps be said about alternative theories of individual differences, particularly those of Klein and Krech (1952) and of Wertheimer (1954, 1955, 1956). Klein and Krech argue as follows: 'Köhler and Wallach restrict satiation to the set of events issuing from the isomorphic impression which a stimulus (described as a *figure*) has on the brain. We would hold to a less restrictive conception. We would maintain, merely, that *any neural activity induces heightened resistance within the area stimulated* and that the degree of resulting distortion of a new stimulation pattern would not necessarily depend upon strong figure-ground differentials. Thus we would re-phrase the argument as follows: the current flow initiated by stimulation of a defined cortical area results in a heightened resistance, *within that area*, to further electrical activity. Should further stimulation occur, the resulting pattern of electrical activity would, as a consequence of this increased resistance, be 'dampened', distorted, or re-routed. In

---

[1] Jaffe (1955) has made amends for reporting observations counter to our theory by showing evidence of stronger tactile adaptation effects in brain-damaged subjects, a finding predictable from our theory. Adaptation, in so far as it is of central rather than of peripheral origin, is essentially inhibitory in nature, and should therefore be stronger and quicker in extraverts and brain-damaged.

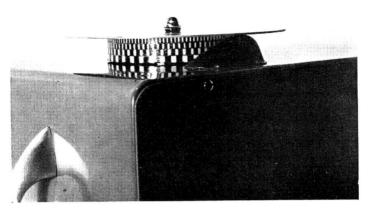

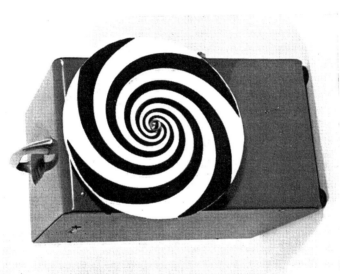

16. Archimedes spiral, as used in drug study.

17. Attachment to Archimedes spiral apparatus, to ensure rotation at exact speeds.

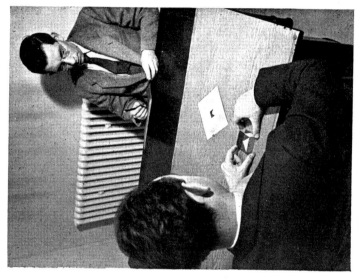

19. Block-design rotation experiment.

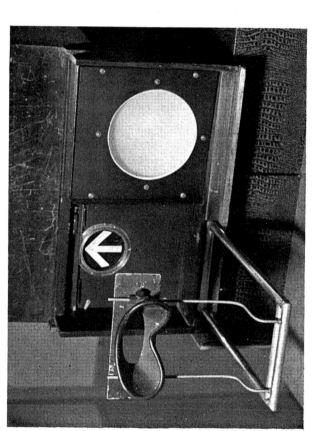

18. Dark-vision apparatus, with light-adapting field on right.

this event we can then speak of *reactive* or a temporary condition of decreased cortical conductivity, i.e. in one specific area and for a finite time cortical conductivity is reduced. For this temporary and localized condition we would assume that the degree of decrease in cortical conductivity is a function of the amount of original stimulation, such that the more stimulation, the greater the drop in cortical conductivity (within certain limits). However, we would postulate another factor which contributes to the extent of drop in cortical conductivity: we would assume that the *over-all state of the cortex* helps to determine the initial or *basal* value of cortical conductivity and the degree of drop *possible*. For example, individuals may be thought of as having high or low cortical conductivity *prior to any stimulation*, i.e. the basal or characteristic level of cortical conductivity. A person with high basal conductivity may be thought of as one whose neural substratum will offer relatively little resistance to the transmission of neural patterns from one area to another and who will suffer a relatively small drop in conductivity as a consequence of a given amount of local stimulation; a person with low basal conductivity may be thought of, conversely, as one whose neural substratum will offer relatively greater resistance to the transmission of neural patterns from one area to another, and who will suffer a relatively large drop in conductivity as a consequence of the same given amount of local stimulation. This postulated relationship between *reactive* and *basal* cortical conductivity permits us, of course, to get some indication of an individual's 'basal' level of cortical conductivity by measuring his 'reactive' cortical conductivity, i.e. by measuring his reaction to localized stimulation or his '*satiationability*'.

The distinction between reactive and basal cortical conductivity is not in the writer's view a useful or even a permissible one. It provides the same kind of prediction as our own hypothesis, but it introduces a postulated relationship between *reactive* and *basal* conductivity which is incapable of verification. It is admitted that all we can measure is reactive conductivity; to postulate (*a*) the existence of a basal cortical conductivity and (*b*) a monotonic relationship between this hypothetical basal conductivity and reactive conductivity, merely in order to enable one to measure basal conductivity by means of reactive conductivity, appears an unnecessarily complicated chain of concepts. If an independent measure of basal conductivity could be found, the concept might obtain empirical justification. As put forward at present it does not add anything on the theoretical level, but merely complicates and confuses the issue. In the absence of such independent evidence therefore, we shall prefer our own formulation to that of Klein and Krech.

The view put forward by Wertheimer constitutes yet another type of theory. According to him, 'individual differences (in figural after-effect) must reflect differences in the ease with which a modification in cortical processes can be brought about. Such a view implies that figural after-effects could be used to measure general cortical modifiability in an individual.' Proceeding from this general hypothesis, he goes on to argue as follows: 'Localized stimulation produces a modification in a localized area of the cortex; this change in the cortex is presumably an alteration in the chemical and/or electrical properties of the neural tissues involved. Hence a large figural after-effect would reflect a relatively extensive change in these physico-chemical properties of the tissues, while a small figural after-effect would reflect a relatively small change. If a given amount of stimulation induces a large figural after-effect in one individual and a small figural after-effect in a second, then the physico-chemical modifiability of the cortex of the first is assumed to be greater than the physico-chemical modifiability of that of the second. Since physico-chemical changes in tissues are metabolic in nature, the first individual may be said to have a greater metabolic modifiability; this greater modifiability is attributed to a more efficient functioning of general metabolic processes. Hence a *large figural after-effect is considered indicative of relatively greater metabolic efficiency.*'

Wertheimer links up, as had Köhler, phenomena such as speed of ambiguous figure reversal with figural after-effects, and provides some experimental evidence regarding the correlation between satiation phenomena and 'metabolic efficiency'. His group of subjects is too heterogeneous to make this demonstration very convincing; nevertheless the possibility cannot be ruled out that some such relationship as is postulated by him may be found on larger and more homogeneous groups. If that were so it might be argued that metabolic efficiency was related causally to the excitation/inhibition balance, and that satiation phenomena reflected this relation. (Such a theory might link up with Pavlov's rather vague notions of 'strong' and 'weak' nervous systems.) However, to date Wertheimer's hypothesis is too scantily supported on the experimental plane to make evaluation easy. It does not seem to contradict our own hypothesis, but, if true, may supplement it in fruitful and interesting ways; more than that cannot be said at the moment.

We may now turn to another, rather different, satiation phenomenon, namely the duration of sensory after-effects. In an unpublished paper by Klein, referred to by Klein and Krech (1952), it is reported that 'where persistence of after-image was measured as a function of the duration of stimulus-exposure, it appeared that for longer exposures the duration of the after-images of brain-injured fell off significantly as compared with non-brain-injured. This could be interpreted to mean that among brain-injured neural activity in regions which had previously been exposed to prolonged excitation is "dampened" as compared to "normals", i.e. consequent upon the same amount of original excitation there is a greater degree of satiation in the brain-injured than in the non-brain-injured. That satiation in the brain-injured is not only greater in extent than in "normals", but that it also persists for a longer time is suggested by another finding of Klein's: the *rate of decrease* in after-image duration upon repeated exposures was more rapid in the brain-damaged than in the controls. In general, then, Klein's studies are congruent with the hypothesis that in the brain-injured successive, prolonged exposure to stimulation induces *satiation* attributes . . .'

After-images, as so studied, are peripheral phenomena, although there are of course central processes involved also. It would appear that the general theory outlined by Klein and Krech, which in essence is not dissimilar to that here advocated, should also apply to more purely central phenomena, such as for instance the class of illusions typified by the waterfall illusion and the Archimedes spiral after-effect (Wohlgemut, 1911). The apparatus used in our studies of the spiral after-effect is illustrated in Plate 16; it consists of a motor-driven spindle, the speed of which is governed by a variable rheostat. On the spindle is mounted a four-throw 180° spiral which is being rotated in a clockwise direction. (The direction of rotation can also be reversed.) A four-speed strobe attachment, illustrated in Plate 17, allows of accurate adjustment of speed. Rotation of the spiral for more than five seconds is followed either by a stopping of the spiral or by instruction to the subject to direct his gaze away from the fixation point (the centre of the spindle on which the spiral is mounted) on to some surface or object in the environment; the consequence is a pronounced after-image, similar but contrary in direction to the originally perceived motion of the spiral. This after-image lasts for an appreciable time, depending almost entirely on the period of original stimulation; exploratory studies have shown angle of regard, size of visual angle, brightness of illumination, and various other factors to have little influence within quite wide limits (Holland, 1957). Length of after-image is monotonically related to length of stimulation, approaching an asymptote after about 90 sec. The phenomenon is of central origin, because if one eye is stimulated, the after-image is perceived by the other eye, although in our experience not quite as strongly as by the eye originally stimulated.

No acceptable theory exists regarding this phenomenon, but we are probably not wrong in stating that the original stimulation sets up certain unspecified cortico-neural events which are perceived as the illusion. According to satiation theory, these cortico-neural events must produce inhibition in the structures mediating the effects, so that eventually the after-image is brought to a stop. The amount of inhibition produced, according to our theory, would be proportional to the position of the subject under examination on the extraversion-introversion continuum, so that much inhibition and short duration of after-image would be expected in the hysterico-psychopathic, the extraverted, and the brain-damaged group. We would also hypothesize that the slope of the regression line of length of after-image on length of stimulation would be less steep for the extraverted groups, i.e. it is maintained that additional periods of stimulation produce proportionally less increase in after-image duration in extraverts than in introverts.

Some evidence is available on this prediction in the work of Freeman and Josey (1949), Standlee (1953), Price and Deabler (1955), and Gallese (1956), more particularly the two last-named studies. Price and Deabler tested 40 normals, 40 non-organic psychotics, and 120 brain-damaged subjects on the spiral after-effect, giving four separate tests and simply determining whether or not an after-effect was perceived. (This method, which was also followed by Gallese, is very rough and ready, and should almost certainly be replaced in future studies by a more systematic exploration of the length of after-effect as a function of length of stimulation. However, the fact that positive results can be achieved even with this very crude technique suggests that the differences are very pronounced indeed.) Their results are given in Table XII below, in which are reported the percentages in the various groups which saw after-effects on 0, 1, 2, 3, or 4 occasions; it will be obvious that the brain-damaged group is very significantly differentiated from the normal and functional groups.

TABLE XII

Number of Archimedes Spiral after-effects demonstrated by Normals, Functionals, and Brain-damaged in four trials

	0	1	2	3	4
Normals	0%	2·5%	0%	5%	92·5%
Functionals	0%	0%	2·5%	2·5%	95%
Brain-damaged	60%	10%	20%	8%	2%

These very striking differences were to some extent verified in the study by Gallese, who scored his test in terms of a cut between two or less and three or more reports of seen after-images, calling the former an 'organic' and the latter a 'normal' score. In 30 normal subjects he found exclusively normal reactions, while in 41 schizophrenics he found 95 per cent of normal reactions, thus substantiating previous findings that this test does not differentiate between normals and functional patients. An organic group consisting of 47 patients suffering from disorders other than those diagnosed alcoholic and convulsive disorders showed only 34 per cent of normal reactions; another organic group consisting of 50 patients suffering from alcoholic and convulsive disorders showed 72 per cent of normal reactions. Twelve lobotomized schizophrenics showed only normal reactions. The retest reliability of the score was found to be high, the fourfold point correlation between first and second testing on 34 organic patients being ·84, for two different examiners.

Gallese concludes that 'with this method of inquiry, and of scoring, the test almost always indicates organicity when organic scores are obtained, although the converse is not true'. He adds the observation that 'it is . . . the author's belief that among the organics who obtained high scores the duration of the negative after-effect was considerably less than among the non-organics'. Altogether, there appears to be considerable support for our deduction. It should perhaps be mentioned that promising but somewhat less spectacular results than those of Price and Deabler have been found in extensive use of the test in this Department; these findings have not yet been published.

One further experimental situation which permits of prediction from our general theory is that of dark adaptation. As is well known, there are considerable individual differences in dark adaptation (Granger, 1957), and as there is considerable information about this phenomenon on the physiological-neurological side, it seems likely that inhibition phenomena should be demonstrable here also. Granger (1957), who has made a thorough study of the field, has put forward the following deductions. In the first place, he points out that 'the dark adaptation situation is one in which, following light adaptation, the recovery of visual sensitivity is plotted over the subsequent period of time spent in darkness. Now light adaptation is . . . a period of "continuous stimulation" which lasts in the present experiments for as long as five minutes. During this period "inhibition" is presumably being generated in the visual system. When the light-adapting field is cut off this "inhibition" will "dissipate" during the subsequent period of non-stimulation. It would seem therefore that . . . the curve of dark adaptation may to some extent represent a "recovery curve" from the effects of "inhibition" by light, and individual differences in the "dissipation of inhibition" should be reflected in various properties of the dark adaptation function.'

Granger goes on to argue that if inhibition is 'a function of the duration and intensity of previous stimulation one would expect individuals susceptible to strong inhibitory stimulation to behave like normal subjects whose eyes had been exposed either to a more intense light-adapting field for the same duration or to one of the same intensity for a longer duration. A considerable amount of work has been done on the effects of varying the intensity and duration of the pre-adapting luminance upon the course of dark adaptation (Haig, 1941; Hecht et al., 1937; Mote et al., 1953; Wald & Clark, 1937), and it is known that increasing the intensity or duration affects the resulting curve in the following way: the initial threshold tends to be higher, the slope of the curve decreases and the time taken to reach a final steady value increases.' Typical curves illustrating this effect are shown in Fig. 36. 'The curves shown have been drawn on the basis of psychophysical data obtained in the experiments referred to in the previous paragraph to be as comparable as possible to the conditions of the experiments under discussion. The top curve results from the greatest intensity or longest duration of light adaptation, the bottom curve from the least intense or shortest pre-adaptation.'

Granger discusses the implications of this theory in some

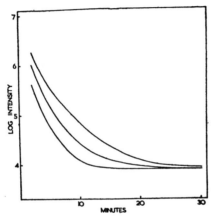

FIG. 36. Dark-vision adaptation after exposure to different pre-adaptation intensities of light, illustrating dissipation of temporal inhibition.

detail, and then argues that spatial inhibition also may be hypothesized to play a part. 'It would seem . . . that light adaptation should exert some effect on a real interaction in the visual system which would also show itself in various properties of the subsequent dark-adaptation curve. From his discussion of "satiation" effects in vision it would appear that Eysenck would postulate as one effect of light stimulation in a given area of the visual field a depression of sensitivity in adjacent areas due to negative induction. . . . It would seem that on this type of theory one might expect lateral interaction in the extravert and hysteric to give rise to strong inhibitory effects. The greater persistence of the effects of previous light adaptation in subjects might be expected to exert some influence on the effective area of the test-field during subsequent dark adaptation. It might in fact tend to reduce spatial integration of light stimuli so that

167

extraverted subjects would behave like normal subjects viewing a test-field of reduced size. Now the effects of using test-fields of different sizes are known fairly well (Hecht *et al.*, 1935; Wald, 1938; Wolf & Fisher, 1950), and typical curves are shown in Fig. 37. The top curve represents the effect of the smallest area of test-field, the bottom the largest. It will be noted that reducing the size of the test-field has the effect of elevating the dark-adaptation curve along the intensity axis, but unlike the effects of increasing the duration of previous adaptation, the

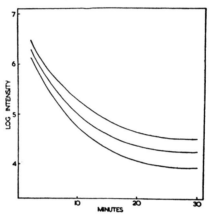

FIG. 37. Dark-vision adaptation as a function of size of test-field, illustrating effects of spatial inhibition.

curves for different field sizes do not tend to converge to the same final threshold value.'

Having outlined Granger's deductions in terms of temporal and spatial inhibition from our general theory on to the special set of phenomena appearing in dark vision, we must now turn to his experiment, which was carried out on 10 hysterics, 10 dysthymics, 10 extraverted normals, and 10 introverted normals; the neurotic subjects were selected on the basis of psychiatric diagnosis, the normal ones on the basis of questionnaire responses. The test used consisted of a 3° circular test-field displaced 7° horizontally into the left visual field of the subject's right eye. Fixation was controlled by means of a red fixation light maintained at a luminance just above the subject's threshold throughout the experiment. Subjects were given light-adaptation to a luminance of 270 ml. for a period of five minutes, and intensity threshold was obtained over a thirty-minute period of dark adaptation. Subjects were asked to report immediately they could detect the presence of light in their visual field to the left of the fixation point. Several checks of the usual kind were introduced to detect malingering and gross cases of inattention; no instances were found. (An apparatus similar to the one used is shown in Plate 18.)

Results are shown in Fig. 38, which records the mean dark-adaptation curves showing decrease in intensity threshold as a

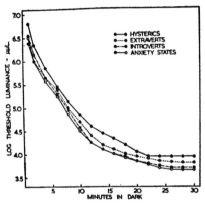

FIG. 38. Dark-vision adaptation of hysterics, normal ex-traverts, normal introverts, and dysthymics, showing greater inhibition effects in extraverts and hysterics.

function of time in the dark. Thresholds have been plotted in logarithmic units of luminance measured in micromicrolamberts. The curves 'follow the form to be expected of a dark-adaptation curve when previous light adaptation has been to moderate or low intensities (Haig, 1941; Hecht et al., 1937; Mote et al., 1953). . . . Following an initial rapid increase in sensitivity the rate of change becomes progressively less and less as the function approaches a final steady value asymptotic with respect to the abscissa.' It will be noted that throughout the course of the curve, the hysterics have higher thresholds than the dysthymics, as predicted. The two normal groups are inter-mediate between the neurotic groups and, except for the initial portion of the curve, extraverts have higher thresholds than introverts. There is no doubt that the results are in agreement with prediction, although this agreement is less pronounced for

THE DYNAMICS OF ANXIETY AND HYSTERIA

the first few readings than for the later ones. This may in part be due to residual effects of pre-light-adaptation stimulation, to residual differences in pupil size, and other artefacts not sufficiently controlled in the experiment; Granger gives a full discussion of the possible causes of such artefacts. Only a repetition of the experiment under even more stringently controlled conditions can tell us whether these hypothetical factors have in fact played any part in giving rise to these results.

One possible objection to the general theoretical approach discussed above is rejected by Granger, namely the argument that dark adaptation can be explained on a purely photochemical theory, without the involvement of central phenomena. He quotes Lythgoe (1940), Granit et al. (1939), Elsberg and Spotnitz (1938), Baumgardt (1950), Rushton (1954), Arden and Weale (1954), Thomson (1949) and many others in support of his conclusion that 'present-day evidence indicates that in addition to any photochemical changes that occur, changes must also occur in the nervous system'. He summarizes his discussion of the physiological basis for any such theory as that here advocated by saying: 'As far as visual research is concerned the value of Eysenck's theory may be similar to that of studies of anoxia and various physiological stresses. Such studies suggest the need for a broader basis for visual theories by making explicit factors which are implicit and regarded as constant or only of secondary importance in the theoretical equations of Hecht and others.'

Many other examples of satiation phenomena could be given in addition to those dealt with so far; only one further set of experiments will, however, be discussed here in order to prevent this chapter from becoming too long. This example has been chosen for two reasons. In the first place, it brings the concept of brain damage more definitely into the picture than could be done in the figural after-effect field by the Klein and Krech study; in the second place, it leads over from our discussion of temporal inhibition to a discussion of spatial inhibition. The phenomenon concerned is the so-called phi phenomenon, i.e. the perception of 'apparent motion'. As is well known, movement can be seen when two stationary stimuli are presented to the eye in succession, provided the time-interval between the presentation of stimulus A and stimulus B is suitably chosen. Wertheimer (1912) has put forward the following hypothesis to explain the occurrence of this perception along the lines of isomorphic gestalt theory. Visual stimulation is followed by the irradiation of excitatory effects from the cortical site of the stimulation. A second visual stimulus in another part of the cortex, appropriately placed and timed, results in irradiation effects which combine with those produced by the first stimulus and produce visual perception of movement which is the perception, in fact, of neural transactions between the two irradiations. It would appear that an increase in inhibition, either over the whole cortex or specifically within the area in which irradiation took place, should weaken or destroy this irradiation thus leading it to a rise in threshold for the perception of movement.

This hypothesis, which has been advanced by Shapiro (1956), would lead us to expect in the field of individual differences that hysterics, extraverts, and people with brain-damage would have higher thresholds. The only group for which such effects have been demonstrated has been the last named. Werner and Thuma (1942) found that out of 20 brain-damaged subjects only two saw movement when presented with successive exposures of two vertical black lines by means of a modified Dodge tachistoscope; with presentation at the same speed all but one of 20 normal subjects saw movement. Both groups were of low I.Q., the average of the brain-damaged group being 69, and that of the non-brain-damaged group being 72. (Apparently the brain-damaged group did not suffer from any gross motor defects or visual agnosias.) Similar findings have been reported by Bender and Teuber (1949). Brenner (1953), using a control group of 12 mental defectives, and an experimental group of 12 post-encephalitic patients and 11 cerebral palsy patients, matched for I.Q., found that only two out of 23 brain-damaged subjects saw apparent movement in exactly the same way as the control subjects. It would appear, therefore, that the hypothesis is substantiated in the case of brain-damaged subjects. (See also the quite recent study of Saucer & Deabler, 1956.)

Shapiro (1954) has shown experimentally that satiation effects set up in the path of the apparent movement had the same effect as brain-damage, i.e. increase the apparent motion threshold. (A similar demonstration has been given by Detherage & Bitterman (1952).)

'The apparatus used consisted of a modified Dodge tachistoscope copied from the model given by Werner and Thuma

(1942); the timing device was electronic, and had continuously variable speeds for the time interval from 0·110 to 0·86 sec. Exposure time was kept constant at 0·09 sec.

'The apparent motion figures consisted of two white lines $\frac{1}{20}$ in. wide and $\frac{5}{8}$ in. long, making an angle of 70°. The lines were made of white sellotape mounted on black velvet cards, 6 × 6 in., and viewed at 20 in. from the subject. The lines were so placed that the one side of the angle was horizontal, and the angle pointed to the left (*see* Fig. 39).'

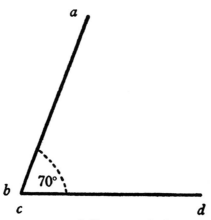

FIG. 39. Arrangements of lines used for measurement of inhibition effects on apparent movement. (Line *ab* was first exposed, followed by line *cd*.)

For continuous stimulation a figure was used consisting of a black circle, 2 in. diameter, mounted on a white screen, 3 × 3 ft. It stood at eye level, 6 ft. away from the subject, so as to occupy the same visual angle as the two lines. The area of continuous stimulation was thus placed in the path of the apparent motion.

'A chin rest was used during fixation, and the experiment was carried out in a semi-darkened room. To avoid complication from the after-image, and to make sure we were dealing with central and not peripheral functions, the continuous stimulation and apparent motion were done monocularly, using a different eye for each—the dominant eye being used for tests of apparent motion.' The subjects for the experiments were 26 normal, intelligent adults, roughly equated for age and sex and divided into an experimental and a control group.

The following procedure was used. First, the threshold for apparent motion for each subject was established on five trials, using the limiting method. 'Then, a second test was carried out on each subject between 24 and 48 hours later. In this test, the experimental group was first treated with continuous stimulation in the appropriate part of the visual field. This was done by fixating a cross in the centre of the circle described above for 3 min. The subjects kept as still as possible while doing this.

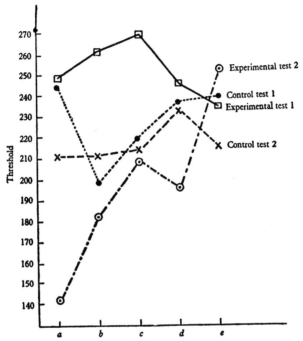

FIG. 40. Satiation effects on apparent movement
threshold.

Immediately afterwards, the threshold for apparent motion was established in the same way as in Test 1, with the same instructions. The time between the two procedures was not measured, but the one followed immediately upon the other in the literal sense of the word. The subjects of the control group had their thresholds for apparent motion established without prior fixation.'

The results are shown in Fig. 40. It will be clear from this figure that the experimental group on the occasion of their second testing show a much higher threshold on Trial *a* than they did on the occasion of their first testing, and also higher than the control group on either the first or the second testing. It will also be seen that the experimental group quickly recovered from the after-effects of continuous stimulation so that on their fifth trial (Trial *e*) their threshold is in no way different from that of the control group. Both these effects are fully significant statistically and show the equivalence of continuous stimulation and brain-damage as far as the threshold for apparent motion is concerned.

This type of experimental inhibition is clearly of the temporal variety and can indeed be seen to dissipate quickly after the cessation of the inhibiting stimulus (*see* Fig. 40). This, however, is clearly different from the position obtaining in the case of brain-damage where it is difficult to conceive of temporal inhibition being responsible for the raising of perceptual thresholds for apparent movement. The possibility must therefore be envisaged that the proper analogue for brain-damage is not temporal but spatial inhibition, i.e. that the inhibition responsible for the raising of thresholds is not produced by *previous stimulation* of the *same* cortical area but rather by the *simultaneous stimulation* of *other* parts of the cortex. Some experimental evidence to show that spatial inhibition does work in this way has been presented by Brenner (1953). This is her description of the experiment carried out to investigate this point: 'Fifteen normal young adults of high average intelligence were presented with apparent-movement stimuli using an inverted V-figure exposed in a viewing box. Exposure-time was 75 m.sec., and the time intervals between alternate exposures were equal. The time-interval was varied continuously from 24 to 600 m.sec. Viewing was binocular and no instructions regarding movement were given. The *S*'s were re-tested half an hour after the initial test. Four types of continuous stimulation were given each *S* at half-hourly intervals. These were:

(*a*) visual—fixating a circle of light in the viewing box;
(*b*) auditory—an electric buzzer;
(*c*) voluntary movement—pacing up and down the room; and
(*d*) simple mental arithmetic.

Each form of continuous stimulation was given for 2 min. and the order varied for different *S*'s. Re-tests were given immediately prior to and after continuous stimulation, and a final re-test was given half an hour after the last test. The thresholds for simultaneity and succession were recorded and the difference between these thresholds represents the range of time-intervals over which apparent movement was perceived.'

Brenner found that each type of continuous stimulation resulted in a highly significant *decrease* in the range over which movement was perceived, which returned to normal during the half-hour rest periods. 'Every *S* showed this decrease, and the order of presentation did not affect the results.

'In all cases, the decrease in the range is a result of simultaneity being perceived at longer, and succession at shorter time-intervals. Some *S*'s reported that simultaneity changed directly to succession and no intervening movement could be perceived. This, as well as alteration in the path and pattern of movement, occurred regardless of the type of continuous stimulation employed.' The effects of *spatial* inhibition are thus seen to be similar to those of *temporal* inhibition.

Brenner rejects the simple satiation hypothesis as an explanation of her findings but does not take into account the possibility of spatial inhibition. She believes that the preoccipital area (Brodman area 19) is the locus for the neural processes underlying the effects of continuous stimulation of apparent movement, 'since this part of the cortex is concerned with visual elaboration and receives impulses from the entire cortex (Bonin *et al.*, 1942). This hypothesis, at the same time, provides a basis for explaining perception of apparent movement between two points which are represented in opposite striate cortices (Smith, 1948).' Whatever may be the value of these speculations it does appear that Brenner has succeeded in demonstrating the postulated effect of spatial inhibition in raising the thresholds in figural after-effects phenomenon.

Having thus demonstrated experimentally that the effects of temporal and spatial inhibition are identical—at least with respect to the phenomenon under observation—we may proceed on the hypothesis that quite generally individual differences in one type of inhibition will be found to go hand in hand with individual differences in the other. In other words, we would expect a person with high temporal inhibition (extravert, hysteric, brain-damaged) also to show high spatial inhibition, and vice versa. We must now turn to the experimental and clinical literature to see whether this hypothesis is in fact borne out, or whether we have allowed ourselves to be misled by a mere analogy without any causal basis.

There is no doubt about the venerable antiquity of the phenomena of spatial inhibition, in spite of their relative neglect at the hands of psychologists. Over 2,000 years ago Hippocrates observed that 'of simultaneous pains, in two places, the lesser is obliterated by the greater'. Among more modern writers Heymans (1927) actually postulated a law of perceptual inhibition to the effect that simultaneous stimuli 'mask' each other. Duncker (1937) experimentally verified Hippocrates' observation quoted above, and Ischlondsky (1930, 1949) has shown in some experiments already quoted that the pain threshold as measured by pupil dilation is raised systematically by different degrees of pressure exerted on the dynamometer.

Most work, however, has been done in the visual field. A thorough review has been undertaken by Granger (1957) and we will here mention only a few of the phenomena which appear to be relevant. Schouten and his collaborators (1939) have produced evidence for a rapidly occurring inhibitory effect in their experiments on 'indirect adaptation'; this extremely rapid process has been called Alpha adaptation. Another spatial inhibition phenomenon is that of simultaneous contrast as studied, for instance, by Graham and Granit (1931), and the simultaneous stimulation threshold effects studied by Beitel (1936). Successive contrast phenomena (Baumgardt & Segal, 1947), although not strictly simultaneous, do appear to involve interaction effects of a spatial kind and are therefore likely to be relevant in this context. These investigators have shown that when two successive flashes were used as stimuli, the one creating a small circular field on top of a larger circular field produced by the other, then, depending on the precise time interval between stimuli, the larger field would inhibit the smaller one, so that, with an interval of 50 m.sec., the smaller field appeared as a black spot in a lighter surround. Another relevant contrast phenomenon is that of metacontrast as studied by Stigler (1913) and Alpern (1953). Experiments on contour formation also are relevant here. Thus Werner (1940) has shown that if exposure of a small black circle is followed at an interval of about 150 m.sec. by that of an annular ring, this causes the small black circle to disappear entirely. These are only a few of the many experiments which have been carried out in the perceptual field to substantiate Hering's original notion of 'induction' but they will perhaps serve to show the reality of spatial inhibition phenomena in perception.

In the mutual interaction of perceptual stimuli, inhibition is not of course the only result. Under certain timing conditions facilitation may also be observed. However, from the theoretical point of view, inhibition phenomena are much more interesting and relevant to our general theory. It should be noted, perhaps, that the very exact quantitative relationships found in this field should make possible a more precise formulation of our general theory. Unfortunately, experimentalists in this field have shown almost no interest in individual differences; thus this very promising approach still remains to be exploited.

Interaction effects of the kind under discussion are of course not peculiar to the perceptual field but are also found in motor behaviour. One of the earlier experimental studies in this field was that of Bowditch and Warren (1890), who made a quantitative study of the influence of various time relations between the application of a secondary stimulus (S_2) and a specific stimulus (S_1) to the patellar tendon. The reinforcing agency most often used in their experiments was the clenching of the right hand in response to a bell. The reinforcement was found to be greatest when the two events were nearly simultaneous. At an interval of 0·4 sec. there appears to be no effect, but during the next 0·6 sec. the height of the kick is actually diminished (inhibition). The work of Yerkes (1904) on frogs, that of Zwaardemaker and Lans (1900) on visual reflexes, and of Dodge (1913) on responses to auditory stimuli are also relevant in this connection, as is the experiment reported by Hilgard (1931) on the reflex response of the eyelid to two unlike stimuli. Reaction time experiments, beginning with the work of Bliss (1893), also show mutual interaction between near simultaneous stimuli. Here, too, the typical finding is that the nature of the influence of S_2 on S_1 depends on the exact timing. Thus in an experiment using a light stimulus (S_1) preceded at varying intervals by electric shock (S_2), Todd (1912) found normal reaction times when the shock preceded the light by 45–90 sigma. When the two were separated by 180 sigma there was a definite retardation of the reaction to light. Altogether, similarities are considerable between this type of work and that on perceptual interaction discussed above, showing again the fundamental similarity of underlying cortical processes.

On the clinical side, methods of simultaneous and near-simultaneous stimulation have been employed for many years, particularly in relation to the diagnosis of brain damage. The work of Oppenheim (1885), Jones (1909), Maas (1910), Head and Holmes (1911), Poppelreuter (1923), Best (1917), Goldstein (1942), Riddoch (1955), Schilder (1935), and many others may be mentioned. A brief review is given by Bender (1952), who refers to the general phenomenon under discussion as that of *extinction*. We shall use his term in preference to alternative ones suggested by other writers, such as inattention, repression, suppression, local adaptation, sensory eclipse, dynamic field, and so forth. The method used to produce extinction effect is defined by Bender as follows: 'In speaking of double simultaneous stimulation, it is employed when two discrete stimuli are applied synchronously or in close succession in two different parts of the sensory field . . . extinction of sensation is defined as a process in which the sensation disappears or a stimulus becomes imperceptible when another sensation is evoked by simultaneous stimulation elsewhere in the sensory field.' Typical of the kind of test used by Bender is the 'face-hand' test. 'It was found that on simultaneous stimulation of the face and hand the subject frequently reported sensation on the face but not on the hand. In this test the subject is not informed of what is to be done. There is no questioning as to whether one or two sensations are perceived . . . this effect, which is apparent on the first examination, occurs either on double tactile or double pin prick stimulus.' This extinction of sensation from the hand can be found in normal people, but according to Bender is much more frequent in patients suffering from cerebral damage. This double stimulation method is claimed to be much more diagnostic than are methods of single stimulation.

Extinction phenomena are not the only consequence of double stimulation. 'When one studies the sensory areas in which extinction could occur, one finds a variety of concomitant changes. Some of the more frequent alterations in sensation are: (*a*) a rise or fluctuation of threshold; (*b*) inability to localize the stimulus; (*c*) decrease or increase in after sensation, and (*e*) effects on perception of size, shape and movement of objects. All of these changes can be made more apparent with the method of simultaneous stimulation as employed.' Bender has also investigated the conditions responsible for the occurrence of the effect and considers as most important the intensity of the stimulus, the timing of the stimulus, the repetition of the stimulus, the type of stimulus, the stimulus background and the effects of attitude and expectancy states. Altogether his work and that of the many others quoted by him leaves little doubt that two deductions from our general postulates are in actual fact verified experimentally. (1) *Spatial inhibition effects occur in perception.* (2) *Spatial inhibition phenomena in perception are much more pronounced in cases of brain damage than they are in the absence of brain damage.* It is interesting to note that there is some evidence in Bender's book for a third deduction from our postulate system, which might be phrased as follows: (3) *Spatial inhibition effects in the perceptual field are stronger in the case of extraverts and hysterics than in the case of introverts and dysthymics.* Bender points out that 'extinction on one side of the body may be found in patients with psychoneurosis, who show hysterical features, but in these cases the sensory changes do not conform to the type or pattern usually found in somatic disorders of the nervous system'. He also adds that 'some of the unusual sensory phenomena which we see in the neuroses, such as hysterical anaesthesia or blindness, can be interpreted in terms of phenomena of extinction'. It would be of exceptional interest if direct and systematic experimental evidence could be provided on this point; in its absence we must leave the verification of our third deduction as an open question.

One further point is worthy of mention. The importance of inhibition for the explanation of hypnotic phenomena in Pavlov's system is well known. If hypnosis is related to an increase in inhibitory potential, then extinction phenomena should be easier to obtain under hypnosis. Bender finds that 'there is also some evidence that extinction of sensation may be induced by hypnosis. In patients with decreased sensation induced by hypnosis double simultaneous stimulation results in extinction in the hyperthetic area. (The only suggestion under hypnosis was that there was to be decreased sensation on one side of the body. There was no suggestion to the patients that extinction was to occur.)'

The work of Bender is clinical rather than experimental and

lacks a firm theoretical framework. In considerable contrast to it are the studies by Shapiro (1951, 1952, 1953, 1954, 1956), which are experimental and which are based on a very definite theory. The basic observation with which Shapiro starts is the fact that when subjects attempt to reproduce a coloured design by means of coloured blocks of wood, they sometimes succeed in reproducing the design correctly but rotating through an angle which may be as much as 45°. Fig. 41 illustrates such an occurrence; the drawing of the design on a white piece of cardboard is shown at the top, the correctly completed but rotated design is shown at the bottom. (Plate 19 shows test in progress.)

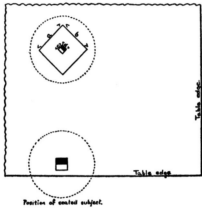

Fig. 41. Design rotation effect. The dotted circle indicates the area of clear perception of a subject presumed to be subject to exaggerated spatial inhibition.

This curious effect is occasionally found with normal, neurotic or psychotic patients, but it is relatively rare in these groups. Hanvik (1953), Hanvik and Anderson (1950), Yates (1954), Williams et al. (1956) and Shapiro himself (1951, 1952, 1953, 1954) have shown that among brain-injured patients rotations of this kind occur quite frequently, and the angles through which the designs are rotated tend to be much larger than they are in normal groups. It appears, therefore, that the block design rotation effect is specifically linked with brain-damage (Yates, 1954). Shapiro has made a thorough investigation of the conditions determining the appearance of this effect and has succeeded in bringing it under experimental control;

he has also provided a theory to account for its occurrence which is essentially an application of the notion of spatial inhibition to this phenomenon. (Shapiro prefers to retain the Pavlovian term 'negative induction', but in our account we shall continue to use the term 'spatial inhibition' in order to bring it in line with the rest of the book.)

Shapiro first established the laws according to which the rotation effect tended to appear. He succeeded in finding three such laws. 'The first one is that the angle of the line of symmetry of a design will affect the amount of rotation. The line of symmetry is the line which divides the design into two

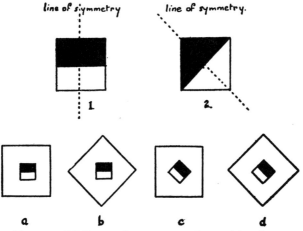

FIG. 42. Different figure-ground combinations.

mirrored halves, as in 1 and 2 of Fig. 42. When the line of symmetry is at an angle to the vertical axis of the total visual field, as in c and d in Fig. 42, the tendency to rotation will be increased. When the line of symmetry is parallel to the vertical axis of the visual field, then the tendency to rotate will be lessened. The second law is concerned with *figure* orientation. 'Figure' is the technical word used in this research when describing the design. When the design is in a square orientation, as in a and b of Fig. 42, then the tendency to rotate will be decreased. When the design is in a diamond orientation, as in c and d of Fig. 42, the tendency to rotate will be increased, except when in conflict with the angle of line of symmetry, which is stronger (*see* 2 in Fig. 42). The third law is concerned

181

with what is called *ground* orientation. 'Ground' in this paper is the word used to describe the 6 in. × 6 in. card on which the figures were placed. The findings are that when the ground is in a diamond orientation, as in *b* and *d* of Fig. 42, the tendency to rotate will be increased, and when it is in a square orientation, as in *a* and *c* of Fig. 42, the tendency to rotate will be decreased, except when in conflict with either symmetry or figure effects, which are both stronger. There are further interactions between these three laws but they do not appear to affect the above laws markedly.

It must be remembered, of course, that these laws have been shown to hold only in a specific experimental situation in which a special form of the block design test was used. This consisted of a series of 40 cards such as those shown in Figs. 41 and 42. Each card is 6 in. × 6 in. in size and the design of each card is 1 in. × 1 in. The subject is required to reproduce the design with four 1-in. blocks such as those shown in Fig. 43. When

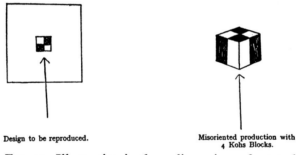

Design to be reproduced.   Misoriented production with
                                        4 Kohs Blocks.

FIG. 43. Illustration in three dimensions of rotated
design.

he has completed the design the subject is asked, 'Is that correct?' The design is accepted as completed only when he says 'Yes.' Each trial is timed from commencement to this point. Patients having completed the design with their four blocks, frequently leave it in a rotated position, as shown in Fig. 41. In this illustration the design is rotated by 45 degrees. This amount of rotation is rarely exceeded, though it occurs frequently. The amount of rotation produced by the subject for each trial was recorded and measured by photographic means.

Having established these laws, Shapiro goes on to formulate

his theory which is essentially based on the hypothesis that 'one of the effects of brain-damage is to increase inhibitory effects in the functioning of at least some of the remaining brain tissues. This generalization can now be regarded as established and is supported by the work of Head (1920), Bender (1946) and Pavlov (1927).' The theory itself is developed as follows:

'First of all it was postulated that in the brain-damaged patients the inhibitory aspect of the negative induction effect is exaggerated. Therefore, when he was attending to an object, additional and surrounding perceptions which would be available for the normal subject would not be available for the brain-damaged. In fact, one could say that the brain-damaged person's perception of an object would be similar in quality to that of a normal person in a dark room in which only the perceived object was illuminated. Thus it is envisaged here that, in the brain-damaged person, the inhibitory aspects of the negative induction effect are intensified, resulting in a relative restriction of content of consciousness. The second postulate is that the factors of *ground* orientation, *figure* orientation and angle of line of symmetry exercise their influence on the rotation effect because they have directional value in space perception. Thus the card in a diamond-oriented position would, if there were no conflicting cues, tend to be seen as a square. Similarly, the diamond-oriented *figure*, if there were no other cues, would also tend to be seen as a square. Which of the two upper sides would be taken as the top cannot be decided in terms of the present theory, and therefore each side must be regarded as having an equal chance of being looked upon as the top of the square. Finally, the line of symmetry must, in a single figure, be assumed to have directional properties. Thus the figure in card *d* of Fig. 42 . . . would tend to be seen as a square not only because of the figure shape but because of the directional value of the line of symmetry. On the other hand, card *b* would possess conflicting directional properties. If the line of symmetry and *figure* orientation have a preponderant effect at the moment of perception, the figure will be seen as a square. If the *ground* orientation preponderates, the figure will be perceived as a diamond, and so on. In a similar way one can make varying combinations of all three factors of *ground* orientation, *figure* orientation, and angle of line of symmetry. How these three sets of directional values interact with each other and how these interactions vary with different individuals will not be analyzed here.

'On the basis of these two postulates it is possible to formulate a description of what happens in the two main perceptual phases of doing the block design test: the perception of the card and the making of the blocks. It will be remembered that the restricted area of clear vision is thought to make impossible a clear simultaneous perception of both the blocks and the card. Let us suppose that the card as shown in Fig. 41 is the one involved. Let us also suppose that the negative induction effect is working in such a way that all that is available to the patient's perception is the card. The supposed area of clear perception is marked in the illustration by a dotted line. Now we can carry out an analysis of the interrelationship of the three factors. The ground will be seen as a square with either side "a" or side "b" as the top. Similarly, the figure will tend to be seen as a square, with either side "c" or side "d" as the top. Finally, the directional value of the line of symmetry would tend to produce the perception of a square with line "d" as the top. When the subject looks down to make the design with the blocks directional cues would appear to be the table edge, the parts of his own body visible to the subject, and the graining of the table. These would therefore provide directional lines of reference which were different to those provided by the card above. Here the perceived "top" would in actuality be 45 degrees to the left of the perceived "top" in the figure. Having previously perceived in the card a square figure whose top was line "d", he would proceed to make himself such a figure in the new frame of reference near the edge of the table, and the figure he would thus make would be the one shown in Fig. 41. Thus to the normal observer the subject would be seen to have "rotated" the blocks in an anti-clockwise direction.'

If this explanation were correct then it would follow that under appropriate experimental conditions it should be possible to induce rotation in normal people. This Shapiro attempted to do by reducing the number of external available cues. By putting black homogeneous material on the table, he reduced the positional cues produced by the graining of the table top. By making his subjects wear field reducers, i.e. half-sections of ping-pong balls with tiny holes which were fastened over the eyes and permitted only very restricted vision, he made it impossible for them to obtain cues simultaneously from the blocks they were manipulating and the design they were rotating. By varying the size of the room in which the experiment was conducted, he tried to alter the availability of directional cues for walls and ceilings. In this way he and Yates (1954) succeeded in producing the rotation effect in the normal group, thus giving experimental support to the general theory of block design rotation effects as being produced by spatial inhibition.

It is not only in block designs, of course, that distortions of this kind occur. Yates (1956) has found that when brain-damaged patients attempt to reproduce designs by drawing, rotations can also be observed, although the effect is as strongly marked as in the case of block designs reproduced by actual coloured blocks. (See also Beech, 1956, and Shapiro & Beech, 1958.)

Shapiro believes that the theory for spatial inhibition tested in connection with this single perceptual anomaly has much wider implications. These can best be described by quoting his own account '. . . it seems that the general theory which was tested in the experiments reported in this paper has some general explanatory value, and a number of observations found in the literature on the psychological effects of brain-damage can be linked together. For example, Patterson and Zangwill (1944) quote Schilder and Goldstein on a "notable tendency to react to a very limited aspect of the perceptual field, and a visual incapacity to relate perceived objects to their wider settings" in cases with a profound degree of mental confusion.'

Another example is the apparently contradictory observation that brain-damaged patients are both more rigid and more distractible than normals. We can assume that when a patient is paying attention to a task, a certain set of cortical arrangements is being stimulated and is in a state of excitation. According to the principle of exaggerated negative induction the surrounding arrangements will, in the case of the brain-damaged patient, be in a relatively intense state of inhibition. If now a new and different stimulus reaches another set of cortical arrangements, the threshold will be much higher than would normally be required for excitatory processes to develop into conscious processes and this new stimulus will have no observable effect. Hence the patient will appear to be 'rigid'. Should, however, the stimulation be strong enough it will reach consciousness, and because of the exaggerated negative induction effect, it might completely inhibit the excitatory processes in the cortical arrangements which were previously in a state of excitation. Thus the patient would appear to be 'distractible'.

The educational methods developed by Strauss and Lehtinen (1947) are also explainable in these terms. It will be remembered that they advocate that the brain-damaged child should be taught to read under conditions which minimize distracting stimulation. They recommend that the child should face a plain wall, that the material to be learned should be broken up and presented within a framework and that teachers should not wear too bright clothing or jewellery. Equally relevant is the practice of some doctors of giving brain-damaged patients excitatory drugs to lessen their 'rigidity'.

Much of the general explosiveness and impulsiveness reported of patients suffering from diffuse brain damage also becomes explainable in these terms. The excitation of any feelings would result in the inhibition of sentiments and attitudes which should normally have a controlling effect. Bleuler's (1950) remarks on page 313 are of interest in this respect: 'The disturbance of associations in organic cases manifests itself in the fact that their number has been reduced; the psychic horizon has been narrowed. The limitations that take place are most striking with respect to the instinctive drives or the effects which are essentially the same . . .' The paretic 'will want to appropriate some object in his ward; he will steal it with a sly expression on his face and hide it carefully under his clothes—all this before the very eyes of the attendants and of the other patients who, at the moment, have ceased to exist for him. The old man wants to satisfy his sexual drives. He sees in a little girl only the woman. He does not stop to consider the moral reasons which forbid sexual intercourse with children; he abuses the first child he happens to meet. Thus the registration of events to which the patient's immediate attention is not directed suffers badly, and with it the orientation . . .

' "*The paretic peeps at the world through a small hole.*" (Our italics.)

'From these considerations it seems reasonable to conclude that we have in the formulation of the exaggerated negative induction effect the beginnings of a general theory of the psychological effects of brain damage. It possesses the essential requirements for such a theory; it is based on experiment, and itself opens up the possibilities of further research. Furthermore, the possibility emerges of directing such research towards increasing therapeutic control.'

As a postscript we may perhaps add that the generalizations put forward by Shapiro with respect to brain-damaged patients should also, if our theory is correct, be applicable to hysterics and psychopaths, as opposed to dysthymics. There is some

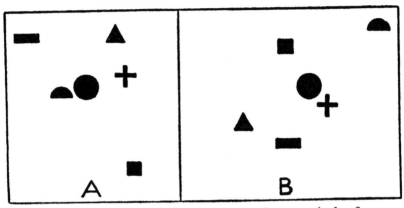

FIG. 44. Two stimulus figures, exposed successively for 5 seconds each.

experimental evidence of this effect in the work of Brengelmann (1955, 1956). The test used by him is rather different from that used by Shapiro, and an illustration of it will be found in Fig. 44. The subject is shown one or the other of two figures, A and B, each of which contains five drawings grouped round a central circular fixation point. Presentation is for 5 sec. and twelve such presentations are made successively. After each, the subject has to reproduce the design from memory. Scoring is in terms of the rotation of the stimuli, as shown in Fig. 45; measurement is carried out by means of a large perspex glass on which the degrees of rotation are engraved, the triangle and the square in the figure representing the objective position of these two stimuli in the original figure and the numbers representing the degrees of rotation (Fig. 46).

This test was given by Brengelmann to 40 normal subjects, 28 psychotics, 61 dysthymics, and 39 hysterics. Our expectation would be that the central figures, i.e. those nearest to the fixation

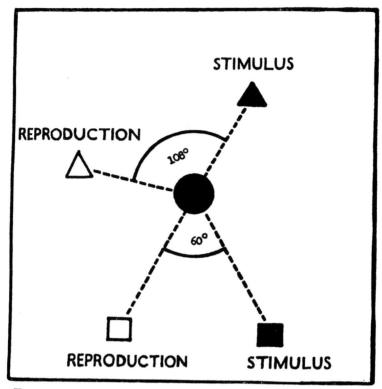

FIG. 45. Measurement of degree of rotation of two repro-
ductions of square and triangular stimulus figures.

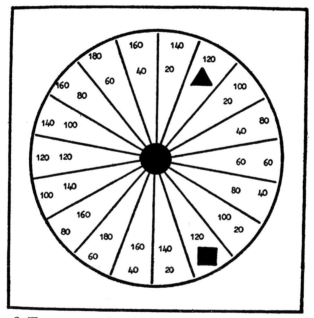

FIG. 46. Transparent drawing for measurement of degree of
rotation of drawing reproduction. Triangle and square
represent true positions of stimuli, numbers indicate degrees
of rotation.

point, would be learned more quickly than the peripheral figures by hysterics as compared with dysthymics. The reason for this prediction, of course, is simply that spatial inhibition would be particularly strong in hysterics as compared with dysthymics and would therefore inhibit peripheral learning as compared with central learning. Fig. 47 shows the results obtained. It can be seen that for all positions normals learn best, psychotics worse, with the neurotic groups intermediate.

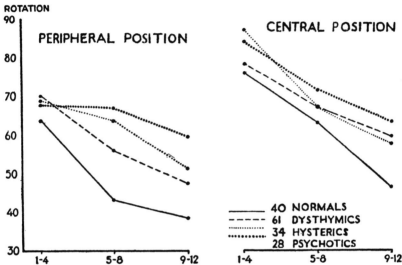

FIG. 47. Rotation values for various groups of subjects during 12 trials, shown separately for central and peripheral positions of stimuli.

It will also be noticed, however, that, as predicted, the hysterics learn *less quickly* as regards the *peripheral position* and *more quickly* as regards the *central position* when compared with the dysthymics. As Brengelmann (1955) puts it: 'Extravertierte—normale wie abnormale—machten zu Beginn in der zentralen Position die meisten Fehler and gegen Ende die wenigsten, während die Introvertierten zu Beginn in der Peripherie die meisten Fehler machten und am Ende die wenigsten ... Es ist nicht so sehr die Lernkapazität oder das Fehlerniveau als solches, sondern die individuelle Lernmethode, welche Extravertierte und Introvertierte trennt.' Similar findings have been reported by Brengelmann with respect to two other scores, namely size of drawing and variability of size of drawing. A detailed discussion of these findings, however, would take us too far away from our main topics; we will merely summarize the results discussed above by saying that as far as they go they support the hypothesis that rotation effects similar to those found in brain-damaged subjects will be found in hysterics.

We have now considered a number of phenomena related theoretically to temporal and spatial inhibition, and we have shown that our prediction linking these phenomena to extra-version, hysteria, psychopathy, and brain-damage have been verified in the great majority of studies. We must now turn to a final topic which, as will be seen later, constitutes a fitting ending to a chapter dealing with visual-perceptual phenomena, namely the topic of the physiological basis of inhibition.

It will have been evident to the reader that the terms inhibition and excitation have been used entirely as molar constructs. It has been suggested that the hypothetical physiological processes underlying these molar concepts are likely to be cortical in origin, and to lie within the central nervous system, but no specific theory has been suggested. In this our account differs very much from that given by Pavlov (1927) and by Köhler (1944), both of whom include in their monographs a considerable amount of theoretical discussion devoted to the hypothetical physiological correlates of the observed effects and processes. Neither account appears to be readily acceptable to physiologists, and Konorski (1940), on the one hand, and Osgood and Heyer (1951) on the other, have attempted to bring the experimental contributions of Pavlov and Köhler in closer relation with orthodox physiology.

Altogether there has been much debate about the use of physiological concepts in relation to personality and behaviour theory. Klein and Krech (1951) and Hebb (1949, 1951) favour the use of neurological models as useful ways of systematizing explanations of behaviour. As Brand (1954) points out, 'they argue that there is no question that the functioning of the brain subsumes behaviour. Therefore they ask, why not use the explanation employing neurological concepts? It may be that the concepts are mistaken . . . but it is unlikely that they will be any more mistaken than non-neurological explanations. In contrast, Kessen and Kimble (1952) advocate the development of conceptual explanations by defining the terms in the explanations through the operational definition of antecedent conditions. In other words, the concepts are tied to the empirical operations in an experiment. Kessen and Kimble object to a physiological or neurological theory because such a theory has little empirical validity.'

The position favoured by the present writer is probably somewhat intermediate between these extremes. It seems unreasonable to postulate psychological variables, the nature or function of which runs counter to physiological or neurological facts. It seems reasonable to formulate hypotheses on the basis of neurological and physiological knowledge, *provided that deductions can be made from these hypotheses which are testable in the molar field*. Conversely, it also appears likely that the molar concepts and theories could be of use in guiding the search of neurologists and physiologists for molecular counterparts of these molar conceptions. Neurologizing only becomes a vice in psychology when it fails to include an operational referent and becomes idle speculation, not leading to any verifiable deductions.

Our failure to deal with neurological and physiological facts in previous chapters therefore is not to be accounted for in terms of any opposition in principle to such notions; it is due rather to lack of relevant and well authenticated facts at this level. It is possible, of course, to point to such work as that carried out by Eccles (1953) and others, who were the first to show conclusively that repeated stimulation produces measurable alteration at the synapse and that this alteration may persist for relatively long periods of time. We may agree with Eccles that the increased effectiveness of transmission is brought about by a swelling of the presynaptic fibre and knob, or by the knobs coming into closer apposition to the post-synaptic membranes, and it is extremely valuable to find evidence, as in the work of Brock, Coombs and Eccles (1952), of the occurrence of molecular events paralleling molar inhibition phenomena, and opposite in direction to molecular events accompanying molar excitation phenomena. These facts regarding depolarization and hyperpolarization in the surface membranes of motoneurones do seem to support in a striking fashion the conclusion based on molar evidence that inhibition is a separate and independent process which is not identical with the fading away of excitatory processes (Malmo, 1954). Yet, however interesting and relevant these facts may be, they do not of themselves hold out any direct promise of improving our theoretical framework for the study of molar processes; neither could they be said to make possible correct deductions confirming or infirming widely-held hypotheses. Until investigations of this type have advanced to a considerable extent beyond their present level, the conclusions can only confirm in the most general way some of the more obvious and widely-accepted concepts in the vocabulary of the behaviour and personality psychologist.

For this reason we shall not go into a discussion of the neural correlates of inhibition and excitation. There would be relatively little to add to a summary given by Dodge in 1926, in which he said: 'Conjectures with respect to the specific neural conditions of inhibition are almost as numerous as the investigators who have studied these phenomena. Most of them, however, fall under one or more of the relatively few phenomenal hypotheses which may be read, as follows: (1) Specific inhibitory nerve centres (Setchinow, Langendoft, Oddi, Wundt); (2) Wave interference (Cyon and Brunton); (3) Artificially stimulated anabolism or an anabolic phase of self-regulated metabolism (Gaskell, Hering, Wundt, Verworn); (4) Drainage of neural energy (Alexander James, William James and McDougall); (5) Refractory phase (Verworn, Froelich, Lucas and Forbes); (6) Chemical theories (depressing drugs, humors, gland secretions, fatigue toxins, etc.). Some of these hypotheses seem, on further consideration, merely to emphasize different states of the same fundamental process.'

From this decision to leave excitatory and inhibitory processes as operationally defined molar terms there is, however, one possible exception which has caused this discussion to be placed just after the section on perception. It would seem that, physiologically, the retina may be regarded not only as a sense organ, in the strict sense of that term, but also as a 'true nervous centre' which ontogenetically is part of the central nervous system. 'When it is studied as a true nervous centre with ample provision for convergence, it is not surprising that the retina should display effects of interaction such as are met with in any spinal reflex activity. One such effect, the basic property of the central nervous system, is inhibition' (Granit, 1951). It is in the perceptual activity of the retina, and perhaps only here, that we may look with some hope of success for an integration of physiological and psychological laws and phenomena. What we have to say here can only be sketchy in the extreme, if for no other reason than the lack of studies relating phenomena in this field to personality and to learning. However, the promise held out by the possibility of such an integration may compensate for the brevity of the treatment given it here.

We may begin with the electrical variations consequent on the stimulation of the eye by light and recorded by placing one electrode upon the cornea and the other close to the exit of the optic nerve. The typical pattern of discharge is as follows: (1) A slight negative deflection of short duration, known as an a-wave; (2) a rapid but much larger positive deflection, known as a b-wave, which reaches a peak and then declines; (3) if the stimulation continues for one or two seconds in the adapted eye, there is another positive deflection of a much more prolonged kind, known as a c-wave; (4) switching off the light results in a momentary positive deflection, so-called d-wave and a slow return to the base line. On the basis of detailed studies Granit has analysed the E.R.G. into three components, called P.I, P.II and P.III. P.II has been correlated with excitation, and the height of the b-wave, with which P.II is associated, is often taken as an index of the optic nerve response. Conversely, P.III appears to be associated with inhibition. The evidence as reviewed by Osgood (1953) and by Granger (1957) suggests that P.III 'is in a sense a process which during illumination prepared the retina for an off-effect, the off-effect itself being a kind of release from inhibition due to the return of P.III to the base line. On analogy with spinal reflex phenomena, the off-effect may be regarded as a *post-inhibitory rebound* in the sense that an optic nerve discharge is released from inhibitory control. Interesting parallels have been drawn by Granit between the analysis of the E.R.G. into two potentials of opposite electric signs and events elsewhere in the C.N.S. He points out that in peripheral nerve, in the spinal cord, and in the superior cervical ganglion, there are opposite potentials like those in the retina which have been correlated respectively with excitation and inhibition.'

There have been several attempts to link these physiological analyses with the results obtained by sensory methods. Thus Schouten and Ornstein (1939) and Wright and Granit (1938) have mentioned a striking parallelism between the time course of the development of alpha adaptation and the development of P.III. 'Taking into account the excitatory component P.II, it becomes possible to analyse a typical sensation-time curve in terms of the E.R.G. record, the primary response, unaffected by inhibition corresponding to P.II and the curve itself being the resultant of the two components P.II and P.III interacting with one another.' Similarly E.R.G. changes have been related to the phenomena of light and dark adaptation, to simultaneous contrast, to after-image formation and flicker fusion. All this work has been reviewed in detail with respect to its bearing on the concept of retinal inhibition by Granger (1957). He comes to the conclusion that it is 'very significant indeed, for it provides a broader framework within which to study retinal activity. No longer should the retina be regarded merely as a highly specialized sense organ; it now becomes a means of eliciting some of the *general* properties of nervous functioning. Apparently sensory activity follows some of the same general laws as motor activity, as Sherrington suggested, and just as inhibition seems to be as essential as excitation for finely adjusted behaviour on the motor side, it seems to be equally essential for precise discrimination on the sensory side.' Indeed, as Granit (1951) has pointed out, it would be difficult to '. . . conceive of any central mechanism of discrimination without thinking of it in terms of inhibition and excitation co-operating towards a common goal. Our primary model of thinking has long been the nervous machinery governing the incredibly finely regulated somatic motor activity, and Sherrington showed how this was achieved by excitation and inhibition in close collaboration.'

We see then that on the whole there is considerable evidence on the physiological level for the proposed integration of perceptual and learning phenomena in terms of common concepts such as those of excitation and inhibition. There is also evidence on the molar level of satiation and excitation phenomena corresponding to those of temporal and spatial inhibition in the learning and motor fields. Thirdly, there is evidence of relationship, as predicted in our typological postulate, between the sensory events studied and personality structure. It seems possible to postulate that similar relationships will eventually be found between personality variables and the physiological processes directly measurable on the E.R.G., particularly P.II and P.III. At the moment it might be more feasible to make precise predictions with respect to phenomena such as dark adaptation, alpha adaptation and so forth, and their postulated relationships with extraversion and introversion. If we postulate hyperactivity of P.III and hypoactivity of P.II in the response systems of extravert, hysterics, and brain-damaged patients, as opposed to hypoactivity of P.III and hyperactivity of P.II in introverts, dysthymics, and non-brain-damaged people, then the theoretical link with sensory phenomena mentioned above would generate testable predictions in considerable number.

Only in one connection has there been any serious attempt to forge such a link. That has been the field of critical flicker fusion. We may perhaps briefly indicate the relationships predicted in terms of our hypothesis, and consider a few isolated studies which have been carried out in this connection. It is reasonably clear that fusion becomes possible owing to the existence of an 'after-effect' resulting from each stimulus, such that succeeding stimuli fall upon the retina while it is still in a state of response to the previous stimulus. On a photo-chemical hypothesis we would expect that the minimum time between the two stimuli required to ensure that the second stimulus should affect the retina while it was still responding to the first stimulus should be greater with more intense stimuli. This would lead one to suppose that the CFF should be *lowered*. In actual fact, however, the CFF is *raised* after the more intense stimulation, and this suggests that there must be some inhibitory mechanism operating to suppress the after-effect of the previous stimulus.

A physiological explanation may be made in terms of the so-called 'pre-excitatory inhibitory', and is closely related to Grant's P.III component of the electroretinogram. The relation of this type of inhibition to flicker fusion has, to some extent, been established by the analyses of Granit (1951) and Enroth (1952). Its function appears to be to inhibit stimulus after-effects so that flicker may still be experienced even with very rapid flash rates, because the after-effect of one stimulus is *suppressed* by the first effect of the second stimulus. In a retina with a strong P.III component, CFF will be high and will increase with increasing intensity of the stimulus because the after-effect of one stimulus is inhibited more readily by the greater P.III component resulting from the more intense second stimulus. On the other hand, in a retina with only a small P.III component CFF will be low and will depend on there being a long enough interval between successive flashes of light to allow the primary excitation wave produced by the first stimulus to decay sufficiently to allow the next stimulus to evoke a new wave of excitation. It follows directly from this argument that extraverts, having constitutionally higher inhibitory potentials, should show a *higher P.III component* and consequently *higher CFF*. We would therefore predict in extraverts and hysterics *lower thresholds of temporal discrimination.* Does the experimental evidence bear out this prediction?

The first relevant research appears to have been that of Krugman (1947). He used 50 normal air-crew returnees and 50 anxiety reaction cases (dysthymics), and determined their flicker fusion thresholds, using two testing conditions. He reports correlations of ·62 and ·45 between anxiety and flicker fusion on the two conditions, using biserial correlation coefficients. When other variables, such as hours of sleep, time of day, age, and alcoholism were held constant by the use of partial correlations, the relationship between CFF and psychiatric diagnosis reached even higher values (·68 and ·55). He summarizes his findings by saying: 'It is apparent that the mean scores made by normals are significantly higher than those made by anxiety reaction cases, though there is considerable overlapping of the distributions. It is also evident that results for testing Condition A (fusion to flicker) seem to be somewhat more related to anxiety reaction diagnosis than the traditional testing condition, Condition B (flicker to fusion).' These results are in line with our prediction, although they cannot be regarded as conclusive. The experimental group differed from the control group, apparently, by being more neurotic as well as by being more introverted; indeed, the criticisms made of the Spence-Taylor studies would apply to any attempt to use Krugman's results as verifying any dimensional theory such as ours. Scores for a hysteric-psychopathic group would be required in order to put the issue beyond doubt.

The same comment applies to the somewhat similar study reported by Goldstone (1955). This author worked on 35 high-anxiety and 39 low-anxiety subjects, most of them patients and their relatives at an out-patient psychiatric clinic. Using an electronically activated 'glow-modulator' tube he determined '(a) FFT, or sensitivity to flicker, (b) slope or precision of judgment (intra-S variability), (c) decline in FFT, which was defined as the difference in flicker fusion threshold between the first ten and last ten runs of the flicker test (a decline in FFT would reflect a reduced sensitivity to flicker associated with continued exposure to the flicker test), and (d) decline in slope, which was defined as the difference in slope between the first ten and last ten runs of the flicker test'. With respect to the results, Goldstone reports as follows: 'With regard to the mean FFT, one observes a lower flicker threshold for those groups designated high anxiety than for the groups designated low anxiety. These group differences in all cases appear reliable at better than the ·005 level of confidence and indicate a reduced sensitivity to flicker in the high-anxiety groups.' There also appears to be a higher 'slope' or index of scatter for the high-anxiety groups, differences again being fully significant.

The groups showing high anxiety have a greater drop in sensitivity to flicker than groups designated low anxiety. Again the statistical significance of the data is assured, showing that the reduction in flicker acuity associated with continued exposure to the flicker test is greater in the dysthymic group. Goldstone thus agrees with Krugman in finding reduced sensitivity to flicker associated with high anxiety, supporting our hypothesis, but not in any sense *proving* it to be correct. The same may be said of the work of Friedl (1954), who demonstrated a correlation of − ·34 between CFF and anxiety in 63 normal subjects.

Further support for our hypothesis comes from the work of Biesheuvel and Pitt (1955) and of Mundy-Castle (1955). These authors follow the Heymans and Wiersma temperament classification originated by Gross (1902), in which 'emotionality' is the term used to denote what we have labelled 'neuroticism', and 'primary *vs.* secondary function' is the term used to denote what we have labelled 'introversion-extraversion'. A very full description of this historically very important set of theories has been given elsewhere (Eysenck, 1953), and we will not discuss either the terminology or the theories again here. Let us merely note that phenomena analogous to the CFF have from the first figured very prominently in the experimental programme of the

Dutch school (Wiersma, 1932; Biesheuvel, 1938). Doubts about the technical aspects of flicker measurement in these studies make the writer somewhat doubtful about accepting them in evidence, however, although the Biesheuvel study, at any rate, appears to give some support to our theory. (The Wiersma studies are difficult to evaluate because they were done on psychotic subjects, where no confident predictions would be made from the present theory.)

Somewhat indirect evidence comes from studies relating the alpha rhythm on the EEG to CFF scores, as in the work of Chyatte (1954) and Friedl (1954). Quite high correlations have been reported between CFF and proportion of alpha rhythm present (Chyatte gives the astonishing figure of ·855!), so that EEG studies would appear to be relevant here by virtue of their close relationship to CFF. In a more direct way, Mundy-Castle postulates that 'alpha frequency is a reflection of degree of the temperament variable secondary function, and that this is associated with a central nervous excitability characteristic'. (It will be remembered that the term 'secondary function' is equivalent to 'extraversion' in our terminology—Eysenck, 1953.) His definition of 'alpha frequency' is in terms of the mean number of cycles per second; as he points out, the alpha rhythm usually possesses two or more separate components (Walter, in Hill & Parr, 1950; Cohn, 1948), so that averaging becomes necessary. Reuning (1955) has provided evidence that this score also correlates significantly with CFF, the actual correlation being ·545.

Mundy-Castle subjected his hypothesis to experimental verification by applying the EEG to a group of subjects who had formed part of an experiment conducted by Biesheuvel and Pitt (1955), in which they had been rated very carefully for extraversion, and in which they had been administered a large battery of objective performance tests. The results of the experiment strongly supported the theory underlying the selection of the tests, demonstrating a correlation of over ·6 between tests and ratings. Mundy-Castle made use of the ratings and scores of these subjects and showed that extraverted individuals have a relatively high alpha frequency (10 to 13 c/sec.), while introverted individuals have a relatively low alpha frequency (8 to 10 c/sec.). These results reached a reasonable level of statistical significance. They also agreed with the findings of Gastaut et al.

(1951), who found that subjects with high alpha rhythms could be described as 'nerveux, actifs, agités, excités, hypomaniaques', while those with low alpha rhythms could be described as 'tranquilles, calmes, lymphatiques'. It is of course difficult to translate these descriptive terms into factor language with any degree of certainty, but at least we may say that they do not contradict the Mundy-Castle findings.

These studies do no more than open up a field of investigation; results obtained with both CFF and EEG measures are notoriously even more unreliable than those obtained with more orthodox personality tests. Too much should therefore not be made of the agreements with prediction reported by Krugman, Goldstone, and the South African group. Altogether, these few paragraphs are perhaps the most speculative in this whole chapter. They have been included in the main because the predictions made here would, if verified, provide the most direct link we could forge at the present time between the work of electro-physiologists and that of students of personality. Any such link between the molecular and the molar level will be of such importance to the development of an integrated psychology that the writer has overcome his general dislike of speculation in the absence of ascertained facts to suggest the relationships outlined above. It is strongly hoped that the next few years will see experimentation either confirming or infirming these hypotheses.

Chapter Six

SOCIALIZATION AND PERSONALITY

IN the preceding sections we have outlined a general theory of extraversion-introversion, implied in which was also a general theory of hysteria and dysthymia. It has been shown that this theory has certain properties which characterize scientifically useful and acceptable theories; in other words, we have been able to predict phenomena previously unknown, such as lack of conditionability of extraverts, the large satiation effects observable in hysterics, the small reminiscence effects found in introverts, and so forth. To those who value a scientific theory in terms of its predictive capacities, these facts may make this general theory more acceptable. However, scientific theories must also fulfil another function, namely that of accounting for all the known phenomena. This means, in brief, that our theory ought to be adequate to explain the experimentally observed facts relating to hysterics and dysthymics, such as the greater persistence of the dysthymics (Eysenck, 1947), their higher level of aspiration (Himmelweit, 1947; Miller, 1951), their greater verbal I.Q. as compared with non-verbal I.Q. (Himmelweit, 1945; Foulds, 1956), the preference of hysterics for sexual and aggressive jokes (Eysenck, 1947), and their tendency to disobey instructions on the Porteus Maze test and to cross lines, retrace, etc., although enjoined not to do so (Hildebrand, 1953; Foulds, 1951).

At the same time we must be able to account for the predominant features of hysterical and psychopathic, and of dysthymic personality as clinically described. Most readers will be familiar with the clinical description of these groups; only a few brief excerpts will therefore be quoted. Here is a description given by Henderson (1939) in his book on *Psychopathic States*.

This term, he says, 'is a name we apply to those individuals who conform to a certain intellectual standard, sometimes high, sometimes approaching the realm of defect and yet not amounting to it, who throughout their lives or from a comparatively early age, have exhibited disorders of conduct of an anti-social or asocial nature, usually of the recurrent or episodic type, which in many instances have proved difficult to influence by methods of social, penal and medical care and treatment . . . the inadequacy or deviation or failure to adjust to ordinary social life is not a mere wilfulness or badness which can be threatened or thrashed out of an individual so involved but constitutes a true illness for which we have no specific explanation'. Henderson also quotes Maudsley (1896) as saying that 'such a person has no capacity of true moral feeling, his impulses and desires are egoistic, his conduct is governed by immoral motives', and Mercier (1902) as saying that 'there are persons who indulge in vice with such persistence, at a cost of punishment so heavy, so certain and so prompt, who incur their punishment for the sake of pleasure so trifling and so transient that they are by common consent considered insane although they exhibit no other indication of insanity'. Similarly, in relation to hysterics we may quote Kahn (1931) to the effect that 'The hysterical personality is in a sense a psychopath in pure culture. They have an egocentric craving for prestige, they want to shine, to be the centre of the stage, their hypertrophic egos need continual inflation by shallow shows for their own satisfaction . . . from the psychiatric point of view social maladjustment is the ultimate crux of the psychopath as regards man and his environment.'

This stress on the lack of moral standards, on the failure of higher regulative, inhibiting and restraining mechanism to prevent the immediate gratifications of instinctive appetites and lusts, recurs over and over in the clinical description of hysterics and psychopaths. Thus Bianchi (1906): 'If it be true that the end justifies the means, the hysterical subject makes the most ample and insane application of this doctrine. To execute his intention, which is generally egoistic, he indulges the strangest ideas, and hatches most dangerous plots, which he thoughtlessly puts into effect.' Bianchi goes on to say: 'Tardieu, Lasegue, Legrand de Saulle, Schüle and Jolly, among others, who have made a profound study of the moral character of hysterical subjects and of their psychic constitution . . . all express the same opinion. The predominant note is one of exaggerated affective excitability, which resolves itself into a series of acts through circuits, upon which the inhibiting power that emanates from the higher centres has no effect. Those centres, very little developed originally, are absolutely pre- vented from performing their functions by the lower centres, which are overcharged at high tension. The activity of the latter is altogether put at the service of the inferior ego (ego- centric), and the inferior ego, exposed to all influences, uncon- trolled and uncontrollable . . . is changeable by reason of the non-operation of the regulative centres, which are the true depositories of historical experience.'

Similarly, Sadler (1936) reports that 'constitutional psycho- paths change work frequently. They try numerous occupations, abandoning their jobs on the slightest provocation. In the presence of repeated failure they frequently develop a defence mechanism of neuroticism. They suffer from poor judgment . . . They yield easily to alcoholic and sexual temptation and are also much given to gambling and, as a result of these latter influences, are frequently led unintentionally into crime. Large numbers of such individuals are observed by psychiatrists, social workers, and others who deal with the delinquent and criminal classes.' Bumke (1948), talking about the egocentric orientation of hysterics, maintains that: 'Dieser Egoismus, frei- lich in einer ganz spezifischen Färbung, ist einer der wichtigsten Grundzüge des hysterischen Charakters.' And Krafft-Ebing (1906), in a famous passage, characterizes the hysteric person- ality thus:

'Das Gebiet des freien Wollens erscheint durch die sittliche und Willensschwäche, durch die Flüchtigkeit und Oberfläch- lichkeit des Vorstellens, durch die formal und inhaltlich geänderte Empfindungsweise, durch Zwangsvorstellungen jedenfalls eingeschränkt und die Kranke ist vielfach nur mehr der Spielball ihrer Launen, Gelüste, Impulse, Einbil- dungen. So kann es geschehen, dass die wichtigsten Pflichten vernachlässigt, die heiligsten Gefühle verletzt werden und den absurdesten Einfällen und Motiven Folge gegeben wird.'

Delgado (1953), in his Curso de Psiquiatria, maintains that 'hysteria is the psychoneurosis *par excellence* . . . Emotional excitability . . . and egotism are usually apparent from child-hood.' Henderson and Gillespie (1947) point out that 'the line to be drawn between psychopathic states as a medical problem and delinquency as a penal problem is sometimes very narrow indeed, and almost inevitably a certain amount of confusion in differentiation must exist. There are a large number of delin-quents who may be described as having psychopathic person-alities, but many people who are psychopathic may never become delinquent.' Rosanoff (1938) says: 'I could not better define the hysteric personality . . . than by saying that it is characterized by total lack of the first principle—ethics of prudence; and that it is, in its typical manifestations, actuated entirely by the third principle—imposed ethics, i.e. in so far as its conduct has any ethical quality at all. This places the hysteric individual in close relation to the criminal. A desire to lead a parasitic existence; to be a burden on relatives, em-ployers, the government; to live on a pension and do no work, is the characteristic of many of these patients. They would, and often do, steal anything conveniently within reach, lie, cheat, make work and trouble for others, wantonly destroy government property. . . . An essential feature of the psychological mechan-ism of hysteria is the existence of a concealed, illicit, ethically untenable motive. . . . There is a highly significant correlation between hysteria and various social maladjustments: behaviour difficulties in children observed at school, at home, or else-where; delinquency and criminality; dependency and pauper-ism; marital troubles; prostitution, etc.'

Through all these quotations—which could be multiplied almost *ad infinitum*—there thus runs a main thread of failure of the socialization process in hysterics and psychopaths, a failure which leads to criminal activities, to anti-social acts, and to generally unethical behaviour. Descriptions by these same authors of the dysthymic group of disorders completely lack any reference to anti-social behaviour; unfortunately such an absence cannot be documented by references in the same ways that its presence can! If anything, dysthymics are reported to display over-socialized reactions, showing guilt and worry over relatively slight and unimportant actions whose anti-social or unethical character is more apparent than real. Their main characteristic, outweighing all others, is that of over-strong fear or anxiety reactions; these may occur even in connection with relatively mild or even quite neutral stimuli or situations.

Sadler, in his *Theory and Practice of Psychiatry,* puts the point well. 'Anxiety is classified as a neurosis *when the anxiety reaction is altogether out of proportion to the stimulus,* to the situation or the experience which calls it forth; and of course, when the anxiety is based on fictitious fears, it is clearly a neurosis. Anxiety, then, is an earmark of a neurosis when it becomes morbid. When fear is translated into dread, and when it becomes acute and severe, it may be spoken of as anxiety state. Because anxieties are usually the fruition of other and preceding chronic worries and dreads, and because there is often such a complexity of factors, together with the unwillingness of most anxiety patients honestly to seek to discover and face the facts, it is often very difficult to run down these anxieties to their original sources.' It is important to stress that emotional reactions of anxiety and fear become chronic and are aroused quite often by situations which appear neutral to most people. It is not merely that dysthymics have strong emotional reactions, but that these reactions are easily aroused by irrelevant stimuli. Strong emotional (autonomic) lability is characteristic of neurotics as a whole; it is the proliferation of emotion-arousing stimuli which distinguishes the dysthymic from the hysteric.

The fact that strong emotionality is characteristic of neurosis as a whole, and therefore of hysterics also, is strongly supported by psychiatric observation. Perusal of the classical sources also points up another difference between hysterics and dysthymics, and their emotional reaction, viz. the *dissociation* which appears in the minds of the hysterics, preventing the emotion from occupying the whole attention of the patient, and also preventing it from developing the positive kind of feed-back which seems to characterize the dysthymic. Thus Delgado talks about '. . . the physiological syndrome of the violent emotions' which afflicts hysterics; similarly Henderson and Gillespie: 'The emotional constitution of the hysteric is shown in his tendency to react much more intensely than the normal to an emotional stimulus; he reacts in a specific region, i.e. in a particular organ or group of organs; the psychic representation of the function has a peculiar tendency to become dissociated from the rest of consciousness; and there is a peculiar passivity in his attitude to the dissociated function.' And again Krafft-Ebing:

'Grunderscheinungen sind das labile Gleichgewicht der psychischen Funktionen, die enorm leichte Anspruchsfähigkeit und die ungewöhnlich intensive Reaktion der Psyche und der rasche Wechsel der Erregungen (Reizbare Schwäche). Im Vordergrund stehen die Anomalien des Gemütslebens. Die Kranken sind durch innere und aussere psychische Reize enorm affizierbar . . .'

Bumke may also be quoted in support:

'Es ist klar, das die Erklärung der bis her besprochenen Charakterzüge in einer *Störung des Gefühlslebens* gesucht werden muss, mit der auch die erhöhte Suggestibilität zusammenhängt. Die Affekte bei der Hysterie sind labil, werden leicht—oft ohne erkennbaren Anlass—ausgelöst und schwellen häufig fast explosionsartig zu sehr groser Stärke an. Darauf beruht das Sprunghafte, Unausgeglichene und Unvermittelte im Leben dieser Kranken, die sich von dem Ideal eines seelischen Gleichmases so weit wie nur möglich entfernen.'

So also Kraepelin (1904):

'Beim Zustandekommen aller dieser Störungen sind vor allem die Schwankungen der Stimmung massgebend. Sie sind es, welche in hohem Grade das gesamte Seelenleben der Kranken beherrschen. Ihr Einfluss ist weit stärker, als derjenigen der vernünftigen Überlegung oder der sittlichen Grundsätze. Die Kranken sind ungemein erregbar; ihnen fehlt die Dämpfung, die beim gesunden Menschen allmählich die raschen und starken Gefühlschwankungen der Kinderjahre abschwächt . . . Ihnen ist nichts gleichgültig; sie sehen sich veranlasst, zu allen Ereignissen in ihrer Umgebung persönlich Stellung zu nehmen. Daher ihre ausserordentliche Empfindlichkeit, die Heftigkeit der Gefühlsausbrüche bei den geringfügigsten Anlässen, daher ihre Neigung, sich überall getroffen zu fühlen, alle sachlichen Beziehungen und Überlegungen sofort mit persönlichen Zutaten zu durchsetzen.'

There is agreement, then, among psychiatric observers that both hysterics and dysthymics are strongly emotional, labile people; and the evidence seems to suggest that this condition is largely due to an inherited autonomic lability which predisposes neurotics as a whole to over-react to emotion-arousing stimuli. Some of the evidence regarding this generalization has been reviewed elsewhere (Eysenck, 1953), and as we are not concerned with neuroticism as such in this volume, we shall not discuss this point any further. What requires elucidation are not those points on which hysterics and dysthymics agree, but those on which they differ, i.e. those characteristics which are related to extraversion-introversion. What we have to explain in terms of our theory, therefore, are the following points:

(1) The failure of socialization in the hysterico-psychopathic group as compared with the dysthymics;

(2) The development of anxiety in relation to neutral stimuli on the part of the dysthymics, as compared with the hysterico-psychopathic group. In other words, what we need is a link between the concept of an excitation/inhibition balance, as developed throughout this book, and the experimental and clinical personality descriptions quoted above.

Such a link is provided by Mowrer (1950) in his theory of the socialization process, which will be briefly outlined below. As is well known, Mowrer agrees with several other writers (Miller & Konorski, 1928; Hilgard & Marquis, 1940; Schlosberg, 1937; Skinner, 1938) in postulating a two factor theory of learning. If, for the sake of simplicity, we refer to classical conditioning as conditioning and to instrumental conditioning as learning, then, Mowrer points out, we find that learning is concerned with *behavioural* responses, conditioning with *physiological* responses. In the second place, this distinction corresponds roughly to that between the *central nervous system,* which is concerned with the transmission of impulses to the skeletal muscles, and the *autonomic nervous system* which mediates responses of the glands and the smooth muscles, and is concerned with the expression of emotion. These distinctions also correspond very roughly to the familiar difference between *voluntary* and *involuntary* responses. The visceral-vascular responses mediated by the autonomic nervous system are beyond direct voluntary control, whereas practically all the skeletal responses are under voluntary control. This distinction between conditioning of smooth muscles and glands, activated through the autonomic system, and learning, mediated by skeletal muscles through the action of the central nervous system, has led Mowrer to suggest the following hypothesis:

206

'Under ordinary circumstances, the visceral and vascular responses occur in a smoothly automatic fashion, and serve what Cannon has called the "homeostatic", or physiological, equilibrium-restoring function. These same responses may, however, be made to occur, not only in response to actual physiological needs, but also in response to conditioned stimuli, or signals, of various kinds. And when the visceral and vascular responses occur on the latter basis as *anticipatory* states, they *produce*, rather than eliminate, physiological disequilibrium and are consciously experienced as an *emotion*. As such, they play enormously important motivational roles, roles so important to the survival of the organism that it is easily understood why the learning of these responses should be automatic, involuntary, distinct from the type of learning whereby ordinary habits are acquired. Biologically, it is clearly necessary that living organisms be equipped with a nervous system which will cause those skeletal responses to be fixated which reduce drive and give pleasure. But it is equally evident that living organisms must also be equipped with another nervous system which will cause emotional responses to be learned, not because they solve problems or give pleasure in any immediate sense, but because without such responses the organism would have slight chance of survival. There are grounds for believing that all emotions (including fear, anger, and the appetites) are basically painful, (i.e. all have drive quality); and it is hard to see how they could be acquired by the same mechanism which fixes those responses (of the skeletal musculature) which are problem solving, drive reducing, pleasure giving. The latter are learned when a problem is resolved, ended; whereas it is often necessary that emotional responses become conditioned to signals which are associated with the *onset*, not the termination, of a problem.'

This is a very important distinction, which appears to be of considerable usefulness. Some types of learning are directly useful and produce results which are pleasant. We learn to ride a bicycle, play cricket, or make love, and the resulting pleasure 'stamps in' the actions which have produced this result. On the other hand, we are afraid when we see a bear in the woods, or hear bullets whining overhead, or find a bus bearing down on us. These reactions are unpleasant; however, they are also exceedingly useful. As Mowrer puts it, learning is parallel to what Freud has called the *pleasure principle*, whereas conditioning is more closely related to the *reality principle*. 'In other words, living organisms require conditioned responses or emotions, not because it is pleasant to do so but because it is *realistic*.' It is certainly not pleasant to be afraid, for example, but it is very helpful from the standpoint of personal survival.

Mowrer develops this distinction between learning and conditioning further by referring to child upbringing and education. As he points out, anthropologists tend to define 'culture' as accumulated and transmitted problem solutions. It is certainly true that some items of culture do in fact help us to solve problems; others, however, actually seem to make problems—problems of cleanliness, problems of conformity, problems of repression of sexual and aggressive impulses, and so forth. We must distinguish between problem solutions which are individually useful and which are learned, and problem solutions which are socially necessary and which are conditioned. 'By and large, the solutions to individual problems involve the central nervous system and the skeletal musculature, whereas the solutions to social problems involve the autonomic nervous system and the organs which mediate emotional responses.' This differentiation is recognized in the common-sense distinction between teaching and training. 'Teaching may be defined as a process whereby one individual helps another learn to solve a problem more quickly or effectively than would be likely on the basis of that individual's own unaided, trial-and-error efforts. Here we are dealing with "items of culture" which are individually helpful. Training, by contrast, may be thought of as involving learning whose primary objective is social rather than individual. In this connection one naturally thinks of "items of culture" which are associated with such words as "morality", "character", "social responsibility", etc.'

The view presented here, in broad outline, gives us the following picture. A child born into this world has a number of imperative needs which require satisfaction. Similarly, society has certain needs it must impress on the infant. The infant *learns* the methods which most satisfy his needs and in most societies undergoes a process of *teaching* in order to acquire the necessary skills. Society, on the other hand, *conditions* him to act in conformity with its precepts and he undergoes a process of *training* in order to become socialized. The infant learns walking, the multiplication table, the English language, and so forth; he becomes conditioned to use a pot, and suppress the direct and immediate expression of his aggressive and sexual urges.

So much for Mowrer's theory. There is no intention here to re-fight the battle of learning theories let loose by the publication of Mowrer's paper (cf. Mowrer, 1951; Birch & Bitterman, 1951; Sheffield, 1951; Kendler, 1951; Miller, 1951; and Ritchie, 1951; see also Mowrer, 1956, for his latest views). We do not feel that the case for a dualistic or pluralistic type of learning theory has been made out sufficiently strongly to give up the very real advantages of a monistic theory. We do not feel that Mowrer and the other 'dualists' have always borne in mind the fact that the majority of laws established in the field of 'conditioning' can also be applied to 'learning', and *vice versa*, a feat unlikely of accomplishment on any but a monistic hypothesis. Lastly, we feel with Hebb (1956) that some of the alleged distinctions between 'classical' or Pavlovian and 'instrumental' or Skinnerian conditioning do not stand up to close scrutiny. Until more compelling evidence is produced, therefore, we would hold that the distinction between learning and conditioning pointed out by Mowrer is not in any sense an absolute one. The main difference between the classes of facts he subsumes under these two categories would, in our view, appear to lie in the nature of the learned response, rather than in the character of the learning process. This difference has been alluded to already on an earlier page, in connection with our discussion of learned drives. What we are proposing is simply that there are important differences between learned activities which are also drives and learned activities which are not. This distinction is not conceived as an absolute one; there are presumably gradations from one extreme to another; but heuristically the difference is of immense importance, and has many interesting consequences. Condition the eyeblink to a tone, and the new C.S. (1) does not motivate new learning, i.e. does not act as a general drive, and (2) easily extinguishes when there is no reinforcement forthcoming. Condition fear responses to a tone, i.e. by coupling the tone with a severe electric shock, and the new C.S. (1) motivates new learning, i.e. acts as a general drive, and (2) extinguishes only with great difficulty, because it provides its own reinforcement (through reduction of the conditioned autonomic drive). (Representative references, in addition to those given in previous chapters, are,

Brown & Jacobs, 1949; Farber, 1948; Hall, 1955; May, 1948; Mowrer & Lamoreaux, 1946; Schoenfeld, 1950.)

Particularly clear examples of the strength and persistence of conditioned fear drives are given in some studies by Solomon *et al.* (1953), Solomon and Wynne (1954), and Wynne and Solomon (1955). These workers conditioned dogs to a light-shock combination, and taught the animals to escape from the shock by jumping over a hurdle from the electrified grid into another room which was 'safe'. The dogs soon learned to jump to the light stimulus, and *without further reinforcement* jumped six hundred and more times, evidently ready to go on jumping as long as the experimenter was willing to go on with the experiment. The mediating role of the autonomic, i.e. the conditioned response-drive combination, was dramatically demonstrated by carrying out sympathectomies on some of the dogs. It was shown that such dogs were all capable of acquiring the conditioned escape response, but the majority *extinguished spontaneously* after learning had once taken place, i.e. after they had learned to jump to the light, thus escaping from the shock which followed 10 sec. later. 'This has never occurred in any of the 30 control dogs which had been trained under the same conditions.' Figs. 48 and 49 show clearly the course of extinction in an operated dog, and the failure to extinguish in a normal dog. These curves are fairly typical, and illustrate the mediating role of the acquired drive properties of the light-shock combination.

Without, therefore, following Mowrer all the way in his two-factor type of theory, we may agree with him that a good case can be made out for the proposal that *the socialization process is mediated to a considerable extent by conditioning reactions of an autonomic kind (anxiety)*. If this general point be accepted, and Mowrer's arguments are certainly strong and well based on available experimental evidence, then we are immediately led to a chain of deductions which runs something like this:

(*a*) Socialization is mediated by conditioning.
(*b*) Extraverts condition poorly.
(*c*) Introverts condition particularly well.

Therefore under conditions of equal environmental pressure we would expect extraverts to be under-socialized, introverts to be over-socialized, with people in less extreme positions on

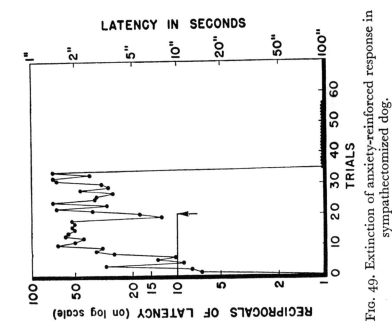

Fig. 49. Extinction of anxiety-reinforced response in sympathectomized dog.

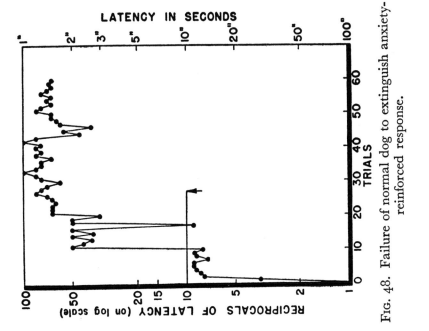

Fig. 48. Failure of normal dog to extinguish anxiety-reinforced response.

the extravert-introvert continuum showing intermediate degrees of socialization.

Roughly speaking, this is precisely what we did find in our experimental results and in the psychiatric descriptions which we have quoted above. There is a considerable degree of social pressure in the direction of persistence of activity and a high level of aspiration; both of these are found in introverts, but are largely lacking in extraverts. Social pressure leads the introvert to learn more words (reading) than the extravert, thus obtaining a higher verbal I.Q.–non-verbal I.Q. ratio. The socialization process emphasizes honesty and the desirability of obeying instructions, hence such results as those reported on differences found on the Porteus Maze Q test score. Here also we would appear to have an explanation for the observation that 'social maladjustment is the ultimate crux of the psychopath' and that these individuals have, from a comparatively early age, exhibited disorders of conduct of an anti-social or asocial nature, and that they have proved difficult to influence by methods of social, penal, and medical care and treatment. The individual's failure to condition easily, on this view, accounts for his failure to become fundamentally socialized, and thus is responsible for these many-sided behaviour patterns. This would appear to be a truly dynamic account of the genesis of hysterical, psychopathic, and criminal behaviour patterns.

Precisely the opposite picture is predicted, and found, among introverts and dysthymics. Here we have, in the ethical realm, an excess of socialization leading to preoccupation with social duties, ethics, guilt, and similar moral notions. Guilt feelings appear easily where ethical levels of aspiration are unduly high, and these levels are high because of excessively quick conditioning in response to parental and social pressure. Quite generally, the theory accounts also for the main feature of dysthymic personalities, namely their excessive anxiety reactions. Strong autonomic-emotional lability and reactivity produce excessive fear reactions to painful and harmful stimuli; through unusually strong and responsive conditioning mechanisms these fear reactions become attached to accidental, irrelevant, neutral stimuli which happen to precede or accompany the fear-producing occasion.[1] Through their connection with these con-

[1] See Shoben's (1949) definition of anxiety as 'either a fear of "nothing" or a fear of something which is objectively irrelevant'.

ditioned fears or anxieties, the previously neutral stimuli now acquire drive properties, such that avoidance of these stimuli becomes rewarding through reduction of the conditioned fear or anxiety attaching to them. There is thus nothing mysterious about the fears, phobias, and anxieties of the dysthymic patient; they are the product of excessively high drive and excessively high conditionability ($D \times {}_sH_R$). It should perhaps be added that in this account we are assuming the experimentally demonstrated phenomena of verbal conditioning (Cohen *et al.*, 1954; Greenspoon, 1955; Sidowski, 1954; Taffel, 1955) and of subception (Lazarus & McCleary, 1951; Miller, 1939; McCleary & Lazarus, 1949; Eriksen, 1956; Lowenfeld *et al.*, 1956; Rubenfeld *et al.*, 1956) to play an important part. Their precise *modus operandi* is not known in this connection, but such knowledge is not indispensable to our general theory. We are also assuming that single-trial conditioning occurs; this is implicit in any kind of traumatic theory. Fortunately this notion is theoretically respectable (Guthrie, 1952), and has experimental support (Hudson, 1953). It may be concluded, therefore, that such mechanisms as are made use of in our theory are not *ex post facto* creations, but have substantial empirical backing.

How does the concept of sociability fit in with our picture? Extraverts are traditionally the more social group, and it may be asked if this fact can be derived from our theory. Such a derivation is possible, although it must be admitted to be somewhat speculative. The introvert, as we have seen, is *socialized*, i.e. he has acquired a conditioned fear mechanism which acts in such a way as to provide immediate punishments and rewards (by drive reduction accompanying withdrawal from socially disapproved acts). Such mechanisms act in response to those stimuli to which they have become conditioned, and consequently the individual's behaviour becomes in part independent of outward and immediate rewards and punishments. It makes his personality (in part at least) autonomous and enables him to withstand group pressure. Conversely, the extravert, not having acquired these conditioned fears to anything like the same extent, is not so independent from immediate rewards and punishments. Now the source of most of these rewards and punishments, in so far as these are not automatic and mechanical consequences of our actions such as *fire-burn*, is the immediate social group, and it would seem to follow that the extravert would become unduly responsive to group opinion, group standards, and group approval. If this immediate group is 'good', i.e. has socially desirable opinions, then he will acquire a tenuous hold upon a second-hand moral outlook; any change in the composition of the group, however, and in particular any change towards the 'bad' end of the scale, would find him less able to resist the group outlook than the introvert. This dependence on the group would be likely to lead him to place great value on it, to seek its approval in all things, and thus to behave in a *sociable* manner.

A direct consequence of this hypothesis would be the prediction that in experimental situations in which the perceptions or attitudes of the individual are opposed to group pressure, as for instance in the work of Ash (1952, 1955) and Crutchfield (1955), introverts should be more likely to resist this pressure than extraverts. There is some very indirect evidence to this effect (see discussion in Eysenck, 1954), but a direct test would be easy to arrange and very relevant to our theory.

There are of course certain complicating features. In the first place, although introverts condition more easily, the social pressure to which they are exposed may not always be in a socially desirable direction. Fagin's school for thieves may produce introverted children conditioned to crime (Franks & Willett, 1956; Franks, 1956). Thus we must pay attention to the direction taken by the conditioning process, as well as the individual's susceptibility to conditioning. In the second place, lack of sociability is characteristic not only of the introvert, but also of the neurotic; Eysenck (1957) has shown that socially abient reactions correlate with both introversion and neuroticism. The reasons for these abient reactions, however, were shown to be quite different. Introverts do not care much for social intercourse, but if necessary can effectively partake in it. Neurotics, or normals with high neuroticism scores, may want to be sociable but are afraid, anxious and worried about making contact, and therefore shy away from doing so. In combination we therefore get the dysthymics as the most unsociable group, being unsociable on two counts. We also get a situation of conflict in the hysterics, whose extraversion would lead them in the direction of sociability, and whose neuroticism would lead them in the opposite direction. It is not unlikely that this conflict may be responsible for the often-noted ambivalence in the social relations of hysterics and their curious social behaviour noted in some of the psychiatric observations quoted earlier in this chapter.

Persistence is another trait found to discriminate between extraverts and introverts, a difference which demands to be derived from our theory. This can be done along two lines. In the first place, as already mentioned, there is social pressure in the direction of persistent behaviour at home, in school, and at work; this is part of the socialization process, and would consequently lead to greater persistence in introverts. But there is another point. Persistence involves nearly always some degree of repetitive work, some long-term exposure to identical stimuli, and would thus be predicted to lead to more rapid build-up of reactive inhibition. This line of argument would lead us to predict that extraverts would be found lacking in persistence. Both arguments lead to the same prediction, and may thus be considered to reinforce each other.

It may also be possible to account, in terms of our theory, for the dissociative features of hysteric behaviour; such behavioural patterns can be predicted in terms of the greater inhibitory potential generated in extraverts. This inhibition thus fulfills very much the same role as did the 'short secondary function' in the Gross-Heymans-Wiersma theory, the main difference being that inhibition has a sound experimental and theoretical basis, and is independently measurable, while 'secondary function' is an *ad hoc* concept of purely descriptive value. As an example of the application of the concept of inhibition to dissociative symptoms we may perhaps take the phenomenon of 'repression'. If we assume that temporal inhibition is monotonically related to the number of neural impulses passing through a given set of synapses in unit time, and if we assume that strongly emotionally charged events and their ideational replications give rise to larger numbers of neural impulses than do more neutral events, then we would expect to find stronger inhibition for precisely those events, and their neural representations, for which 'repression' is reported. (We are making the additional assumption that the appropriate mental analogue for inhibition in this context is forgetting; Köhler has shown to what extent the precise indexing of satiation and inhibition phenomena depends on the experimental context.) And we would also predict 'repression' to occur most strongly in those groups, i.e. hysterics and extraverts generally, in whom clinical and experimental evidence agree in finding it. (Cf. Carlson, 1953; Eriksen, 1952, 1954; Eriksen & Davids, 1955; Eriksen & Kuethe, 1956. Smith and Daygar (1956) may also be relevant, although difficult to interpret. Kogan (1956) finds a correlation between authoritarianism and repression; this is predictable in view of the relation between authoritarianism and tough-mindedness.)

The extension of the concept of 'inhibition' or 'satiation' to so-called mental phenomena, such as thought process, memory, and the like, may not appear at first sight to be admissible. It should be remembered, however, that mental processes on any reasonable hypothesis must have a neural substratum, and that the rules of inhibition must apply just as much to these as to perceptual or learning phenomena. Again, Köhler specifically included memory processes in his discussion of satiation and brain dynamics (1940). Also, there is experimental evidence for the occurrence of satiation in thought processes; Wertheimer (1956) reports that the loss of meaning which often accompanies the repetition in thought of any particular word chosen at random for the purpose occurs more quickly in those subjects who show strong satiation phenomena on perceptual-type tests, while subjects with weak satiation need more repetitions before the word loses its meaning. In this connection, then, 'loss of meaning' is the mental analogue of inhibition, and the predicted relationship with other inhibition phenomena is demonstrated. It would seem to follow that hysterics, psychopaths, brain-damaged, and extraverted subjects generally should show loss of meaning after fewer repetitions than would dysthymics and introverts; no evidence is available on this point.

It need hardly be said that these arguments are highly speculative. Far more experimental evidence is required before we can with any degree of confidence assess the value of this particular application of the general theory of inhibition. The few results and observations available do not rule out of court the hypotheses suggested; but they cannot be said to lend more than tenuous support either. It is perhaps inevitable that our theory should be weakest and most speculative at the two extremes, as it were: at the physiological end, where molar merges into molecular, and at the gross behavioural end, where psychology merges into sociology. Perhaps the hypotheses put forward in these regions can best be regarded as emissaries sent into strange and alien lands, suggesting links and alliances where previously there was blank suspicion and isolation. To what extent these overtures may be fruitful cannot be decided at this early stage.

There is one further deduction from our general theory, however, for which there appears to be considerable support from a large group of experimental investigations. Reference here is to an extension of our nomological network to the phenomena of social attitudes, their structure and organization. The argument on which this extension is built has been discussed in detail in *The Psychology of Politics* (Eysenck, 1954). It may briefly be stated here as follows: extraverts, as we have seen, are under-socialized, introverts over-socialized. Socialization in our particular cultural pattern stresses the *inhibition of overt aggressive and sexual activities*. We would therefore expect extraverts and introverts respectively to differ with respect to such activities. However, there are considerable difficulties in the way of testing a hypothesis of this kind. Activities such as those mentioned are sometimes illegal and nearly always frowned upon by society; consequently they are often indulged in secretly and therefore not easily investigated. We can overcome this difficulty by studying *attitudes* rather than *actions*. As the author has argued at some length in *The Psychology of Politics*, an attitude has the status of a *habit* in our behaviour system, and as our hypothesis of extraversion-introversion specifically deals with habits, it should be possible to make certain predictions in this field. Indeed, one such prediction follows immediately from what has been stated so far. *Extraverts on the whole should have attitudes favouring the overt expression of aggressive and sexual impulses, whereas introverts should have attitudes strongly supporting those ethical and moral agencies and conceptions which act in such a way as to inhibit overt aggressive and sexual behaviour.* Before turning to the evidence in this very clear-cut point, let us consider a complicating factor in our argument.

The prediction just made was mediated through our notion of *conditioning* leading to socialization. Other attitudes are also mediated, however, in terms of *learning* as defined by Mowrer. This second principle of attitude acquisition would in our particular type of society lead us to an additional prediction. As is well known, our society is divided into social classes which have

217

interests which, to some extent, conflict with each other. Ordinary reward learning would lead us to predict that different social classes would hold social attitudes favourable to *them* and unfavourable to their opponents. It would also seem reasonable to suppose that they would create political parties or other instruments in order to put these policies into action. Under the

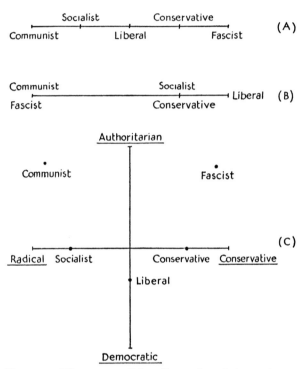

FIG. 50. Three possible dimensional hypotheses regarding the five main political parties in Great Britain.

special circumstances of the present culture pattern in Europe and North America, where the main conflict is between middle-class and working-class groups, we would therefore expect the emergence of sets of radical and conservative attitudes opposed to each other. There is no reason to assume any relationship between the sets of attitudes mediated through *conditioning* and the sets of attitudes mediated through learning, so that our theoretical analysis would lead us to postulate two orthogonal factors. The first of these, mediated through learning, would be the radical-conservative factor; the second mediated through conditioning would be what the author has called the tough-minded (extraverted) versus tender-minded (introverted) factor.

These analyses, *mutatis mutandis*, should also apply to the political organization set up to represent the attitude structure of the voting public. When we look at popular conceptions of the relationships between political parties, we find indeed that there is some evidence for such a belief. On the one hand we have those who postulate a radical-conservative factor, arranging the political parties from Communist, through Socialist to Liberal, and then to Conservative and Fascist. Other people point out certain similarities between Communist and Fascist beliefs and arrange the parties in a rather different sequence, with Communist and Fascist together at one end, Liberals at the other end, and Conservatives and Socialists in between. If we assume that both these conceptions have some truth in them then we come to a two-dimensional picture very much as shown in Fig. 50 which illustrates these three conceptions. The hypothetical authoritarian-democratic factor in the political field corresponds to the tough-minded–tender-minded factor in the social attitude field.

A large number of attitude studies carried out by the writer and others, and summarized in *The Psychology of Politics*, shows that the deductions made in the previous paragraphs are in fact borne out. Fig. 51 illustrates the relationships between a variety of attitudes objectively determined by means of a series of factor analytical studies. It will be seen that we do find a clearly marked radicalism-conservatism factor, but that, in addition to this, we also have our hypothetical tough-minded factor. As postulated, the main characteristic of the tough-minded part of our second factor is the insistence on overt gratification of sexual and aggressive impulses (attitudes favourable to flogging, companionate marriage, the death penalty, easier divorce laws, harsh treatment of criminals, abolition of abortion laws, and capital punishment). The main characteristic of the tender-minded, on the other hand, is an insistence on ethical and religious ideals opposed to those overt gratifications (making birth-control illegal, pacificism, making religious education compulsory, giving up national sovereignty, going back to religion, regarding conscientious objectors as worthwhile people, and so on). These results and many others reviewed in *The Psychology of Politics* leave little doubt about the verification of this particular deduction.

There is also to be found strong verification of our two other hypotheses. There is a highly significant relationship between tough-mindedness and extraversion, and between tender-mindedness and introversion. This relationship also extends in ways which can easily be deduced from our general theory to the value-systems of individuals, as tested by the Allport and

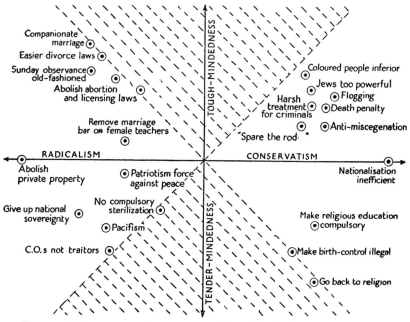

FIG. 51. Diagrammatic representation of relationships between attitudes.

Vernon *Study of Values*. Lastly, the predicted relationship between political party structure and social attitude organization is indeed found to be as postulated, the autocratic parties showing tough-minded attitudes, the democratic parties showing tender-minded attitudes.

This set of studies completes our chain of deductions leading from the physiological notions of an inhibition-excitation balance, through conditioning, individual differences, personality types, and through socialization to the structure of social attitudes and the formation of political parties. The discussion has, perforce, been too brief to allow of digressions which would have filled in the picture in more detail. Thus in our theoretical discussion we made the assumption that social pressure would be equal for different groups, so that their ultimate degree of socialization would be determined exclusively by the excitation-inhibition balance. This is clearly an untenable simplification, and evidence is given in *The Psychology of Politics* to show that social pressure differs from one class to another, and that this amount of pressure is related to the degree of tough-mindedness shown by members of these classes. (Cf. also Oppenheim, 1956.)

However, it cannot be denied that much further evidence is desirable in relation to the precise way in which the socialization process works. It is curious that, with all the emphasis on the importance of child up-bringing, particularly in the early years, which has been so characteristic of psychoanalytic speculation, there has been practically no detailed observation or follow-up work relating behaviour patterns in later life to early methods of training. In the absence of such detailed evidence a direct verification of the Mowrer hypothesis would be extremely difficult to procure, and until such time as evidence of this kind will be available, it must be regarded as the weakest link in our chain of deduction.[1]

In closing this chapter we may fittingly return to the difference in opinion we noted in our second chapter between Mowrer on the one hand and Miller and Dollard on the other. It will be remembered that in their theories of neurosis these writers were in sharp contradiction, Mowrer advocating a theory according to which the Id was too powerful as opposed to the Super-Ego, while Miller and Dollard advocated a theory according to which the Super-Ego was too powerful as opposed to the Id. We can now see that these theories are relevant, not to neurosis, but to extraversion-introversion. What we have called excessive degree of socialization, due to strong conditionability, these writers call Super-Ego; what we have called insufficient degree of socialization, due to weak conditionability, these writers call Id. Mowrer appears to be dealing exclusively with the extraverted symptoms and syndromes, Miller and

---

[1] Readers interested in a review of the evidence may care to consult Mussen and Conger (1956). This book on *Child Development and Personality* is reasonably thorough in its coverage, but somewhat uncritical in its easy acceptance of Freudian dogmas. It should be regarded as a guide to the original sources rather than as an adequate account of facts and theories in this field.

Dollard with the introverted symptoms and syndromes. If there is any truth in our theory, then it will be clear that both sides fail to come to grip with the problem of neurosis, or excessive emotionality, i.e. that which is in common to both hysterics and dysthymics, and deal rather with a continuum which is orthogonal to neuroticism. Thus our theory appears to reconcile the apparently contradictory observations of these men in a larger synthesis. It also succeeds in getting away from the reification inevitable in the use of such concepts as Id and Super-Ego, and it provides a mechanism causally responsible for individual differences in these respects which has a solid experimental foundation and whose laws of functioning are reasonably well known. For all these reasons we venture to offer this theory as not only an alternative to, but as an improvement on, those of Mowrer, Miller and Dollard.

Chapter Seven

DRUGS AND PERSONALITY

MUCH can be said of the relationship between personality study and various fields outside psychology. In order to keep this book within manageable bounds, only one such field has been chosen, namely that of pharmacology, and even as far as that science is concerned, only a brief discussion will be given. Our aim in this chapter will not be that of reviewing the very considerable literature on the psychological effects of drugs, a task adequately performed many times already (Berg, 1949; Darrow, 1929; Gray & Trowbridge, 1942; Meyer, 1922; Poffenberger, 1914, 1916, 1917, 1919; Reifenstein & Davidoff, 1939; Hollingworth, 1912, 1923; Shock, 1939; Spragg, 1941; Boor; 1956); we will be concerned rather with the following points of interaction:

(1) Pharmacological effects are usually studied on a purely empirical level. A certain drug is given to a group of subjects, and various tests, chosen more or less at random, are then applied. Results usually show either an increment or a decrement of performance as compared with other groups who have been given some form of placebo treatment. While such results are obviously of some interest, they do not form part of any kind of theoretical system and do not lead to any sort of rational prediction. Our first task therefore will be to show that by adopting the general system of postulates here developed it becomes possible to rationalize at least a part of this general field; to make predictions going beyond the vague kind of hunch that a person working in this field tends to develop; and to select certain types of tests and experiments in preference to others on a rational, rather than on a chance basis. In part, the solution here

suggested has already been adumbrated by Hull and McDougall. However, we propose to extend the former's postulate system and bring it into closer relationship with a number of investigations not considered at all by him and his followers.

(2) The prime interest of the student of personality in this field is the fact that drugs are among the few influences which can be brought to bear experimentally on human subjects in an endeavour to change their performance and possibly even to shift their position on one of the personality continua. Mescaline and lysurgic acid appear to produce an increase in psychoticism; adrenaline appears to produce an increase in neuroticism. As we shall argue later, the so-called depressant drugs increase central inhibition and produce a shift towards extraverted behaviour patterns. Thus there is a two-way relationship between pharmacology and personality study as envisaged here: psychological theory helps to rationalize the ordering of drugs in terms of their effects, and the administration of drugs helps us to produce an experimental shift to alter a subject's position on various personality continua.

The theory which will be proposed here has certain important similarities to one proposed almost 30 years ago by William McDougall (1929) and, as a comparison of these two theories will be instructive, a brief outline of McDougall's hypothesis may not be out of place. He began by accepting the existence of a continuum or dimension of personality corresponding to Jung's factor of extraversion-introversion: 'I suggest that all personalities can be arranged in a single linear scale according to the degree to which this factor is present in their constitution . . . such a distribution of a temperamental trait is most naturally explained by the influence of some chemical factor generated in the body and exerting a specific influence upon the nervous system in proportion to the quantity that is produced and liberated into the blood stream.' McDougall confessed himself puzzled by the problem of which was the positive and which the negative state. He finally came to a somewhat arbitrary decision: 'In all probability extraversion is the positive state, introversion the negative, that is to say, extreme introversion represents a defect, a minimal quality or minimum rate of secretion of the postulated substance (let us call it X); and extraversion in its various degrees is a consequence of correspondingly large quantities or rapid rates of secretion of X.'

How is this secretion supposed to act? McDougall begins by explaining his theory of introversion: 'The introvert . . . is the man in whom the lower levels of the nervous system are constantly subjected to a high degree of inhibition by the higher cortical activities, and of the lower inhibited functions the most important are the affective or emotional-conative functions of the thalamic region. . . . Thus the introvert, by reason of the predominant activity of his cortex and in virtue of its restraining or inhibitory effect on the outflow of thalamic excitation in its normal or direct channels of emotional expression, is a man in whom thought seems to flourish at the expense of emotion . . . introversion seems then to be the natural consequence of the great development and free activity of the cortex.'

McDougall then goes on to postulate that there is an increase in introversion as children grow up into adults corresponding to the greater functional dominance of the cortex. However, 'Nature has provided an antidote against such increasing and excessive introversion. It has generated in the tissues, or in some tissue unknown, an extraverting hormone, or endocrine substance, the function of which is to prevent, to diminish in some measure this inhibiting, paralysing influence of the cortex upon the more primitive, lower level functions of the nervous system. The man who is constitutionally provided with a large amount of this antidote to cortical inhibition is the extravert.'

We now come to the pharmacological aspect of McDougall's theory. 'How . . . may we conceive the postulated internal secretion X to work upon the brain to maintain various degrees of extraversion, to antagonize and moderate the inhibiting influence of the cortex? I suggest that we may find the clue to a simple, intelligible and adequate hypothesis in consideration of the influence of alcohol upon the brain functions (and of ether and chloroform), and that the phenomena of alcoholic intoxication go very far to justify the hypothesis . . . I have observed in a number of cases that the markedly extraverted personality is very susceptible to the influence of alcohol. A very small dose deprives him of self-restraint and control and brings on the symptoms of intoxication, all of which are essentially expressions of diminished cortical control over the lower brain levels. The introvert, on the other hand, is much more resistant to alcohol. He can take a considerable dose without other effect than that he becomes extraverted. . . . Alcohol, in short, seems to be an extraverting drug pure and simple so far as its influence on the nervous system is concerned.'

McDougall now formally states his hypothesis. 'In order to explain extraversion I make, then, the simple assumption that in the extravert some tissue (or tissues) normally and constantly secretes the extraverting substance X, a substance whose action upon the nervous system is very similar to that of alcohol (ether and chloroform); that is to say, I assume that the extraverting internal secretion X acts directly upon all synapses, raising their resistance to the passage of the nervous current or discharge from neurone to neurone. I make also the highly probable assumption that the synapses of the various levels of the nervous system are in the main solidly and stably organized in proportion to the philogenetic and ontogenetic age of the levels in which they occur. In other words, I assume that the synapses of the high levels are the less solidly organized, have higher resting resistances, and are less stable, more subject to variations of their resistance by a variety of influences, including the chemical ones of strychnine, alcohol, and the postulated substance X.'

Having stated this formal hypothesis, McDougall goes on to explore some of the theoretical connections with abnormal mental states. He argues that extraverts are more prone to hysteria, hypnosis, trances, automatic actions, crystal visions and so on, while introverts are more prone to neurasthenia, schizophrenia and insomnia. All these differences seem to mean the greater liability of the extravert to suffer dissociative effects in the nervous system, whether local, as in local functional paralyses and anasthesias, or general, as in general amnesia, trance, hypnosis and sleep. And this is to be expected; for, just as alcohol is a dissociative drug, which acts first and most intensely upon those most delicately organized synapses that are involved in the latest acquired and highest-level processes of the cortex, subserving self-conscious control and self criticism, and involving the reciprocal play of one cortical system of highest level neurones upon another, so also the extraverting substance X may be supposed to affect most markedly those higher-level synapses, maintaining during waking life an incipient state of dissociation and rendering easier the onset of all more pronounced states of cerebral dissociation, from normal sleep and of alcoholic intoxication to hypnosis and functional paralyses and amnesias. In short, the introvert is liable to disorders of continuing conflict, because conflict cannot readily be obviated by dissociation; while the extravert finds relief from internal conflict through the onset of some complete dissociation between conflicting systems and tendencies.

This, then, is a brief outline of McDougall's hypothesis, which to the writer seems plausible, ingenious and extremely fruitful.[1] It has been almost completely neglected by psychologists and psychiatrists alike for a variety of reasons, some of which may be worth stating. In the first place, McDougall does not provide objective measures of extraversion-introversion which might be used to identify any given person's position on the continuum, and which might be used to measure the shift of that person's position on the continuum subsequent to the administration of the given drug. His argument is confined to observational methods whose unreliability was becoming more and more apparent in the 1930's as a result of psychological investigation. As we shall have occasion to point out later in connection with the methodology of drug research, objective methods are absolutely essential in the testing of a hypothesis such as that advocated by McDougall. Thus the work of Shagass (1954, 1956) is a striking confirmation of McDougall's observation quoted above that 'the markedly extraverted personality is very susceptible to the influence of alcohol', while 'the introvert, on the other hand, is much more resistant to alcohol. He can take a considerable dose without other effect than that he becomes

---

[1] From the point of view of the theory here developed, McDougall's hypothesis is of course superseded by the inhibition theory. It should be noted, however, that with respect to brain-damage McDougall's notion may still be retained as an important adjunct to our own. It will not have escaped the reader that there is a certain contradiction in the development of our theory as far as brain-damage is concerned. An increase in inhibition following cortical insults of any kind accounts well enough for the phenomena of extinction, lowered conditionability, and increased figural after-effects; but how does it make the person affected more extraverted? In terms of our theory, extraversion arises through failure of socialization due to lack of conditionability; but by the time brain-damage occurs socialization has already been accomplished in most cases. Consequently we need another type of mechanism, activated by inhibition but not working through the medium of conditioning, which is responsible for the de-socialization of the brain-damaged person. McDougall's suggestion of impaired control of the higher centres, which presumably in some unspecified way are the substratum of the laboriously acquired socialization products, applies to the effects of depressant drugs like alcohol, but would seem to apply with equal force to brain-damage. A more detailed theory might with advantage be worked out on some such basis; at present there is not sufficient evidence to enable us to say very much more than that this line of argument, though vague, is probably not entirely mistaken.

extraverted.' But this demonstration had to await the elaboration by Shagass of an objective method for measuring the
intoxication threshold, or 'sedation threshold' as he calls it.

The second reason for the failure of McDougall's hypothesis
to be widely accepted lies in the mysterious nature of his substance X. This appears purely *ad hoc*, is not integrated in any
way with the existing body of psychological knowledge, and
does not conform with the rules science lays down for the introduction of hypothetical constructs and intervening variables.
In the third place, McDougall was rather half-hearted in his
specification of the relation between temperament and drugs.
His main interest obviously being in substance X, drugs are only
being introduced into the paper by virtue of the hypothetical
similarity in action between alcohol and X. A last reason may
be found in the general tendency of psychologists at the time
McDougall's article was written to disown higher-order concepts
implying generality in the personality field (such as extraversion-
introversion), and to seek instead for specific stimulus-response
connections. All these reasons working together may explain,
but cannot justify, neglect of McDougall's contribution.

A link between drug action on the one hand and learning
theory on the other (and therefore between learning theory and
personality theory), was adumbrated by Hull (1935) in a pioneer
paper on the influence of caffeine on rote learning. Basing himself on a quotation from C. L. Evans (1930) to the effect that
caffeine had a marked tendency to eliminate internal inhibition,
Hull made certain predictions on the molar effects which should
follow in human rote learning from the administration of this
drug. Thus he argued that if, as Lepley (1934) had shown, the
bowing of the serial learning curve is due to internal inhibition,
then the administration of caffeine, by eliminating such inhibition, would reduce the degree of bowing observed. Working on
only eight subjects, he failed to find the predicted effect, but
found instead that 'the subjects as a group showed a fairly
definite tendency to give more anticipatory reactions after taking caffeine, the mean percentage of increase being 33, with a
probable error of 7, and a satisfactory C.R. of 4.' This effect
can be predicted from the hypothesis that caffeine eliminated internal inhibition; as anticipatory reactions are supposed to be
held in check by these inhibitions, they would therefore be
released by their elimination. However, Hull appears to have

regarded this experiment as a failure, and never returned himself to this vital area.

It is possible to generalize along pharmacological lines the approaches of McDougall and Hull. As is well known, there are two sets of drugs which have antagonistic effects at both the physiological and the psychological level. On the one hand we have the so-called *central nervous system depressants*, such as the anaesthetics, alcohols, hypnotics and sedatives; of these, the best known are probably the alcohols and the barbiturates. On the other hand we have the *central nervous system stimulants*, such as strychnine, picrotoxin and the xanthines; the best known of these is probably caffeine. In addition to these agents, there is a large group of drugs whose effects on central stimulation may be considered as secondary, but important; the best known compounds here included are probably ephedrine, amphetamine and various sympatheticomimetic amines.

Generalizing from McDougall's alcohol and Hull's caffeine to depressants and stimulants generally, we may propose the following postulate: *Depressant drugs increase cortical inhibition, decrease cortical excitation and thereby produce extraverted behaviour patterns. Stimulant drugs decrease cortical inhibition, increase cortical excitation and thereby produce introverted behaviour patterns.* This postulate was informally suggested in a previous paper (Eysenck, 1955) and formally stated two years later (Eysenck, 1957). It should be noted that the terms 'depressant' and 'stimulant' are here used in their pharmacological sense as listed by Goodman and Gilman (1955); it would be valuable to know the chemical and biochemical properties characterizing these drugs and causing the opposing effects, but such knowledge does not appear at present to be available. It should also be noted that in many cases drugs which fall in one or the other of these two groups have side effects which may be so strong as to cancel out the predicted effects; thus many excitant drugs are also sympatheticomimetic. It is important in submitting the postulate to experimental investigation to choose drugs having as few side effects as possible. We shall refer to this problem later on in this chapter.

We may now note some of the ways in which the present theory differs from, and may be said to improve upon, that of McDougall. In the first place, the drug action postulated is stated in terms of two reasonably well-defined groups of drugs whose existence is clearly recognized by pharmacologists and whose contradictory properties are well known. In the second place, the effects postulated can now be deduced directly from a general theory of behaviour. This point can be illustrated by reference to Table XIII, which shows the postulated correspondence between drug effects and the various levels of our behaviour-personality theory. These relationships should be

TABLE XIII

Causal level:	Excitation—Inhibition
Clinical-behavioural level:	Dysthymia—Hysteria
Test level:	Introversion—Extraversion
Drug effect:	Excitant—Depressant

borne in mind during our discussion of the methodology of drug research which forms the next section of this chapter, and which amplifies this point in considerable detail. In the third place, we do not have to rely, as did McDougall, on simple observation, but are enabled to test our deductions with reference to objective laboratory procedures in the fields of learning and conditioning, of perception, and of the work decrement. These are important advantages, as by making predictions more precise and more objective, we also make the theory more incisive, and easier to disprove if in error.

The success or failure of any theory depends essentially upon the ability of that theory to enable investigators to make clear-cut deductions and testable predictions. It is part of the duty of anyone proposing such a theory to indicate the types of prediction which he would regard as crucial to the correctness or incorrectness of his theory. It is this task to which we must now turn.

Roughly speaking, we have open to us three avenues corresponding to the three levels (causal, clinical, and test level) indicated in Table XIII. Thus at the clinical-behavioural level our theory would imply the prediction that *excitant drugs produce dysthymic symptoms and behaviour patterns, and a reduction in hysterical symptoms and behaviour patterns. Conversely, depressant drugs produce an increase in hysterical symptoms and behaviour patterns, and a decrease in dysthymic symptoms and behaviour patterns.* This is probably the least useful type of prediction because of the great observational difficulties which impede objective determination of the predicted results.

At the test level, we would predict that *any test which has been shown to differentiate reliably and validly between introverts and extraverts will, when applied to subjects who have been administered an excitant (or depressant) drug, show shifts in scores in the direction characteristic of greater introversion (or extraversion).* In view of the large number of tests covered by this deduction and the objective nature of the scores obtained, this is a useful and valuable type of prediction. We might add to it, in parentheses, a similar prediction derived from the fact that brain injury appears to have extraverting consequences, namely that *the effects of depressant drugs are similar to those of brain-damage as far as objective psychological tests are concerned. Conversely, the effects of excitant drugs are opposite to those of brain-damage.*

At the third level, and this may be regarded as the most fundamental of all, we are dealing with the hypothetical causal factors underlying both clinical behaviour and test scores. Our predictions here would therefore be in terms of the theory of excitation-inhibition, and can be applied directly to the field of drug studies without necessarily going through the intermediate state of being applied to the dysthymic-hysteric differentiation, or that between extraverts and introverts. (Hull's (1935) prediction, mentioned above, would be of this type.)

While the last type of prediction is the most advanced theoretically, and the most fundamental psychologically, it is also probably the one presenting the greatest difficulties. The theory of excitation and inhibition is nothing like as rigorous, definite and clear cut as one would like it to be, and the failure of an experiment to satisfy the drug postulate may be due to a mistaken application of the general behaviour theory rather than to an error in the drug postulate itself. This of course should not deter the investigator from making predictions of this kind and testing them regardless of the outcome. The results would almost certainly be of considerable interest from the point of view of learning theory, as well as from that of the study of drug effects. Indeed, one of the most important outcomes of the study of drug effects might be a clarification of certain puzzling features in learning theory, and the growth of a methodology for verifying or disproving certain assumptions of learning theory.

Nevertheless, from the point of view of making predictions which are crucial for our postulate, it would seem advisable to choose tests whose use can be justified at all three levels, i.e. tests whose theoretical derivation at the causal level is clear cut, which are known to differentiate between dysthymics and hysterics, which are known to distinguish between normal introverts and normal extraverts, and which are known to be affected by brain-damage in a certain manner. An example of such a procedure is that of conditioning. Ease of conditioning is clearly determined by the growth of excitatory potential and the relative absence of inhibitory potential, while difficulty in the forming of conditioned reflexes is clearly related to the presence of strong inhibitory potential and the relative weakness of excitatory potential. Thus, on the causal level conditioning techniques present as clear cut a production as we can make.

At the other two levels, work described in a previous chapter has clearly shown that eyeblink and PGR conditioning differentiate at a very high level of reliability and validity between hysterics and dysthymics, and between extraverts and introverts. Similarly, there is in the literature a good deal of evidence to the effect that brain operations tend to have an inhibitory effect on conditioning. All in all, then, the results from those various sources indicate that if our postulate is correct, *depressant drugs should produce a decrease in the rate of conditioning, while excitant drugs should produce an increase in the rate of conditioning.*

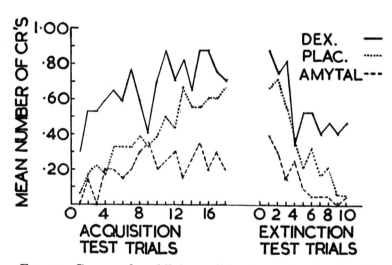

FIG. 52. Course of eyeblink conditioning and extinction in three groups of subjects given different drugs.

232

The evidence regarding this prediction has been reviewed by Franks and Trouton (1957; cf. also Franks & Laverty, 1955; and Laverty & Franks, 1956), who have also performed an experiment using eyeblink conditioning as the dependent variable. By random allocation of subjects they make up three groups, one of which, the control group, received a placebo, while the other two received sodium amytal and dexedrine respectively. The results were very definite and in conformity with our hypothesis as will be seen from Fig. 52. The group

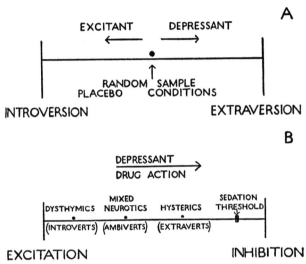

FIG. 53. Research designs for two methods of investigating drug action.

which had been administered the sodium amytal conditioned least well, the group which had been administered the dexedrine conditioned best of all, while the group which had been administered the placebo was intermediate. This experiment may serve as an example of the type of prediction which can be made with the greatest confidence from our postulate.

The research design used by Franks and Trouton has been illustrated in Fig. 53a. It will be seen that it does not depend in any way on the assessment of the personality of the subjects prior to the experiment. Subjects are randomly allocated to control and experimental groups, and what is studied is the *general* effect of the drugs under investigation on what might be called the *standard subject*. This paradigm is of course capable of certain improvements. Thus the same group of persons might be tested three times under placebo, depressant and excitant drug conditions, so that each subject would constitute his own control. This is possible in perceptual experiments, but not in conditioning and learning experiments where nearly all the improvement in performance takes place during the first session. Other improvements in the experimental design contingent upon the one suggested above might include the assessment of the standing of the subjects on the extraversion-introversion continuum, and the calculation of possible interaction effects in an analysis of variance design. However, these refinements do not in any way affect the general principle of this design, which is probably the most widely used of all.

A rather different design is illustrated in Fig. 53b. This design makes use of the known position of groups of subjects such as dysthymics and hysterics on the introversion-extraversion continuum, and thus explicitly contravenes the random sampling technique of design A. This design harks back to McDougall's observation that extraverts need less alcohol to reach a point of intoxication than introverts, who with the same amount of alcohol simply become more extraverted. Such a research design requires an objective *terminus ad quem*, i.e. the terminus of an 'intoxication threshold' which would enable us to ascertain the amount of alcohol required by different groups of subjects to reach the same level of cortical inhibition as defined by this threshold.

The only example of the use of such a technique which the writer has been able to find is a study by Shagass (1954, 1955, 1956) using what he calls the 'sedation threshold' of sodium amytal. The sedation threshold is an objective pharmacological determination, which depends on EEG and speech changes produced by intravenously given amobarbital (amytal) sodium. 'Amobarbital sodium is given intravenously at the rate of 0·5 mg./kg. of body weight every 40 seconds. The patient is tested for slurred speech, and the injection is continued at least 80 seconds after slurred speech is noted. Continuous EEG's are recorded from transverse frontal and sagittal frontocentral placements.' Fig. 54 shows that sodium amytal produces a rather striking increase of fast frequency (15–30 cps. activity). The amplitude of this fast frequency is taken by Shagass as a response to the drug and the dosage-response curve plotted. 'The typical curve has a sigmoid shape and contains a point of inflexion, preceding which there is a sudden increase in the amplitude of the fast activity, and following which the curve tends to plateau. This inflexion point generally occurs within 40 sec. (0·5 mg./kg.) of the time when slurred speech is first noted, and the slur and inflexion point are used together as indicators of the threshold. The threshold is the amount of sodium amytal, in mg./kg., required to produce an inflexion point in the 15–30 c/sec. amplitude curve, which occurs within

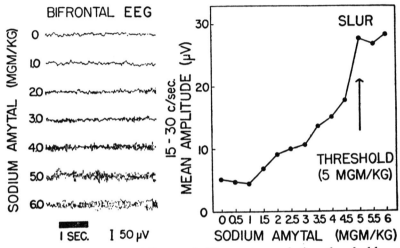

FIG. 54. Bifrontal EEG records illustrating sedation threshold.

80 sec. (1 mg./kg.) of the time when the slur is noted. The slur localizes the threshold roughly, the EEG inflexion point does it more precisely. . . . The measurement is highly reliable; its probable error is not greater than 0·5 mg./kg. of body weight. Age, sex, and previous intake of sedatives in usual psychiatric dosage have not been found to influence the threshold.'[1]

According to the theory outlined in this chapter (which was developed before Shagass's work was known to the writer), we should be able to make a very definite prediction. Sodium amytal, being a depressant drug, would be postulated to

[1] It should be noted that it has been our own experience, as well as that of other workers, that the determination of the sedation threshold is more difficult and less objective than is indicated in Shagass's papers. This difficulty may be due to lack of experience, but it appears to be fairly universal. Possibly not all the conditions requisite for duplication are stated sufficiently explicitly by Shagass.

increase inhibition. An extravert, whose cortex, according to our theory, is already in a relatively inhibited state, should require comparatively little sodium amytal before reaching the critical sedation point; such a person should have a low sedation threshold. The introvert, on the other hand, whose cortex is in a state of considerable excitation and low inhibition, would require a considerable amount of sodium amytal before reaching the critical sedation point; he would be predicted to have a high sedation threshold. If we express this general hypothesis in

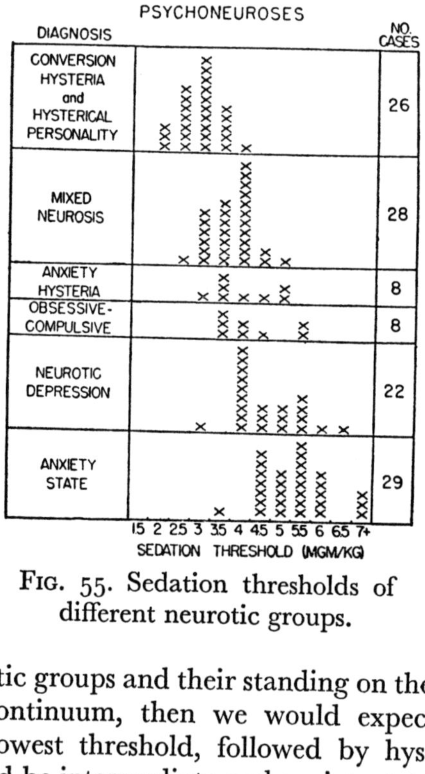

FIG. 55. Sedation thresholds of different neurotic groups.

terms of neurotic groups and their standing on the extraversion-introversion continuum, then we would expect psychopaths to have the lowest threshold, followed by hysterics. Mixed neurotics would be intermediate and anxiety states, obsessionals and reactive depressives would have high sedation thresholds. An experiment along these lines was carried out by Shagass; his results are given in Figs. 55 and 56. It will be seen that these results bear out our prediction in every detail.

This design too, of course, is capable of certain interesting modifications. If something corresponding to the sedation or intoxication threshold could be found at the introverted end of

236

the continuum, we would predict lower thresholds for dysthymics than for hysterics, and quite generally a reversal of the relations found on Shagass's research. Thus the same groups of patients at different times might be given different and opposing drugs as well as placebos. However, such developments depend on the discovery of such threshold effects for excitation drugs, which might possibly be looked for in EEG patterns corresponding to wakefulness as opposed to sleep.

Having given examples of the two main methods of research in this field, we must now turn to a survey of some of the results

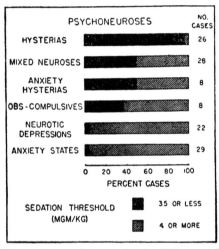

FIG. 56. Proportions of neurotics in different diagnostic groups with high and low sedation threshold.

of work on this topic in relation to our theory. We have argued previously that subjective feelings of boredom, sleepiness, and so forth are the introspective concomitants of inhibition. In terms of our postulate, we would expect such subjective feelings to decrease after the administration of stimulants and to increase after administration of depressants. This deduction has been verified by several writers, in particular Barmack (1938, 1939, 1940). He summarizes his work by saying: 'The interpretation is favoured that the effect of the benzedrine . . . is principally on the inclination rather than on the ability to do continuous repetitive work.' This conclusion is in line with the Hullian notion of I_R as a drive and consequently the growth of a negative drive or 'inclination', as Barmack puts it.

In view of what is known about the growth of I_R and $_SI_R$, we would expect stimulants to be effective after some time rather than immediately. This follows from the simple consideration that their ability to decrease inhibition is dependent on the previous growth of inhibition; during early stages of practice little inhibition has been developed and the drug therefore cannot show any considerable effectiveness in overcoming inhibition. Again, Barmack has shown that this deduction is verified. Here is a typical quotation from him, summing up his results on continuous adding: 'The differences in rate of work obtained for the two conditions (placebo versus drug) were negligible at the beginning, and most striking at the end of the work period.'

Reactive inhibition should be diminished by stimulant drugs according to our postulate, and Tolman (1917) has, in fact, shown in an early experiment that 'We . . . find greater inhibition for the days without caffeine than for the days with caffeine.' Similarly we would expect conditioned reactions to be augmented, inhibitory processes decreased (Wentinck, 1938; Wolff & Gantt, 1935), experimental extinction to be diminished (Grether, 1935), and the rate of responding in the Skinner Box to be increased during extinction (Heron & Skinner, 1937). All these effects have, in fact, been observed. Equally we would expect the latent period of the delayed conditioning reflex to be shortened, an expectation shown to be correct in a study by Switzer (1935).

Another prediction which can be made directly from our postulate is the following: If learning takes place when the subject is receiving treatment by a depressant drug he should produce higher reminiscence scores than subjects subjected to placebo treatment. Subjects receiving a stimulant drug should show the least amount of reminiscence. (Testing for reminiscence would of course have to be carried out after the effect of the drug had worn off. This is necessary because of the distinction between the formation of an S–R band and its elicitation. Cf. Settlage (1936) for an experimental study emphasizing this point.) It might also be predicted that the effects of drugs during a retention interval would be for the depressant drugs to improve retention (by inhibiting effects of external stimuli acting as retroactive inhibitors for the learned material) and for stimulating drugs to have the opposite effect. Both these predicted effects of depressant drugs have been demonstrated in a study by

Steinberg and Summerfield (1955) in which nitrous oxide was used. Three matched groups were given eleven trials on a non-sense-syllable learning task, followed by an interval of 12·5 minutes, after which learning was continued for 40 trials. Group 1 received air throughout; Group 2 received air during the learning trials and the drug during the interval; and Group 3 received the drug during the original learning and during the interval, but air during the last learning period. Results showed significant differences in the amount of reminiscence. Group 1 showed a performance *decrease* during the interval, Group 2 showed no change, and Group 3 showed an *increase* during the interval (positive reminiscence effect).

Equally deducible from our general theory are findings such as that stimulants decrease reaction times (Cheney, 1935, 1936; Gilliland & Nelson, 1939), improve performance on psycho-motor and intellectual tasks (Barmack, 1940; Carl & Turner, 1939, 1940; Kleemeier, 1947; Seashore & Joy, 1953; Thornton *et al.*, 1939), increase tapping rate (Simonson & Enzer, 1941), inhibit ergographic fatigue (Alles & Feiger, 1942; Cuthbertson & Knox, 1947; Seashore & Joy, 1953), and inhibit the work decrement (Hauty & Payne, 1955; Payne & Hauty, 1953, 1954, 1955), while depressant drugs have the opposite effect in each case (Steinberg, 1954; Strongin & Windsor, 1935; Seward & Seward, 1936; Mead, 1939; Marx, 1950; Laverty & Franks, 1956; Seitz & Barmack, 1940; Vanner, 1933; Waldfogel *et al.*, 1950). Particularly impressive in this connection is the very extensive and rigorous work done by Payne and Hauty (1954, 1955) on the work decrement, which methodologically is distinctly superior to most of the other studies mentioned in this section.

It is unfortunate that work in the perceptual field has been very much less extensive. Of outstanding interest is a paper by Trent (1947) showing that 'visual contour clarity is found to be enhanced by nembutal narcosis', suggesting that the effect might be produced through inhibition of lateral summation in the retina.

There are also a few interesting studies on flicker fusion (Robach *et al.*, 1952; cf. reviews by Landis, 1953, 1954), the results of which are conflicting; this is not to be wondered at in view of the great complexity of the phenomenon and the frequent failure to control relevant variables. It would be of very great interest to study the influence of drugs on satiation, where the prediction would be that *depressant drugs would increase satiation while stimulant drugs would have the opposite effect.* Experiments on spatial perceptual inhibition under stimulant and depressant drugs would also appear to be indicated as of great theoretical interest, the prediction being, of course, that depressant drugs would increase and stimulant drugs decrease inhibition effects. Bender (1952, p. 53) has presented some evidence to the effect that alcohol and sodium amytal increase extinction effects.

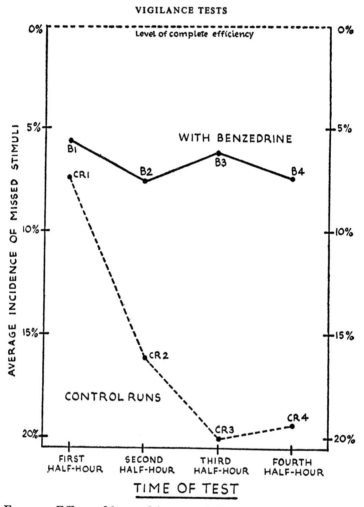

FIG. 57. Effect of benzedrine on vigilance test performance.

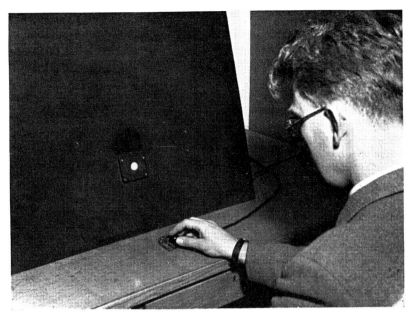

20. Variable stimulus intensity reaction time experiment.

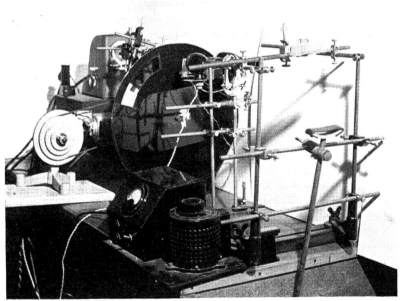

21. 'Bidwell's Ghost': apparatus as seen from subject's side. Chin rest in front, with red light intensity adjustment knob on left. Note viewing tube just visible between two lamps trained on rotating disc (*centre*).

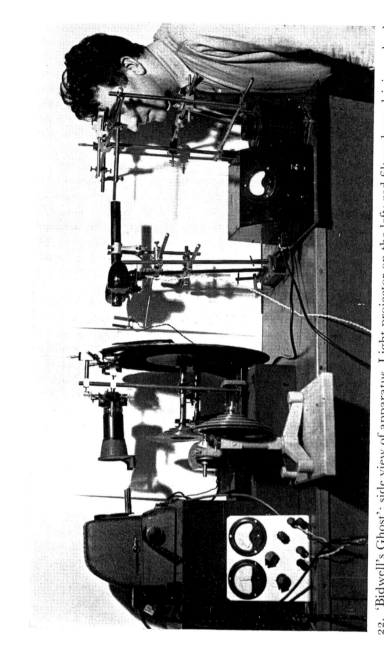

22. 'Bidwell's Ghost': side view of apparatus. Light projector on the left; red filter above driving wheel for rotating disc.

Mackworth (1948) has shown, in some very impressive experiments, how inhibition effects in vigilance experiments can be overcome by the administration of benzedrine. The test used was of the clock-watching type described in an earlier chapter, where occasional changes in the speed with which the hand moves round the clock have to be spotted; the score is the number of such changes missed in the course of four successive half-hour periods. Fig. 57 shows the decrease in accuracy which is the index of inhibition in this experiment, giving a decline from 5 per cent errors in the first period to 20 per cent errors in the other three periods. The benzedrine groups show no such decline.

In addition to the quotation of these few selected references from the literature, it may be worth while to mention results from a few experiments carried out in our own laboratory in an effect to find evidence regarding the theory here outlined. We have already mentioned the Franks's studies in conditioning. The other experiments to be mentioned deal respectively with the after-effects of the Archimedes spiral, with the work decrement, and with Bidwell's ghost, the latter being a rather obscure after-image effect first observed by Bidwell (1897) and named after him. (For reports, cf. Eysenck & Holland, 1957; Eysenck, Trouton & Casey, 1957; Eysenck & Aiba, 1957.)

The apparatus used for the Archimedes spiral experiment is illustrated in Plates 6 and 7, and the theory underlying this phenomenon has been discussed in a previous chapter. It follows directly from our hypothesis that *stimulant drugs should prolong the after-effect*, and that *depressant drugs should shorten it*. Six subjects were used, each of whom was subjected in counterbalanced order to the three treatment conditions, i.e. placebo, sodium amytal and dexedrine. The spiral was rotated for one minute, and the length of the after-effect measured with a stopwatch. The spiral was rotated clockwise and also counterclockwise, and four readings were obtained in each condition.

Analysis of variance revealed highly significant F ratios for 'people', 'drugs' and 'replications'. The last-mentioned simply indicates a tendency for later repetitions of the experiment to give shorter after-effects, a tendency not inexplicable in terms of accumulating inhibition. The existence of highly significant differences between people, i.e. subjects, is not unexpected in view of the large individual differences observable on this test.

The significance of the 'drug' variable at the $p = \cdot 001$ level supports the main hypothesis the experiment was designed to test. Amytal, as predicted, shortens the after-effect, while dexedrine lengthens it. (The interactions in the analysis were insignificant, thus suggesting that the drugs may act in a uniform manner on different subjects.)

The work decrement experiment makes use of the pursuit rotor illustrated in Plates 7 and 8 and the experimental arrangement already discussed in relation to our experiments on reminiscence (p. 126). In other words, five minutes of continuous work are followed by 10 minutes of rest, another 5 minutes of work, another 10 minutes of rest, and a final 5 minutes of work. Four groups of subjects were used, receiving respectively placebos, sodium amytal, and 'long dexedrine' (drug administered at least 250 minutes before testing) and 'short dexedrine' (drug administered approximately 75 minutes before the test). The prediction was that dexedrine would facilitate work and delay the occurrence of work decrement, while amytal would favour the occurrence of work decrement and thus depress the work curve. The results are shown in Fig. 58, and it will be seen

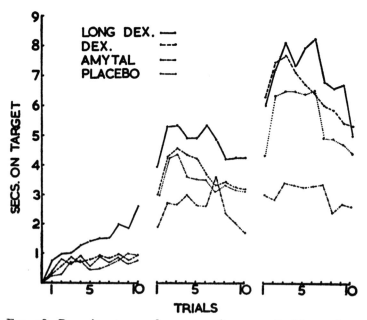

Fig. 58. Pursuit rotor performance of groups of subjects given different drugs.

242

that the predictions are borne out. Statistical analysis shows that the performance of the groups is significantly differentiated at an acceptable level.

The third phenomenon investigated is an objective after-image determination first introduced by Bidwell (1897). If a brief stimulation of the eye with red light is followed by a prolonged stimulation with white light, then what is seen is not a red flash but a green one. This vision of the after-image without awareness of the original stimulus is a somewhat ghost-like, insubstantial phenomenon, and hence the experiment has become known as Bidwell's ghost. The experimental arrangement used by Eysenck and Aiba (1957) is shown in Plates 21 and 22. The light-source on the left throws a shaft of white light through a red filter into a viewing tube on the right; the subject holds one eye close to the other end of the viewing tube. The beam of light is interrupted by a rotating disc, into which a small sector has been cut; this sector allows a red beam to pass for a period of 20 m.sec. before it is interrupted by the solid disc. The red beam is followed by a piece of white paper pasted on to the disc on the side of the subject, and illuminated by a variable light-source. (Duration of exposure of the white stimulus was 125 m.sec.) Starting with a very bright red, the subject's task is to reduce the intensity of the stimulus until he sees only green and no red at all. Six subjects participated, each serving as his own control under placebo, amytal, and dexedrine conditions.

Before discussing the predictions made from our theory, we must find a theoretical basis for the phenomenon under discussion. Such a basis may be postulated by reference to Granit's pre-excitatory inhibition, already discussed in an earlier chapter, and the use made of this concept in accounting for flicker fusion phenomena. (It is noteworthy that Lehman (1950) reports correlations between Bidwell's phenomenon and the CFF threshold which appear to link together individual differences in these experiments.) Briefly, the postulated chain of events is this. The brief red stimulus sets up two chains of events. One of these is photochemical, the other neural. Before the neural message reaches the cortex and is transformed into a red sensation, the white light is exposed and sets up pre-excitatory inhibition which destroys the neural effects of the red stimulus. Thus no red is seen, provided its brightness has not been too strong for

THE DYNAMICS OF ANXIETY AND HYSTERIA

the inhibitory impulse to overcome. At the same time that the red stimulation ceases, the photochemical activity is reversed, and produces the green after-image. This image is now seen simultaneously with the direct sensation from the white stimulation, which thus produces a slight loss in saturation in the after-image. If dexedrine reduces the inhibitory effects postulated while amytal raises them, then we would expect the former to have the effect of lowering the threshold of the original red stimulus, while amytal would raise it. The predicted differences were in fact observed, all differences being significant at the ·o1 level or better, and the placebo group being intermediate between the two drug groups. (Analysis showed differences between days and between people to have been highly significant as well, as might have been expected. These results are not relevant to our theory, however.)

One last experiment may be worthy of mention. McDougall in his theory lays stress on reversible perspective measures as good indicators of extraversion-introversion, and an experiment was therefore carried out in an attempt to trace the influence of dexedrine and amytal on the rate of fluctuation of the Necker Cube, shown in a viewing box. The results of the experiment, which was arranged in a similar manner to those discussed above, were negative, in that analysis of variance failed to disclose any significant differences between the placebo, amytal, and dexedrine groups (Eysenck & Holland, 1957). While the number of subjects involved is not large (N = 6), this number has sufficed in the spiral and after-image studies to produce highly significant results, and in any case McDougall's own studies usually employed even smaller numbers.

In addition to these perceptual experiments, a repetition of Hull's experiment on nonsense-syllable learning was carried out by Willett (1957) with certain relevant and important modifications. Using the same four groups of subjects described in our discussion of the work decrement experiment on the pursuit rotor (placebo, amytal, long dexedrine, and short dexedrine), these writers used the Maudsley Nonsense Syllable Apparatus illustrated in Plates 24 and 25 to present, at a rate of presentation of two seconds each, a series of twelve carefully selected nonsense syllables of roughly equal associative power. Presentations of the series were separated by pauses of six seconds, and learning by anticipation was used until one complete correct reproduction had been achieved. The predictions made follow naturally from our theory, and are as follows:

(1) The number of repetitions needed to reach the criterion of learning is increased by sodium amytal and decreased by dexedrine;
(2) The mean number of anticipatory errors is increased by dexedrine and decreased by sodium amytal.
(3) The bowing of the curve indicative of the serial learning position effect is greater after sodium amytal and less after dexedrine.

TABLE XIV

Number of Trials to Learn List of 12 Nonsense Syllables to Criterion

Group A (Amytal):	40.68 ± 12.05
Group B (Placebo):	$37 \cdot 21 \pm 14 \cdot 08$
Group C (Dexedrine, short):	$34 \cdot 00 \pm 14 \cdot 83$
Group D (Dexedrine, long):	$34 \cdot 47 \pm 17 \cdot 29$

$$F = 0 \cdot 77$$

Results relevant to the first of these predictions are given in Table XIV; it will be seen that the differences between the groups are insignificant, but that the order of groups is as predicted. Results relevant to the second prediction are given in Table XV; it will be seen that long dexedrine, placebo, and sodium amytal give results as predicted, but that the short dexedrine group is out of line. As in our other experiments we had also found this group to behave less clearly according to prediction, the possibility cannot be ruled out that a lengthy period has to elapse before dexedrine becomes fully effective. Results relevant to our third prediction are shown in Fig. 59, where the twelve positions of the nonsense syllables are plotted on the abscissa and the percentage number of errors for each position on the ordinate. The expected greater 'bowing' of the curve for the amytal group, and the expected lesser 'bowing' of the curve for the dexedrine groups, are not to be found in fact; our data are as negative as were Hull's. This failure may mean one of three things:

(1) The drug postulate is in error.
(2) The Lepley theory, according to which the bowing of the serial position curve is due to inhibition, is in error.

(3) Drug effects are too slight to give demonstrable results in this situation.

The first alternative does not seem a likely one in view of the many deductions from this theory which have been verified; choice between the other two hypotheses is at present impossible.

TABLE XV

Mean Number of Anticipatory Errors as Per Cent of Mean Trial Number

	%
Group A (Amytal)	38·99
Group B (Placebo)	41·31
Group C (Dexedrine, short)	36·08
Group D (Dexedrine, long)	48·13

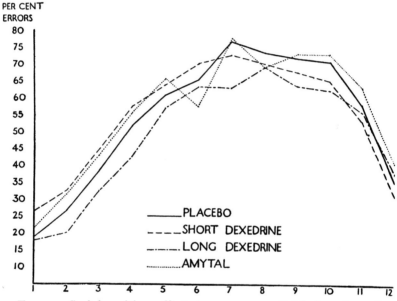

FIG. 59. Serial position effects in nonsense-syllable learning of groups of subjects given different drugs.

These experiments on the whole support the general hypothesis put forward at the beginning of this chapter. The practical usefulness of the successful elaboration of a theory of drug action on personality will be too obvious to require any further comment. The writer would like to stress, however, another point, namely the reciprocal interaction between a theory like that outlined here and general behaviour theory. It is customary in the work of Hull, Pavlov, Spence, and their followers to attribute certain psychological effects to hypothetical constructs and intervening variables like excitation or inhibition, without proving that the inhibition responsible for, say, reminiscence effects is the same inhibition which is responsible for, say, serial learning position effects. While it is very likely that phenomena which obey the same laws do, in fact, depend upon the same hypothetical constructs, a more formal demonstration or proof would seem to be required. Such a proof, in the writer's opinion, can be furnished most easily by reference to the field of individual differences and drug effects.

This general view can perhaps be illustrated best by reference to a hypothetical example. Let us suppose that two experimental phenomena, A and B, are supposed to be produced by the mechanism of inhibition. One method of proving that this was so would be to demonstrate on the physiological-neurological level that the underlying processes in the central nervous system were identical. Such direct proof would of course be the most satisfactory method of dealing with this problem but unfortunately the possibility of such a demonstration is extremely remote at the present time. Consequently we must look for some other method of proof.

To aid us, we have two postulates, which include the factor of inhibition in a manner experimentally independent of phenomena A and B. We have, first of all, the temperamental postulate stating that inhibition is stronger in extraverts than in introverts, and we have the drug postulate stating that depressant drugs increase inhibition whereas excitant drugs decrease inhibition. Proof of these two postulates lies in tying them up with phenomena C, D, E . . . N, which form part of the general inhibition theory. We can now apply these postulates to phenomena A and B and state that if these *are* phenomena produced by the general factor of inhibition, then (a) both A and B should be more pronounced in extraverts than in introverts; (b) both A and B should be more pronounced after the administration of a depressant drug than after the administration of a placebo; and (c) both A and B should be weakened after the administration of an excitant drug as compared with the administration of a placebo. These are testable predictions which enable us to answer our original question regarding the status of phenomena A and B in learning theory, and they at the same time give us information regarding the status of phenomena A and B within personality theory, and within the theory of drug effects. Thus, this mutual interweaving of data from different and hitherto largely isolated fields within the general field of psychology constitutes the main claim of the temperamental and drug postulates to the attention of psychologists and psychiatrists interested in fundamental theory and in the integration of the biological sciences concerned with the study of human behaviour.

These mutual interactions may also be used to solve certain problems in the pharmacological field. Thus it is often found that drugs have very diverse effects on people, so that one and the same dose of a drug given to two people may produce an apparently strong effect in the one and almost no effect in the other. Altogether it has been found impossible to rationalize the amount of drug which ought to be given in order to produce similar results. Pharmacologists of course have worked out certain rules. There is, for instance, the theory of what is called the 'therapeutic ratio', which is obtained by dividing the lethal dose by the therapeutic dose. Then there are such rules as those of Clark, Young and Cowling, relating to age, and the various rules relating dosage to body weight. In practice these rules appear to have very little value, particularly where stimulant and depressant drugs are concerned.

The reason for this follows directly from our postulated system. It appears obvious that in terms of that system, the most important variable in predicting the effects of the drug, and in prescribing the particular dosage required for a specific purpose, would be the excitation-inhibition ratio obtaining within the particular person concerned. This ratio would not be likely to be very highly correlated with weight or any of the obvious surface characteristics which are taken into account by pharmacologists at present. Thus, to provide a given effect, such as the reaching of the sodium amytal sedation threshold, the dosage required is clearly related to the position of the subject on the extraversion-introversion continuum. That position, as Shagass's results show, correlates far more highly with the dose needed than do any of the variables at present used by pharmacologists to assess the amount of drug required. It is likely that we can explain in a similar way the differential effects of various doses of alcohol. It is also likely that the same rule would apply in the opposite direction, such that introverts would require relatively little dexedrine or caffeine to reach a level of excitation (sleeplessness?) which could only be reached by extraverts after a considerably larger dose of these drugs had been administered.

It will be seen, then, that the theory here proposed makes possible the beginnings of a rational solution to a number of problems in drug administration. While the theory is not in any sense quantitative as yet, there is no reason to expect that if our hypotheses have been at all along the right lines, such quantification should prove difficult or impossible. In the writer's view, the next point of advance in the study of the relationship between drugs and personality will be that of developing truly quantitative relationships on the rational basis provided.

Chapter Eight

PSYCHOLOGICAL THEORY AND
PSYCHIATRIC PRACTICE

W E have proposed in the preceding chapters a theory of personality which claims to account for a large number of observational and experimental facts by reference to certain general laws which have received much support in the work of modern learning theorists. In this chapter an attempt will be made to do two things. In the first place, an evaluation will be presented of the strengths and weaknesses of the theory proposed, and an indication given of the precise place which this theory, in the writer's opinion, holds within the framework of general psychology. In the second place, the relationship will be discussed between psychology and psychiatry, or more particularly between psychological theory and psychiatric practice, in so far as it is affected by the results of our work. It will be seen that the implications are quite drastic, and that considerable changes in the present relationship are necessary if psychology is to make its maximum contribution to the alleviation of psychiatric suffering.

In assessing the theory here presented, it is important to be clear about the meaning and implications of the term 'theory'. There are, by and large, three meanings of this term. According to the first of these, a theory is a quantified system of postulates and deductions linking together a very large body of experimentally ascertained facts, and pointing forward to an even larger body of experiments the results of which can be predicted in terms of the theory in a precise and quantitative fashion. No such theory is at present possible in psychology, and there is no pretence that anything of the kind is presented here. Hull in his writings sometimes gives the impression that he conceived of his system as approximating such a quantitative theory, but it is only necessary to recall the extremely arbitrary way in which unknown constants are introduced into equations, or invented to make the data fit the equations, to see that very little in the way of true quantification has in fact been achieved. Koch's (1954) critique has done valuable service in drawing attention to this fact, and indeed Hull's later writings suggest that he was fully conscious of these defects himself. The theory here presented, being in essence an application of Pavlovian and Hullian principles to certain areas of normal and abnormal personality function, cannot be regarded as being any more quantitative than the principles themselves which are being applied, although it is hoped that it has been possible to avoid certain inaccuracies, factual errors, and inconsistencies apparent in the original systems.

In another meaning of the term, theory refers to a vague, speculative system, all-embracing in its implications, and capable of 'explaining' everything after a fashion, but incapable of predicting anything. Various systems of 'dynamic' psychology share these characteristics (Eysenck, 1954); the writer hopes that the present monograph will not be considered to fall into this category.

According to the third meaning of the term 'theory' we may deal with a qualitative system of postulates derived in a non-rigorous way from previous experiments and generalizations, and giving rise to qualitative predictions and deductions in a more or less rigorous fashion. The purpose of such a system is as follows: In the first place, it may be regarded as a first feeble attempt to achieve the aims of a properly quantified and rigorous system. In the second place, it may serve to bring together, in one set of generalizations, large numbers of more or less certainly established facts. In the third place, such a system may give rise to predictions whose main interest will be not only the verification of the system they make possible, but also the fact that they point to areas of investigation which might otherwise have been overlooked. The system here suggested is of this mongrel type. In some parts of it predictions are quite definite and verification has been forthcoming. In other areas predictions are much less rigorous and verification is either partially or quite non-existent. In some fields quantification, if only of an elementary kind, is already a definite prospect, if not an accomplishment; in others, no feasible method has even been suggested for achieving quantification. Of the defects inevitable in such a system the writer is only too aware. It may perhaps be said in extenuation, that anyone familiar with the present state of psychology would not reasonably expect more.

The critical reader of the preceding chapters will have noticed that predictions based on our typological postulate are less clear-cut and precise than one might have wished, not always because of any lack of precision of the postulate itself, but because of the lack of precision found on the side of experimental definition of such variables as reminiscence, figural after-effect, and so forth. The writer has given a detailed account of some of the difficulties which arise in deriving measures of individual differences from work on such phenomena as reminiscence, as reported in the literature (Eysenck, 1956). It is usually not at all clear how precisely the phenomenon in question should be quantified, and even when additional experimental studies solve this question in at least a preliminary fashion, it is often found that the reliability of the measures used is not very high. In other words, while the theory can identify the phenomena for which predictions can be made, with some degree of confidence, the actual testing of the predictions is involved in considerable difficulty because of the failure of experimental psychologists to have evinced any interest in individual differences, or their measurement, as far as the phenomenon in question is concerned. In view of the fact that in very many experiments the variance contributed by individual differences is considerably in excess of that contributed by the experimental variables under investigation, such a disregard of personality effects on the part of psychologists is difficult to understand. When it is realized that interaction effects with personality are also frequently significant, this disregard becomes quite incomprehensible.

Even when a method of measurement has been worked out, however, prediction may not always be easy. As an example of the unexpected complexities encountered, we may take the prediction that extraverts will show greater reminiscence effects on the pursuit rotor, because of the greater accumulation of reactive inhibition in that group. Inhibition produces reminiscence, true, but it also produces other predictable phenomena which counteract the production of reminiscence. Thus when reactive inhibition reaches a sufficiently high level to induce involuntary rest pauses, extraverts tend to turn round and talk to the experimenter, or in other ways dissipate their too-high inhibitory potential. Once dissipated, the inhibitory potential is then no longer available to produce reminiscence effects, so that the predicted effect might not be found due to its place having been taken by a different inhibition-produced effect. Instructions unfortunately are not always successful in preventing extraverts from acting in this fashion, and in any case the precise method of 'disinhibition' adopted may not always be so obvious —some subjects dreamily close their eyes, or cease to focus properly, or start daydreaming. Thus an introvert who grimly follows instructions may show greater reminiscence than an extravert who dissipates inhibition by disobeying instructions; yet this apparent reversal of prediction may in fact be due to behaviour patterns actually explicable in terms of the theory. In a very similar manner, extraverts in satiation experiments frequently fail to fixate the inspection figure properly, possibly because such fixation is made more difficult for them by the postulated greater accretion of inhibition. But this inhibition-induced failure to fixate prevents the inhibition-induced satiation effects from showing, thus again apparently infirming the prediction.

Such extraneous inhibition-induced phenomena do not always or necessarily work against the theory to be tested; equally frequently they may work in the same direction. Thus the prediction that the after-effects of the Archimedes spiral would last less long in brain-damaged subjects than in normals may have been verified in part because brain-damaged patients are liable to cease fixating the spiral more frequently than do normals, possibly because of inhibition induced by constant fixation. Such features of the experimental situation are difficult to control, and equally difficult to measure; nor are they always easy to predict or to detect. Great care must be taken in testing predictions from the theory to exclude as far as possible attentuating or reinforcing behaviour patterns which, while in accord with the theory, are not in fact used to index the phenomenon which is being measured. It is unlikely that we have always succeeded in the experiments reported in this book in overcoming this difficulty.

Another complexity which arises is due to quite definite

ambiguities in the inhibition-satiation theory itself. Two examples will be given. The first relates to the build-up of inhibition in the reminiscence situation. Introverts and extraverts may differ in the rate of build-up of inhibition, or in the asymptote which inhibition approaches before causing voluntary rest pauses, or in the rate of dissipation of inhibition, or in any combination of these three features. The Hullian theory is not specific on this point, and consequently any rigorous deduction or test is impossible. Subsidiary hypotheses become necessary, such as those advanced by Kimble, and the success or failure of the prediction becomes dependent, in part at least, on the proper selection of such subsidiary hypotheses.[1] Again, therefore, the adequate testing of our typological postulate is made difficult because of deficiencies on the side of learning theory.

Our second example relates to the build-up of satiation in the figural after-effect situation. Our prediction was that satiation would build up faster in extraverts, would reach higher levels, and would dissipate more slowly. Satiation theory does not aid us in determining which of these indices, or which combination of them, should be chosen for testing. Worse, it is possible to argue that exactly the opposite deductions would follow from our theory. Extraverts, it might be argued, have been subjected to visual stimulation throughout the day, and consequently have already reached a high level of satiation when the experiment starts; consequently, they would be capable only of little addi-

---

[1] The different possibilities mentioned in this paragraph give rise to different experimental phenomena, and are therefore susceptible to empirical investigation. If it is rate of build-up of inhibition which most differentiates extraverts and introverts, then the number of I.R.P.s is the crucial score to use; this would rule out pursuit-rotors as measuring instruments because they give us no information on this point. Vigilance tests, with certain minor adjustments, would appear much better suited to the task. If it is the asymptotes which differ, then the pursuit rotor is a suitable instrument, and the reminiscence effect the appropriate score, particularly when conditions are so arranged that I_R only is built up, and no $_sI_R$. The experiment reported by Eysenck (1956) is not crucial because length of practice (5 min.) was such as to allow both reactive and conditioned inhibition to appear; thus the observed differences between extraverts and introverts might be due to the extinction of larger amounts of $_sI_R$ during the first post-rest period of practice in the case of the extraverts. (An excess of $_sI_R$ in this group might have arisen because of the greater frequency of I.R.P.s acting as reinforcement.) A recent and as yet unpublished experiment by Star, in which practice periods of 90 sec. were used, suggests that in the absence of $_sI_R$ reminiscence effects do not differentiate between extraverts and introverts, thus favouring the view that it is the speed of build-up, rather than the asymptote, which differentiates the groups. Much more detailed work is clearly required before any kind of definitive statement becomes possible.

tional satiation. Introverts, being less satiated at the beginning, would be capable of much more satiation. Consequently, although the rate of satiation of extraverts, *ceteris paribus*, might be greater than that of introverts, yet being nearer their asymptote they would in fact show less figural after-effect in the experimental situation. (Köhler and Fishback (1950) actually put forward a similar argument.) While such a possibility cannot be dismissed outright, figural after-effects seem to be sufficiently specific to make the argument implausible. In any case, by making a lengthy period of dark-adaptation precede the experiment, semi-permanent satiation effects could be reduced to vanishing point without difficulty; thus it would be possible experimentally to escape from this apparent impasse.

Similar complexities and difficulties appear in connection with the pharmacological and physiological details of the theory. The terms 'excitant' or 'stimulant', and 'depressant' are not used in any very exact sense by pharmacologists, and the writer suspects that drugs having quite different actions—as well as different side-effects—are gathered together under these over-inclusive concepts. If this be true, then our deductions would be expected to hold for some of these drugs, but not for others. Even with respect to those for which our predictions could be verified, there are still many unsolved problems. Dosage is one, and time of maximum action is another. Also, buffer actions are often set up, and by producing a strong counter-reaction a large dose of a drug may actually produce a smaller experimental effect than a small dose which did not produce such a reaction. On the physiological side, theories relating evidence from the electroretinogram to phenomenological effects such as CFF or 'Bidwell's ghost' are still very speculative, and direct proof largely missing. Further, the identification of central inhibition phenomena with pre-excitatory inhibition is little more than a stab in the dark; although there is some evidence in its favour, this evidence is largely indirect.

Along rather different lines, the theory here presented might be attacked as being far too simple and direct to account for the enormous complexity of actual behaviour as observed in the clinic, or even the laboratory. Surely, it might be asked, a much more complex and sophisticated type of theory is required even to begin to explain the phenomena of hysteria and anxiety, of extraversion and introversion, or of brain-damage? With such a criticism the writer would agree up to a point. The theory here presented does not attempt to explain all of behaviour, but only a carefully demarcated aspect; such important features as intellectual ability, for instance, have not been included in our account. The reason for such restrictiveness is not far to seek; psychology simply is not at present in a position to deal with the 'whole personality', but can only advance slowly by formulating much more restricted theories about part-functions which biologically and behaviourally seem to form sub-wholes or action-entities. In due course such modest part-theories of personality will no doubt be integrated into a larger whole, but it would be unreasonable to expect this to happen in the near future. Psychology is a very backward child, and no pretence at grown-upness will alter this distressing fact, although it may succeed in bringing the child into disrepute among scientists as a prospective or actual juvenile delinquent.

More complex theories, such as the psychoanalytic ones, may appear to do more justice to reality, but this apparent advantage is bought at too high a price. Such theories are not, in fact, scientific theories at all, because they do not permit in any real sense of disproof. No incontrovertible deductions can be made from them which can be tested and confirmed or infirmed; loopholes are always left open by failure to specify which of several mechanisms is to take precedence when, as is usually the case, more than one is involved. The writer has a deep-rooted preference for theories, however crude and over-simplified, which allow of relatively straightforward disproof; the capacity of a theory for permitting of having its bluff called is one of the most wholesome features which any theory can possess. Once a theory has shown its ability to predict a reasonably large number of hitherto unknown phenomena, we can set about the task of stating and verifying all the necessary qualifications and restrictions, and of investigating the laws of interaction with other part-theories. Science begins with the notion of clear-cut deduction and disproof; a theory which does not generate such deductions, and which does not allow of disproof, is not a scientific theory.

A criticism quite the opposite to the one just discussed might be made with more apparent justification. It might be said that any attempt to link together the half-formed theories in such

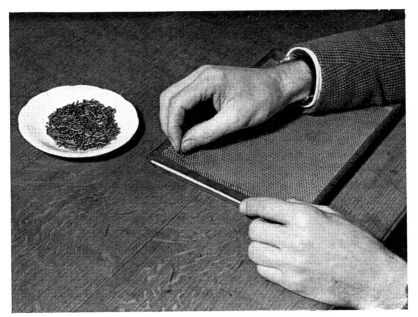

23. Pin-board used for studies into the influence of drives on the productivity of mental defectives.

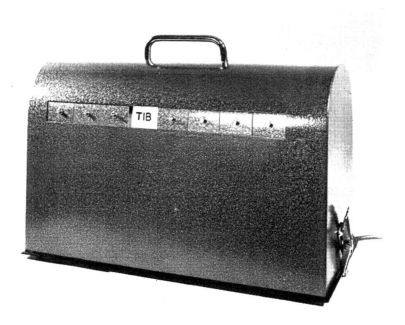

24. Nonsense-syllable learning; Maudsley memory drum.

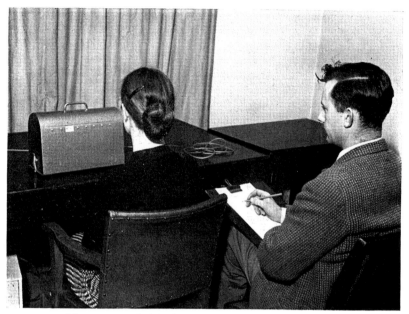

25. Nonsense-syllable learning experiment in progress.

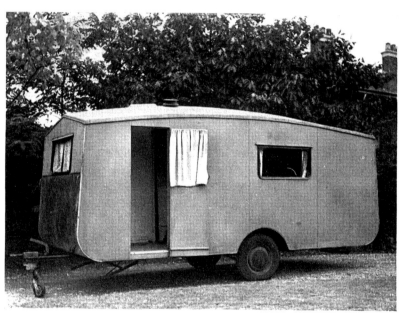

26. Mobile psychological laboratory, used for testing at mental hospitals, schools, mental defective colonies, and other institutions.

diverse disciplines as perception, learning and conditioning, social psychology and attitude formation, physiological psychology, psychiatry, pharmacology, and electrophysiology is doomed to failure, and that the very notion that such theories might be integrated in terms of the nebulous concepts of personality research can hardly be taken seriously. With such a criticism the writer would have much sympathy; indeed, the various hypotheses stated in the preceding chapters were put forward without any great expectations of finding much experimental support for the predictions derived from them.[1] Nevertheless, theories should not be dismissed on *a priori* grounds, and the number of facts which support some such theory as that put forward here is so large by now that it cannot be dismissed out of hand. Many modifications, perhaps of quite a radical kind, will certainly be required in the light of accumulating evidence, and certain parts of the theory may have to be dropped altogether. But, when all is said and done, the critic who wishes to dismiss the whole of this theory would then have to explain in terms of some other theory the observed experimental data. No such theory exists, to the writer's knowledge, and the reader might, for the sake of amusement, try to deduce the reported facts relating to satiation, conditioning, reminiscence, spiral after-effects, drug effects, brain-damage, and so forth from some such theory as the psychoanalytic: he will soon realize how very remote these speculations are from the facts of the experimental laboratory. In fact the writer has at various times asked well-known psychoanalysts to make predictions with respect to various experiments in progress which involved hysterics and dysthymics; the batting average was slightly but not significantly worse than chance!

All these points are relevant to another question which is likely to occupy the critical reader. The relationships observed between variables which according to our hypothesis should be

[1] Seward (1954) has a paragraph which is relevant to this discussion. 'To settle the most pressing systematic issues Hull outlined an experimental program of staggering proportions. Realizing that he could direct only a relatively small part of it, he was anxious to stimulate others to undertake the task. At one time he remarked that he had discovered the best way to do this. Few students or colleagues had ever bothered to do the experiments he suggested. But all he had to do was to make a clear, unqualified statement on a point of theory, and half a dozen experimenters would run to prove him wrong.' The writer can confirm the efficacy of this method, and it is in this spirit, rather than one of dogmatic certainty, that most of the predictions offered in this book have been made.

correlated are not usually very close; correlations of the order of
·3 to ·4 are the rule, and values of ·2 or even ·1 are more frequent
than values of ·7 or ·8. Thus on the average the variables
correlated with each other only share between 10 per cent to
20 per cent of the variance. Psychometricians used to rather
higher values in connection with intelligence tests may feel
disturbed by the low level of correlation so apparent in this
field. Yet it would not be reasonable to expect anything else,
and if higher values than these were in fact observed at this
early stage of development of our theory, one might reasonably
feel suspicious about the lack of contamination of the data. An
example may make this reasoning clearer. Our hypothesis
maintains that *conditionability* should correlate with *introversion*,
and on the assumption of equal environmental pressure this
correlation ought to be unity. However, environmental pressure
clearly is not equal, as pointed out in a previous chapter, and
consequently the correlation would be expected to decrease
from unity to something more like ·8 or ·7. Next, we must note
that our measure of conditionability is far from being perfectly
reliable and perfectly valid. Reliabilities are difficult to establish
in this field, but it is doubtful if the eyeblink test would show a
test-retest correlation much above ·7. Equally, the eyeblink test
is only one of many possible measures of conditioning, and these
cannot be presumed to correlate together perfectly, due to the
influence of specific factors. Thus the validity of the eyeblink
test, i.e. its factor loading on a general factor of conditioning, is
likely to be well short of unity. This would lower the probable
correlation with introversion to perhaps ·6 or ·5.

But equally our measure of introversion, whether questionnaire or diagnosis or a combination of both, is neither perfectly
reliable nor perfectly valid. This again must lower the observed
correlation, so that it would be unreasonable to expect anything much in excess of ·3. Add to this the large probable errors
or correlation coefficients when small numbers of cases are
involved, and results to be expected are likely to vary from ·1 at
the low end to ·5 at the high end. Values much higher than ·5
would not only be unexpected, but would suggest contamination, or other failures in experimental technique or sampling.
When dealing with extreme groups rather than with total
samples, these considerations do not apply quite so forcibly, and
findings such as Franks's success in achieving a perfect differen-

tiation between a group of hysterics and a group of dysthymics become possible. It will be remembered, however, that Franks (1) used a double criterion of classification, and (2) used a combination of two conditioning tests. Improvement in the size of observed relationships is to be expected with experimental arrangements involving larger numbers of tests on the side both of selection and of conditioning.

What is true of conditioning is probably even more true of other tests used in this study. The unreliability of reminiscence tests has already been mentioned. A phenomenon which itself is somewhat capricious and difficult to produce is not likely to give very accurate estimates of individual differences, and unreliable estimates of this kind are not likely to correlate highly with any outside criterion, however valid. The fact that significant correlations can nevertheless be found under these circumstances is therefore encouraging; it is one of the paradoxes of psychometrics that valid but unreliable tests are the most promising ones, more so than equally valid but more reliable ones. This is due to the fact that it is usually easy to improve reliability, and concomitantly validity; where reliability is already high, it is difficult to increase validity.

For these reasons we do not consider the fact that correlations tend to be low to be in contradiction to our theory. Behaviour is determined by many factors in addition to those discussed in these pages; it is possible to isolate one factor without having to demonstrate perfect correlations with imperfect estimates of behaviour. It is only when all the major determining factors have been isolated and measured, and when the estimates of behaviour have themselves been purified, that we can expect much higher relationships to emerge. We are at the beginning, not at the end of this particular quest, and it would be idle to judge the theory here presented as being more final, more advanced, and more definitive than it claims to be.

If there is any considerable degree of truth in the general theory and the specific hypotheses advanced in this book, then it would appear that certain important consequences follow with respect to the relation between psychology and psychiatry, the practice of clinical psychology, the methodology of diagnostic testing, and the application of psychological theory to the cure of neurotic disorders. We may perhaps begin with a brief discussion of the relevance of our findings to the practice of diagnostic testing. Now, as has been pointed out elsewhere (Eysenck, 1957), tests can be of three kinds: they can be based on notional, empirical, or rational grounds. A test is called *notional* when its rationale is based on nothing but a hunch, or a notion, or a clinical impression which has not been verified objectively. As an example of a notional test we may perhaps instance the Rorschach test. This technique originated with the notion that personality would express itself in the perceptual organization of relatively unorganized material, such as ink-blots, a notion which has some *a priori* likelihood, although it has not received any very convincing proof, and the equally important notion that one could argue back from the observed organization to the personality responsible for it, a very unlikely hypothesis (Eysenck, 1957). Thirty years of research now enable us to evaluate the success of these notions in generating a valid and reliable test. The writer may perhaps quote the summarized conclusions from a review of a large and representative number of research papers in the projective field, dealing mostly with the Rorschach (Eysenck, 1957): '(1) There is no consistent, meaningful and testable theory underlying modern projective devices. (2) The actual practice of projective experts frequently contradicts the putative hypotheses on which their tests are built. (3) On the empirical level, there is no indisputable evidence showing any kind of marked relationship between global projective test interpretation by experts and psychiatric diagnosis. (4) There is no evidence of any marked relationship between Rorschach scoring categories combined in any approved statistical fashion into a scale and diagnostic category, when the association between the two is tested on a population other than that from which the scale was derived. (5) There is no evidence of any marked relationship between global or statistically derived projective test scores and outcome of psychotherapy. (6) There is no evidence for the great majority of the postulated relationships between projective test indicators and personality traits. (7) There is no evidence for any marked relationship between projective test indicators of any kind and intellectual qualities and abilities as measured, estimated or rated independently. (8) There is no evidence for the predictive power of projective techniques with respect to success or failure in a wide variety of fields where personality qualities play an important part. (9) There is no evidence that conscious or unconscious conflicts, attitudes, fears, or fantasies in patients can be diagnosed by means of projective techniques in such a way as to give results congruent with assessments made by psychiatrists independently. (10) There is ample evidence to show that the great majority of studies in the field of projective techniques are inadequately designed, have serious statistical errors in the analysis of the data, and/or are subject to damaging criticisms on the grounds of contamination between test and criterion.'

Empirical tests, as contrasted with notional ones, are tests which have been shown to correlate reasonably well with external criteria widely accepted. It is to them that the definition of 'validity' as 'correlation with an outside criterion' applies. Most prominent in this category are miniature test situations, i.e. miniature replicas of the kind of behaviour the experimenter is interested in. Objective studies of traits such as honesty, persistence, punctuality, integration, suggestibility, perseveration, tension, and many others would fall into this category; a thorough review of many of these studies is given by Vernon (1953) and Eysenck (1953). These tests have an important role to play in the assessment of personality, but they usually lack any theoretical background and are of little fundamental scientific interest.

Rational tests are tests which are developed, not on the basis of notions and hunches, but which are firmly based on theory. They form part of what Cronbach and Meehl (1955) call a 'nomological network', and their validity is established by means of what these writers call 'construct validation'. This is how these concepts are defined by Cronbach and Meehl:

'Construct validation takes place when an investigator believes that his instrument reflects a particular construct, to which are attached certain meanings. The proposed interpretation generates specific testable hypotheses, which are a means of confirming or disconfirming the claim. . . . Scientifically speaking, to "make clear what something *is*" means to set forth the laws in which it occurs. We shall refer to the interlocking system of laws which constitute a theory as a *nomological network*. . . . We can say that "operations" which are qualitatively very different "overlap" or "measure the same thing" if their positions in the nomological net tie them to the same construct variable. Our confidence in this identification depends upon the amount of inductive support we have for the regions of the net involved. It is not necessary that a direct observational comparison of the two operations be made—we may be content with an intra-network proof indicating that the two operations yield estimates of the same network-defined quantity. . . . A rigorous (though perhaps probabilistic) chain of inference is required to establish a test as a measure of a construct. To validate a claim that a test measures a construct, a nosological net surrounding the concept must exist.'

The advantages of having psychiatric diagnoses as part of the nomological network, defining by way of observed interrelationships of behaviour patterns such concepts as neuroticism and extraversion-introversion, will now be apparent. We can transfer inferences from one group to the other and make predictions and deductions in terms of the general theory. As an example of this we may consider the series of researches on conditioning reported earlier. We find that hysterics (psychiatrically diagnosed) are less easy to condition than dysthymics (psychiatrically diagnosed). In terms of our general theory it follows that normal extraverts (selected by factor-analytic procedures) should be less easy to condition than normal introverts (selected by factor-analytic procedures). Such predictions, empirically confirmed, considerably strengthen the nomological network, and at the same time anchor more firmly the particular system of co-ordinates chosen in our factorial studies to other sets of empirically derived concepts, systems and laws. In view of the many statistical difficulties and methodological weaknesses inherent in factor analysis, this procedure of aligning factors with theoretically relevant concepts and groupings outside the field of operation of the correlational analysis itself, appears to the writer an essential part of the task of construct derivation.

If these distinctions between notional, empirical, and rational testing procedures be accepted—it should be noted that no absolute validity is claimed for these 'types' of tests, but merely heuristic usefulness—then it would seem to follow that clinical psychologists should attempt to use, as far as possible, rational methods of diagnostic testing, followed, where no such rational methods are available, by empirical ones. Notional methods should never be used in practice, although of course no such ban would extend to their use in research—the notional methods of today may be the empirical methods of tomorrow! This implies a complete reversal of the actual mode of clinical procedure at present in vogue, which uses notional methods almost exclusively, which uses empirical methods very occasionally, and which uses rational methods practically never. To many clinical psychologists it may seem that the procedures discussed in this book are not 'personality tests' at all, in the usual sense of that term. This may be true. Nevertheless, the writer would argue that the unsatisfactory position of clinical psychology and of diagnostic measurement in general on which so many contributors to the Annual Review of Psychology have commented during the past few years, is almost entirely due to the fact that so much stress has been laid on notional and empirical tests, and that so little attention has been given to the integration of personality measurement with psychological theory and experimental practice in general. *The future of the psychological measurement of personality lies in the development of rational tests soundly based on general psychological theories and, inevitably, these tests will assume more and more the character of laboratory investigations.*[1] This development will inevitably necessitate considerable changes, both in the training and the equipment of clinical psychologists. At the moment clinical psychologists are too frequently lacking in the requisite knowledge and training to apply the principles of learning theory to the problems facing them in the clinic, and they are too frequently ill-equipped with apparatus and other facilities to enable them to make use of recent developments in the fields of learning, conditioning and perception for their

[1] This belief is sometimes criticized on the grounds that such laboratory phenomena as conditioning, which apparently require elaborate equipment, soundproof rooms, and lengthy periods of adaptation and testing, surely cannot be of any importance under ordinary conditions of every-day life, where such requirements are not met. This argument completely mistakes the logic of science, and the purpose of 'taking a problem into the laboratory'. The purified and carefully controlled conditions obtaining in the laboratory of the physicist and the chemist at first sight have little similarity to the complex and confused world outside, yet we know that the laws and principles elaborated under these apparently esoteric and highly artificial conditions do in fact govern the behaviour of matter in general, and enable us to make predictions of considerable accuracy. Similarly, the laws and explanatory principles of the psychologist are not likely to be discovered without the possibilities of control and exactness which only the laboratory affords; there is no reason to expect that the laws of conditioning work only in the laboratory, just as there is no reason to expect that the second law of thermodynamics, or Heisenberg's indeterminacy principle, apply only under the precise conditions which led to their discovery. The precise method of application of knowledge obtained in the laboratory, and the interaction of the processes so isolated with other processes, does of course present additional problems which require to be solved experimentally; but here too psychology does not in any way seem to differ from the exact sciences in principle, however much it may differ in achievement.

clinical task of describing personality, evaluating prognosis, and advising on different types of treatment (Eysenck, 1955). No psychiatric hospital would expect an electroencephalographer to carry out his work efficiently and well without a proper supply of apparatus and technical help. Not until it is recognized that the psychologist also requires a considerable amount of apparatus, technical help, sound-proof rooms and so on, to carry out the assessment of relevant personality variables to the best advantage, will all his potentialities be realized and full use be made of the help which he can give to the psychiatrist in this central field of human behaviour.

In brief, the writer would agree with Magaret (1952) that the emphasis during the past 20 years has been faulty. 'If subsequent investigations follow the major trends of the immediate past, . . . then, in this reviewer's opinion, the future looks discouraging indeed. One cannot read in detail the contemporary literature in diagnostics without being overwhelmed by the tremendous expenditure of time, money and labour involved in bringing forth inconclusive or trivial results. It is no accident that, for the past few years, reviewers of this literature have consistently failed to discover in the studies any comprehensive or coherent pattern. Too many investigations are haphazard, isolated or fragmentary; too many stop where they should begin; too many seem to appear in our journals like rejected orphans, with no meaningful past and no promising future.'

The present writer does not feel optimistic that the current approaches, which attempt to improve the botched-up edifice of pseudometrics and psychomagic which constitutes modern clinical practice in personality assessments, are radical enough to improve the situation. The only realistic hope, he would suggest, is a return to the long-neglected principles of scientific work with its stress on the hypothetico-deductive procedure, objective measurement, appropriate techniques of statistical analysis and the realistic restriction of the effort of measurement to something less nebulous and less grandiose than the 'total personality'. The approach initiated by Spence and Taylor, by Mowrer and Miller, and by other learning theorists interested in personality, with all its crudities, exemplifies the type of approach which, in the long run, is likely to yield better dividends than any of the others mentioned, and in so returning to the principles and methods of Pavlov, rather than relying on those of Freud, these writers may have rescued personality testing from a cul-de-sac which threatened to lead it into esoteric absurdity.

No less radical and revolutionary than in the diagnostic field would be the introduction of rational methods in the treatment field. Here also, as the writer has pointed out (Eysenck, 1956), we may distinguish notional, empirical and rational procedures. As an example of the notional type of procedure, we may perhaps cite psychotherapy. The notion that by talking to the patient, by delving into his or her putative 'unconscious' motivations, by directing his suppositious 'transferences' hither and thither, it is possible to rid him or her of neurotic disabilities and symptoms, is one the *a priori* probability of which is difficult to assess. What is certain is that no evidence exists on the basis of which one could confidently assert that this notion has any kind of empirical backing (Eysenck, 1952, 1953). It is less easy to find good examples of empirical procedures, as the efficacy of physical methods of psychiatric treatment (electroshock, lobotomy, etc.) has not really been properly demonstrated in a thoroughly acceptable fashion. Nevertheless, for the purpose of the argument it is probably not counter to fact to say that these methods do have effects, and that these effects are not predictable on any theoretical basis. Thus methods of physical treatment, in so far as they work, must be listed as empirical procedures.

Attempts have been made in recent years to demonstrate that psychotherapeutic procedures, particularly those of the Freudian kind, can be deduced from learning theory, and thus given a sort of *ex post facto* figleaf of rational respectability. An interesting attempt in this direction is that of Shoben (1949). His argument runs as follows: 'The common problem characterizing clinical patients is anxiety and the behavioral defences built up against it. The goal of psychotherapy, regardless of the therapist's theoretical leanings, is to eliminate the anxiety and thereby to do away with the symptomatic persistent nonintegrative behaviour. To accomplish this goal, all therapists use the devices of conversing with the patient about his anxiety and the situations calling it forth both currently and historically, and forming a unique therapeutic relationship. Since all psychotherapies seem to have successes to their credit and since psychotherapy seems to be a process whereby a patient learns to modify

his emotional reactions and his overt behaviour, it is hypothesized that therapy may be conceptualized from the point of
view of general psychology as a problem in learning theory.
Such a conceptualization must account for the changes that
occur in counselees in terms of these factors that are apparently
common to all forms of counseling.'

Shoben goes on to account for the effects of psychotherapy in
terms of three interrelated processes: 'First, the lifting of repression and development of insight through the symbolic reinstat-
ing of the stimuli for anxiety; second, the diminution of anxiety
by counter-conditioning through the attachment of the stimuli
for anxiety to the comfort reaction made to the therapeutic
relationship; and third, the process of re-education through the
therapist's helping the patient to formulate rational goals and
behavioral methods for attaining them.'

Shoben correctly sees that the fact that all types of psychotherapy achieve results not fundamentally different from each
other requires a theoretical explanation in terms of processes
which they have in common; it must also follow that if, as
the evidence seems to indicate (Brill, 1955), spontaneous
recovery and orthodox medical, non-psychotherapeutic treatment produce as marked effects as do the various forms of
psychotherapy, then we must widen the circle of facts to be
explained and cover these phenomena also. It also follows that
those features in psychotherapy which Shoben stresses, and which
play no part in spontaneous recovery or non-psychotherapeutic
procedures, must be eliminated from the theory. As all his three
points are directly related to psychotherapy, we must look for
quite a different type of theory, one which takes into account all
the facts of the situation. (It should be made clear that when
Shoben published his paper, most of the evidence regarding
non-psychotherapeutic improvement was not yet available;
consequently he cannot be criticized in any way for not dealing
with the points raised here.) The position recalls the well-known
story of King Charles and the Royal Society. The King sent a
question to the newly-formed Society asking them why a fish
resting on the bottom of a tank of water weighed less than the
same fish swimming about in the water. Many ingenious hypotheses were advanced until it occurred to someone to carry out
the experiment; he soon found that there is in fact no difference
in weight, and consequently nothing to be explained. Similarly,

explanations of the alleged effects of psychotherapy are some-what premature and might with advantage await the time when such effects had been demonstrated. All we know at the moment is that spontaneous remission and non-psychotherapeutic treat-ment produce improvements in neurotic disorders which follow an exponential curve the formula for which is:

$$X = 100 \left(1 - 10^{-0.00435N}\right)$$

where X stands for the amount of improvement achieved in per cent and N for the number of weeks elapsed (Eysenck, 1957). Psychotherapy, if the published figures are to be trusted, does not appear to improve on this rate (Eysenck, 1952).[1]

Shoben follows in its essentials the Freudian position, accord-ing to which symptoms have symbolic significance, and are indicative of some underlying repressed conflict; symptomatic treatment is useless because it does not cure this conflict. Treat-ment is based on the discovery of historical factors, leading to insight. Verbal methods of extinction and reconditioning are all-important. Concern is mainly with *content* rather than with *function*. The writer would like to oppose to this view another which might be called the Pavlovian, although Pavlov himself never attempted to formulate any comprehensive theory of neurotic behaviour. However, such a view is implicit in his general outlook, and might be presented somewhat like this. Symptoms are learned S-R connections; once they are extin-guished or deconditioned treatment is complete. Such treat-ment is based exclusively on present factors; like Lewin's theory, this one is a-historical. Non-verbal methods are favoured over verbal ones, although a minor place is reserved for verbal methods of extinction and reconditioning. Concern is with *function*, not with *content*.[2] The main difference between the two

---

[1] Some readers may be under the impression that since the writer published these figures, the work of Rogers and Dymond (1954) has produced evidence in favour of psychotherapeutic effectiveness. Unfortunately their book is subject to very damaging criticism (Eysenck, 1955) and consequently cannot be adduced in evidence.

[2] The meaning of this distinction between *content* and *function* can best be illustrated by reference to the word-association test. As is well known, patients suffering from functional disorders often respond very slowly to emotionally arousing words, when compared with normals. Writers of the 'dynamic' school explain this in terms of 'complexes' aroused in the patient which interfere with his adequate responding to the emotionally toned stimulus word; their concern is with the content of these words, and the leads thus furnished to the discovery of these

theories arises over the question of 'symptomatic' treatment. According to orthodox theory, this is useless unless the underlying complexes are attacked. According to the present theory, there is no evidence for these putative complexes, and symptomatic treatment is all that is required.

Fortunately the two theories make different predictions with respect to the consequences of therapy, and these consequences can be verified. Thus it would follow from the Freudian theory that symptomatic cures would be followed by the emergence of other symptoms, by greatly increased anxiety, or some other manifestation of the unresolved complex. It would follow from the present theory that Freudian methods would be much less efficacious in curing the symptoms, and that conditioning methods should not produce the evil after-effects predicted by the Freudians.

The difference between the theories might be phrased like this. According to Freud, there is a 'disease' which produces symptoms; cure the disease, and the symptoms will vanish. According to the alternative view, there is no 'disease', there are merely wrong habits which have been learned and must be unlearned. If such 'unlearning' and 'relearning' is efficacious, and there is no evidence of any 'disease', then surely we must dismiss this additional concept as superfluous.

Much of the available evidence relates to the cure of symptoms such as enuresis (Crosby, 1950; Davidson & Douglass, 1950; Martin & Kubly, 1955; Mowrer, 1950), writer's cramp (Sylvester & Leversedge, 1955), alcoholism (Thompson & Bielinski, 1953; Bugalskii, 1952; Thirann, 1949; Alguero, 1948; Wallace, 1949; Morsier & Feldman, 1949), stammering and stuttering (Cherry et al., 1955; Jones, 1955; Johnson, 1955; Wischner, 1950), and tics (Yates, 1957), i.e. symptoms which are fairly

putative 'complexes'. An alternative explanation would be in terms of function; thus the hypothesis might be formulated that functionally disordered patients tend to be slow in their responses (Babcock, 1933; Eysenck, 1953; Nelson, 1953; Shapiro & Nelson, 1955; Anne Broadhurst, 1956). Word reactions to emotional stimuli would then be regarded merely as one of many different possible responses demonstrating this tendency; there would be no implication regarding the special relevance of the content of these words. An experiment by De (1953) may be regarded as giving support to the functional type of theory. He demonstrated that neutral words, such as table, chair, green, differentiated normal, neurotic and psychotic groups slightly more efficiently than emotional words, such as kiss, breast, death, when speed of response was scored. The difference between neutral and emotional words was not significant, but the results certainly do not support the view that the content of the words is relevant to their differentiating power.

definite and the presence or absence of which can be established without any reasonable doubt. The general impression which one gains from the literature is this: (1) Psychotherapy is particularly ineffective in these conditions. (2) Conditioning procedures are reasonably, and often quite surprisingly successful. (3) Symptom substitution does not as a rule occur, even when psychoanalytically trained investigators are specially on the look-out for it. On the whole the evidence supports the theory here presented, and goes counter to the Freudian view. This conclusion is strengthened by individual case studies, such as one by Gwynne Jones (1956) from this Department, reporting cases where psychotherapy had failed, but where conditioning methods successfully and quickly abolished the main symptoms, improved the general mental health of the patient, and did not lead to any kind of symptom substitution. Even a single case of this kind is crucial, because on the Freudian theory such an outcome should be impossible, and one positive case can infirm a theory which denies the possibility of such a case existing.

The Jones study deals with a 23-year-old girl, somewhat introverted, who complained of frequency of micturition with associated secondary fears, general lack of confidence, and anxiety. Her career as a dancer was made impossible by her having to pass water every half-hour. Psychotherapy, concentrating on a sexual history involving loss of virginity, coitus interruptus, and various other factors, produced very little change in her condition, and was about to be terminated. 'At this stage the psychologist was consulted as to the possibilities of applying learning techniques to the symptomatic treatment of the urinary frequency.'

Jones based his technique on a report by Bykov (1953), who had introduced warm water into the bladders of human subjects, recorded the pressure changes graphically and displayed them on a manometer placed before the subject. This manometer could be disconnected without the subject's knowledge, and since the urge to urinate tends to occur at a definite pressure for each individual, the subjects rapidly developed a 'connection' between the manometer reading equivalent to this pressure and the urge to urinate. 'An intense urinary urge and an associated galvanic skin response could be elicited merely by calling out, via a microphone and loud-speaker, the figure of the critical manometer reading. This response occurred even when the bladder contained practically no fluid. Conversely, and of more direct interest, if the manometer, disconnected without the subject's knowledge, registered zero, it was possible to introduce far greater quantities of fluid than normally produced urination without evoking the urgency response.'

In the light of this report the apparatus illustrated in Fig. 60 was constructed. 'The manometer was fitted with a scale in arbitrary units and, by means of an inconspicuous tap, could

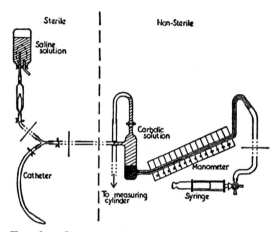

FIG. 60. Cystometric apparatus used in urinary control conditioning experiment.

be connected to a syringe, thus creating a back pressure and decreasing the reading on the scale. By means of this apparatus, with appropriate arrangement of the clips and taps, varying volumes of sterile saline solution could be introduced into the patient's bladder, true or decreased pressure readings could be taken at any stage, and the patient's bladder could be voluntarily evacuated, the outflow being measured in a cylinder. In use the manometer was placed at bladder height and immediately before the subject where she could read the scale.' A conditioning programme was now started along the lines of the Bykov report, to get the patient used to tolerating larger quantities of water in her bladder by presenting her with false (low) manometer readings. The details and complexities of the case are too involved to be dealt with here, and the reader is referred to the original publication; suffice it to say that the treatment, in spite of its brevity, was entirely successful, and that fifteen months after discharge 'her private physician reported that she had remained free of symptoms and had recently married with apparent success'. Anxiety did not increase with the abolition of the symptom, but decreased instead, and no alternative symptoms arose to take the place of the one treated in this fashion.

Reports of this case have at various times been presented before psychoanalytically oriented audiences, and their responses may be of some interest. In spite of the failure of alternative symptoms to develop, speakers nearly unanimously assumed that such symptoms either must have been present, or would develop in due course; for this reason they refused to even consider permitting treatment of this kind for patients under their care. Similar objections have been made to the use of conditioning techniques in the treatment of enuresis, and in spite of its proven value this technique is not used in any child guidance clinic in this country. (There may be a few exceptions to this universal negative, but if so their number must have been very small, and they have not publicized their methods so as to make their use of them known in the profession.) Thus observed facts are subordinated to *a priori* assumptions, and the results of critical experiments argued away because they do not agree with the theory they are designed to test. Under the circumstances, it may be permissible to ask just how the uncommitted scientist is to test the theory that 'symptom-curing' is not enough, and always leads to 'symptom-substitution', when the demonstration that no such substitution does in fact occur is argued away as being due to errors in observation, and when those who advance this argument refuse outright to carry out such experiments and observations themselves, on the grounds that their theory already tells them what the outcome of the experiment is going to be? It is not too far-fetched, perhaps, to recall the historical parallel of the followers of Aristotle who refused to look through Galilei's telescope because they already knew that what he said he saw there couldn't be there, as it would be in contradiction to Aristotelian dogma. The history of science does not deal kindly with attitudes of this kind.

It might be argued that the papers referred to deal with monosymptomatic disorders quite unlike the usual run of anxious and depressed patients who seek help from the psychiatrist. How would a theory of the type here presented fare

271

when applied to patients of this kind? Fortunately we have available the careful work of Wolpe in answer to this question (Wolpe, 1952, 1954). Wolpe deals directly with anxiety, rather than with any of the other symptoms mentioned so far, and he develops a general theory which in no way runs counter to that here developed. He attempts to show in his paper 'that when fundamental psychotherapeutic effects are obtained in neuroses —no matter by what therapist—these effects are nearly always really a consequence of the occurrence of reciprocal inhibition of neurotic anxiety responses, i.e. the complete or partial suppression of the anxiety responses as a consequence of the simultaneous evocation of other responses physiologically antagonistic to anxiety. . . . If a response incompatible with anxiety can be made to occur in the presence of anxiety-evoking stimuli it will weaken the bond between these stimuli and the anxiety responses.'

In producing these 'incompatible' responses, Wolpe is not content with reliance on purely verbal 'on the couch' methods; he makes use of many diverse and ingenious procedures having a sound experimental background. His theory therefore agrees in its major aspects with that presented here, and we may use the success of his method, as compared with the success of orthodox psychoanalysis, as an approximate measure of the value of the two theories. (It should be borne in mind in making such a comparison that Wolpe's method is much less time-consuming than is the Freudian; he gives the mean number of interviews per patient as less than thirty. Type of case and criteria of recovery are quite similar, as far as it is possible to assess such very subjective matters.) Such a comparison is presented by Wolpe himself (1954), based on 122 cases of his own, and a much larger number of cases treated by psychoanalysis, and reported in the literature. Statistical tests of significance were carried out, and the conclusion was reached 'that the probability that the higher proportion of successes in the present series is due to chance is negligible. . . . 90 per cent of the patients in our two series were either apparently cured or much improved, and only about 60 per cent of the cases in the other two series. If the favourable results of the present series are, to the extent of 60 per cent, regarded as due to the non-specific reciprocal inhibition that would occur in any kind of interview situation, the additional 30 per cent of good results appears to be attributable to the special measures for obtaining reciprocal inhibition described above. Furthermore, the small average number of interviews needed suggests that the use of these special measures early in treatment greatly accelerates the improvement of those patients who would have responded to the non-specific factors alone.'

To this we have only one point to add. Wolpe's 'non-specific' factors mediating reciprocal inhibition are apparently to be found equally in psychotherapeutic situations as in ordinary life situations not involving psychotherapists, because the evidence does not show any greater proportion of cures following psychotherapy as compared with spontaneous remissions or exposure to non-psychotherapeutic conditions of medical care. His demonstration of success superior to the spontaneous remission rate is the first, and indeed the only, such demonstration the writer has come across in all the voluminous writings of psychiatrists concerned with the treatment of neurotic disorders, and while the obvious weaknesses of all actuarial comparisons makes it imperative that further trials of this method be arranged under stringent control conditions, and comparisons be made on larger groups of patients randomly assigned to the different treatments, nevertheless the results as far as they go do not seem to be unfavourable to the Pavlovian type of theory. In the absence of further evidence, no more than this can be said at present.

We would take issue with Wolpe on one point, however. He has postulated one particular method of extinction, namely that of reciprocal inhibition, and formulated his theory entirely in terms of this method. Our own theory is somewhat wider, postulating merely the importance of experimental extinction but without specifying the precise method to be adopted. It would appear that circumstances must dictate the choice of method, and that it would not be wise to close the door to procedures other than that chosen by Wolpe. An example from our own Department may make this point clearer (Yates, 1957). The experiment in question deals with the elimination of a set of tics in a 25-year-old woman of high average intelligence, markedly neurotic and slightly extraverted. She was complaining of four clear-cut tics: a complex stomach-contraction/ breathing tic; a nasal 'explosion' (expiration); a coughing tic; and an eyeblink tic. These tics appeared to have started originally following two very traumatic experiences about ten years previous when she felt that she was being suffocated while undergoing anaesthesia; she was terrified and struggled madly. She could not bear the thought of an anaesthetic mask and could not tolerate any object being placed over her face. Superficially, at least, these tics seemed to be conditioned avoidance responses, originally established in a traumatic situation. She also said she felt a 'need' to do the tics and experienced relief when they occurred (i.e. they were drive-reducing).

Yates proposes the following theoretical model. 'It is hypothesized that some tics may be drive-reducing conditioned avoidance responses, originally evoked in a highly traumatic situation. In this situation, intense fear is aroused and a movement of withdrawal or aggression is made. This movement produces (or coincides with) the cessation of the fear-inducing stimulus, hence the movement is performed at the moment when drive-reduction takes place. On subsequent occasions, through stimulus generalization (including internal symbolization), conditioned fear ("anxiety") may be aroused, which is then reduced by the performance of the abient movement. In this way the tic is constantly aroused by a large variety of stimuli and eventually achieves the status of a powerful habit.' Yates quotes Solomon and Wynne (1954), Wolpe (1952) and others in support of the fact that 'animals placed in a highly traumatic situation will develop conditioned avoidance responses which apparently reduce the anxiety associated with the original situation, and which resist extinction'. He also refers to Gerard (1946) in support of the clinically-held view, based on case histories of tiqueurs, that the tic is an avoidance response arising in the first instance in a highly traumatic situation, especially in childhood. (Gerard, of course, offers very different deductions as to treatment from those made by Yates.)

In this theory, then, the tic is regarded as a habit $(_sH_R)$ which is multiplied by the momentary drive to produce the visible and audible symptom $(_sE_R)$, 'i.e. the actual potential frequency of the tic at a given moment will be a multiplicative function of the habit strength of the tic (determined mainly by the number of times it has previously been evoked) and the momentary drive strength (anxiety) which will fluctuate from time to time. One further point needs to be made. Habit strength $(_sH_R)$, in the course of learning, increases as a simple negatively accelerated positive growth function and eventually reaches an asymptote. Beyond this point, further performance of the tic cannot increase its habit strength.'

Yates then proceeds to deduce a method of treatment. 'According to the above model, the tic may be treated as a simple, learned habit, which has attained a maximum habit strength. . . . In terms of the theory, it should be possible, therefore, to extinguish the habit by building up a negative habit of "not performing the tic". This may be attempted in the following way. If the subject is given massed practice in the tic, then, according to Hullian theory, reactive inhibition (I_R) should build up rapidly. When I_R reaches a certain critical point, the patient will be forced to rest, i.e. not perform the tic. This habit ($_sI_R$) of not performing the tic will be associated with drive-reduction (due to the dissipation of I_R) and hence will be reinforced. With repeated massed practice, therefore, a negative habit ("not-doing-the-tic") will be built up and will militate against the positive habit of doing the tic. Furthermore, the repeated voluntary evocation of the tic should *not* serve to increase the habit-strength of the tic itself, since this should already have reached its asymptote and hence will not be affected by massed practice.'

The following method of treatment was therefore adopted. 'It was decided to treat the four tics concurrently but independently. Each tic was given five one-minute periods of massed practice, with one minute's rest between each period. At the end of the fifth trial, a rest of three minutes was given and then the next tic was practised. The subject was instructed to reproduce each tic as accurately as possible and to repeat it steadily during the practice periods, i.e. without pauses. No stress was laid on speed, however. A complete session lasted exactly 45 minutes. One such session was carried out at the hospital each day under supervision; the patient carried out the other on her own. The order of practising the tics was varied at random. The score recorded was the number of tics per minute.'

The following detailed predictions follow from the theory. (1) Successive trials within each five-minute period should produce a slowing down of the tic due to the accumulation of I_R, one-minute rest pauses not being sufficient for its complete dissipation. (2) On successive days the total number of tics produced should be decreasing, due to the accumulation of $_sI_R$. (3)

Cessation of practice for lengthy periods ('holidays') should not produce a reversal of this decline, as $_sI_R$ is a habit which does not dissipate with time. (4) Changes in D ('anxiety') should produce changes in the rate of production of the tic, because D acts in a multiplicative manner upon $_sH_R$. (5) Frequency of the tic, although the easiest aspect of the phenomenon to measure, would not be expected to be the only index of the growth of extinction; a lowering in the vigour with which the tics were

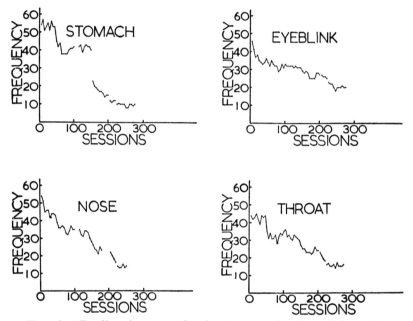

FIG. 61. Decline in rate of voluntary production of four tics during course of treatment by extinction through conditioned inhibition.

formed, and a lessening in their amplitude, would also be expected. (6) The extinction should extend beyond the place and time of the 'training' and reduce the incidence of the tic in the patient's ordinary life.

All these predictions were borne out at high levels of statistical significance. Towards the end of the experiment the subject would be sitting in front of the mirror, which was used to enable her to check the accuracy of her voluntary reproduction of the tics, *unable to produce the tic voluntarily for many seconds on end!* Fig. 61 shows the actual decline in the curves; it will be remembered that these present voluntary evocations of the tic, and thus are not direct measures of the tics themselves.[1] Even when the tic as an involuntary movement has disappeared, we would still expect the subject to be able to produce the movements involved on a voluntary basis. (It is an interesting point whether in due course it might be possible to inhibit a person's power to produce a particular movement voluntarily so completely that he had no further control over the movement. This would require so many repetitions beyond the point where the tics had already disappeared that in the present case the subject would have had no incentive to continue, merely to settle an academic point of this kind. The experiments of Calvin *et al.* (1956), in which the running behaviour of hungry rats towards the food box was extinguished in a similar fashion, suggest that the present experiment, if continued, would have produced complete extinction.)

The tic itself, as produced involuntarily outside the experimental situation, was weakening throughout the period of the experiment, until the subject could take up a new job—with all the increase in D ('anxiety') involved—without betraying the fact that she was a tiqueur, and without being asked 'what was the matter with her?', or any of the other questions usually elicited by her tics. For all practical purposes, the tics were abolished by the treatment; no other symptoms took their place; and no increase of anxiety was observed either. Quite on the contrary, the abolition of the very debilitating and worrying tics had a very positive effect on the mental outlook of the patient.

There is no space to go into the history of this mode of treatment, which has roots in the classical work of Meige and Feindel (1907) and the later studies of Dunlap (1932). These earlier

---

[1] The details of the experiment are too complex to be put down in their entirety; the original publication should be consulted in this connection. Suffice it to say that each dot on the graph represents five sessions, i.e. 25 one-minute trials. Each standard session consisted of five one-minute trials with one-minute rest intervals. Occasional periods of no practice are indicated in the graph by gaps; these were included to test the hypothesis that $_sI_R$ had been generated in the practice periods, so that failure to practice would not lead to dissipation of the inhibition accumulated. The sudden drop in the 'stomach' tic after the 150th period is due to a change in instructions, to the effect that the contraction should be made as *intense* as possible. In the nasal tic, three periods of massed practice were interpolated from trial 101 to 111, from trial 151 to 180, and from trial 221 to 250; these consisted of fifteen-minute periods of uninterrupted practice.

workers, although aware of the learned character of tics, and even of the possibilities of treatment by repetition of symptoms, had not available to them the large body of theory and fact which makes up modern learning theory, and did not succeed, therefore, in integrating their pioneering proposals and methods of treatment with the laws of general psychology. Nor can we go here into the experimental modifications of this treatment, as for instance by increasing the time given to the practice of one tic and reducing the time given to another, which Yates has reported. By and large, these results very much strengthen the theory by showing that the experimenter has succeeded in bringing the phenomenon in question under experimental control, so that any desired change can be produced by suitable manipulation of the independent variables. (Theoretically it would be possible to increase the frequency of the tics again, but in the therapeutic situation this could, of course, not be attempted.)

Not too much should be made of this experiment, or of the related one of Gwynne Jones (1956), or even of the far more numerous ones reported by Wolpe (1952, 1954). We are not claiming that the approach here suggested, and the theory on which it is based, will solve all psychiatric problems overnight, and serve as a quick cure-all or *vade-mecum*. It is possible that the psychoanalytic approach may be applicable to certain cases, and that the Pavlovian approach is better able to deal with others. Indeed, the whole problem of the application of the theory here advocated to the different psychiatric disorders is still in an embryonic stage. What the writer would conclude, however, is this. More and more, in recent years, have the psychoanalytic model and the psychoanalytic type of therapy become monolithic and virtually monopolistic, insisting on 'training analyses' and other indoctrinating devices in all those who set out to deal with psychiatric disorders. This position has not been supported by scientific experiment, by rational argument, or by the demonstration of therapeutic effectiveness; quite on the contrary, on all three scores the evidence is counter to psychoanalytic doctrine rather than favourable. By thus overemphasizing one possible, though as yet speculative, approach to the treatment of psychiatric disorders, they have succeeded in withdrawing attention from many other possible and promising methods. As far as the evidence goes (which admittedly is not very far), the methods for treating tics used by Meige and

Feindel in 1907 are theoretically sounder and practically more effective than those used by modern psychoanalysts; yet almost the only type of theory the budding psychiatrist or clinical psychologist is likely to encounter in textbooks or in lectures is the psychoanalytic!

What is required, clearly, is a much greater concern with facts, with provable deductions from firmly-based theories, with tentative hypotheses rather than with dogmas; a more experimental approach to the actual practical value of different therapies, and a more responsible attitude to theoretical criticism and empirical demonstration. It is the writer's belief that when the theories here advocated are put to the test they will prove of greater value in diagnosis, in prognosis, and in treatment than do those at present current, and some slight evidence to this effect has already been presented. In view of the very great complexity of the issues involved, and the very fragmentary extent of our knowledge, this belief is not held with any great strength of feeling; nevertheless, the evidence on which it is based cannot altogether be dismissed as worthless. Clearly, the time is ripe for comparative studies to enable some preliminary decision to be made; until the outcome of such studies is known, we can do no more than offer the present model as an alternative to the Freudian one.

One further point may require clarification. The individual's position on the neuroticism, extraversion, and psychoticism axes is regarded as largely determined by hereditary factors, and some evidence with respect to the first two dimensions has been given by the writer (Eysenck & Prell, 1951; Eysenck, 1956) that identical twins resemble each other significantly more closely than do fraternal twins when comparisons are made on factor scores derived from test batteries of neuroticism and extraversion. More recently, Shields (1957) tested 38 pairs of identical twins brought up in separation from each other with the Maudsley Personality Inventory, and found correlations of ·52 and ·60 between the twins on neuroticism and extraversion respectively. These correlations are somewhat lower than those found for intelligence (Dominoes test) and vocabulary (Mill Hill Vocabulary Test), which amounted to ·77 and ·74; this may in part be due to the lower reliability and lower validity of personality questionnaires as measures of their respective dimensions. Even as they stand, these figures strongly support the

279

view that heredity plays an important part in the genesis of neurotic and extraverted behaviour patterns.

Consideration of genetic factors is often hindered by fears that it might lead to 'therapeutic nihilism', or a belief that nothing could be done where heredity is concerned. The writer has shown elsewhere (Eysenck, 1954) how untrue this view is, and how it contradicts the logic of genetic analysis. It is not by denying the facts of nature that we can hope to solve the problems of psychiatric disorder, but only by understanding their implications and using them for our purposes. If the factors determining a person's rate of conditioning are largely innate, then we must learn to develop methods of retraining which make use of this fact; if another person's inhibitory potential is innately strong, then again it would be foolish to disregard this fact in planning a course of therapy for him. Genetics may set certain bounds to what we may hope to do, but it also indicates to us the methods we may use to change behaviour patterns. It is never the pattern itself which is inherited, merely the predisposition to react in certain ways; these predispositions can be used to change any given patterns once they are known and can be measured.[1] It is in this way that diagnostic testing can be genuinely integrated with therapeutic endeavours; to know a person's degree of conditionability is more than an item of diagnostic knowledge, it is also an indicator of the direction which therapy should take. Thus the general theory here advocated involves a genuine synthesis between diagnosis and therapy, a synthesis which demonstrably does not obtain in present psychiatric practice.[2]

[1] An interesting clinical observation which is very relevant to this whole argument was made by R. Payne, in the course of the psychological investigation of a male patient with pronounced dysthymic disorders. This patient had an identical twin brother who agreed to come to the hospital, but who showed a pronounced extraverted personality, thus contrasting with his brother both in behaviour and in test performance. This unexpected contrast led Payne to advance the hypothesis that the extraverted brother must have experienced certain events productive of inhibition, and consequently extraverting in nature. The most obvious such event is brain-damage, and indeed electroencephalographic and other studies showed indisputable evidence of brain-damage in the extraverted twin, who had thus been protected from the kind of breakdown suffered by his brother! It is not suggested that brain-damage is a suitable method of therapy for introversion, although of course leucotomy (Petrie, 1952) and ECT, with its probably brain-damaging effects, are used in cases of dysthymic disorders.

[2] The reader may have noticed that Gwynne Jones, working with an introverted patient, made use of a *conditioning* procedure, while Yates, working with an extraverted patient, made use of reinforcement by *inhibition*. It is likely that know-

If the views here presented should prove to be of some value, the question will undoubtedly arise: 'What shall the relation be between psychologist and psychiatrist?' Theoretically, three alternatives are possible. (1) The psychologist might replace the psychiatrist in dealing with all strictly *mental* disorders. This would lead to considerable confusion in view of the necessity of ruling out physical causes before treatment—a task which would require the help of a physician. Other difficulties would arise because of the physical nature of many symptoms, and the involvement in many cases of the autonomic system. The often highly desirable administration of drugs also would involve the aid of a medically trained person. On the whole, it is doubtful if it would be wise for the psychologist to 'go it alone'. (2) The psychiatrist might master the theory and practice of psychology, and particularly of learning theory. While this might be desirable in many ways, there is little prospect on a realistic basis for the addition of another six years' study to the already overcrowded curriculum of the psychiatrist. (3) Psychologists and psychiatrists might co-operate on the basis of absolute equality, but with the psychiatrist retaining responsibility for the *physical* health of the patient. The exact pattern of mutual interaction and respective areas of responsibility would require to be worked out in detail, but it may perhaps be suggested that this solution is the most likely to lead to a fruitful and mutually satisfying collaboration.

In advocating such collaboration, it should of course be understood that the psychologist we have in mind would differ very considerably in training and background from the present-day type of clinical psychologist, with his major interest in psychoanalysis, psychotherapy, and projective methods of personality assessment. We have in mind someone with a good background in the exact sciences and mathematics, with a solid foundation in learning theory and perception, and experience in the use of the experimental method and of statistics in a clinical setting. Only a psychologist so equipped can make the essential contribution to psychiatry which the physiologist makes to general medicine.

ledge of a patient's position on the extravert-introvert continuum will often be of considerable use in determining the type of treatment or re-training which is most likely to prove efficacious in changing his habit-family hierarchy.

BIBLIOGRAPHY AND AUTHOR INDEX

Numbers in italic type at the end of each entry refer to
the page on which the reference is quoted.

ADAMS, D. K. Learning and explanation. In: *Learning theory, personality theory, and clinical research.* New York: John Wiley & Sons, 1954. *78.*

ALGUERNO, P. F. El replejo condicionado de avercion en el alcoholismo cronico. *Bol. Col. med. Camaquey*, 1948, 11, 42-4. *268.*

ALLES, G. A., & FEIGER, G. A. The influence of benzedrine on work decrement and patellar reflex. *Amer. J. Physiol.*, 1942, 136, 392-400. *239.*

ALLPORT, G. W. *Personality.* London: Constable, 1937. *72.*

ALPERN, U. Meta contrast. *J. opt. Soc. Amer.*, 1953, 43, 640-57. *176.*

AMMONS, R. B., & AMMONS, C. H. Bilateral transfer of rotary pursuit skill. *Amer. Psychologist*, 1951, 6, 294. *56.*

AMMONS, C. H. An experimental study of temporary and permanent inhibition effects associated with acquisition of a simple perceptual motor skill. Unpublished Ph.D. Thesis, University of Kentucky, 1955. *56.*

ARDEN, G. B., & WEALE, R. A. Nervous mechanisms and dark adaptation. *J. Physiol.*, 1954, 125, 417-26. *170.*

ARDIS, J. A., & FRASER, E. Personality and perception: the constancy effect and introversion. *Brit. J. Psychol.*, 1957, 48, 48-54. *28.*

ASCH, S. E. *Social psychology.* New York: Prentice Hall, 1952. *214.*

ASCH, S. Studies of independence and submission to group pressure. I. A minority of one against a unanimous majority. Swarthmore: Pre-publication copy. *214.*

AXELROD, H. S., COWEN, G. L., & HEILIZER, F. The correlates of manifest anxiety in stylus maze learning. *J. exper. Psychol.*, 1956, 51, 131-8. *101.*

BABCOCK, H. *Dementia praecox: a psychological study.* Lancaster, Pa.: Science Press, 1933. *268.*

BARMACK, J. E. The effect of benzedrine sulphate upon the report of boredom and other factors. *J. Psychol.*, 1938, 5, 125-33. *237.*

BARMACK, J. E. Studies of the psychophysiology of boredom: Part I, Effect of 15 mgs. of benzedrine sulphate and 60 mgs. of ephedrine hydrochloride on blood pressure, report of boredom, and other factors. *J. exper. Psychol.*, 1939, 25, 494-505. *237.*

BARMACK, J. E. The time of administration and some effects of 2 grs. of alkaloid caffeine. *J. exper. Psychol.*, 1940, 27, 690-8. *237, 239.*

BARTLETT, M. S. Further aspects of the theory of multiple regression. *Proc. Camb. phil. Soc.*, 1938, 34, 33-40. *17.*

BARTLETT, M. S. The general canonical correlation distribution. *Annmath. Statist.*, 1947, 18, 1–17. *16, 17.*

BAUMGARDT, E. Les théories photochimiques classiques et quantiques de la vision et l'inhibition nerveuse en vision liminaire. Paris: Editions de la Revue d'Optique, 1950. *170.*

BAUMGARDT, E., & SEGAL, J. Facilitation et Inhibition. *L'année Psychologique*, 1947, 43–53, 54–102. *176.*

BEAM, J. C. Serial learning and conditioning under real life stress. *J. abnorm. soc. Psychol.*, 1955, 51, 543–51. *101.*

BEECH, R. An investigation of the performance on a perceptual motor task by psychiatric patients, with special reference to brain damage. London: Ph.D. Thesis, 1956. *185.*

BEITEL, H. J., Jr. Inhibition of threshold excitation in the human eye. *J. gen. Psychol.*, 1936, 14, 31–61. *176.*

BENDER, M. B. Changes in sensory adaptation time and after-sensations with lesions of parital lobe. *Arch. Neurol. Psychiat.*, 1946, 55, 299–319. *183.*

BENDER, M. B. *Disorders in perception.* Springfield: C. C. Thomas, 1952. *178, 240.*

BENDER, M., & TEUBER, N. C. Disturbance in visual perception following cerebral lesions. *J. Psychol.*, 1949, 28, 223–33. *171.*

BERG, O. A study of the effect of Evipan on the flicker fusion intensity in brain injuries. *Acta psychiatrica & neurol.*, 1949, Supp. 58. *223.*

BERRIEN, F. K. Finger oscillations as indices of emotion. I. Preliminary validation. *J. exper. Psychol.*, 1939, 24, 485–98. *135.*

BEST, F. Hemianopsie und Seelenblindheit bei Hirnverletzungen. *Arch. f. Ophth.*, 1917, 93, 49–64. *178.*

BIANCHI, L. *Textbook of Psychiatry*, London, 1906. *201.*

BIDWELL, S. The negative after-images following brief retinal excitation. *Proc. Royal Soc.*, London, 1897, 61, 268–71. *241.*

BIESHEUVEL, S. The measurement of threshold for flicker and its value as a perseveration test. *Brit. J. Psychol.*, 1938, 29, 27–38. *198.*

BIESHEUVEL, S., & PITT, D. Q. The relationship between secondary function and some aspects of speed and tempo of behaviour. *Acta Psychol.*, 1955, 11, 373–96. *197, 198.*

BIESHEUVEL, S., & PITT, D. Q. Some tests of speed and tempo of behaviour as predictors of the primary–secondary function temperament variable. *J. Nat. Inst. Personnel Res.*, 1955, 6, 87–94. *197, 198.*

BILLS, A. G. Blocking: a new principle of mental fatigue. *Amer. J. Psychol.*, 1931, 43, 230–45. *64, 67.*

BILLS, A. G. Fatigue, oscillations and blocks. *J. exper. Psychol.*, 1935, 18, 562–73. *64.*

BILLS, A. G. *The psychological efficiency.* New York: Harper, 1943. *64, 67.*

BILLS, A. G., & SHAPIRO, K. J. Mental fatigue under automatically controlled rates of work. *J. general Psychol.*, 1936, 15, 335–47. *65.*

BILLS, A. G., & MCTEER, W. Transfer of fatigue and identical elements. *J. exper. Psychol.*, 1932, 15, 23–36. *66.*

BINDRA, P., PATERSON, A. L., & STRZELECKI, J. On the relation between anxiety and conditioning. *Canad. J. Psychol.*, 1955, 9, 1–6. *125.*

BIRCH, H. G., & BITTERMAN, M. E. Sensory integration and cognitive theory. *Psychol. Rev.*, 1951, 58, 355–61. *209.*

BITTERMAN, N. G., & HOLTZMAN, J. H. Conditioning and extinction of the galvanic skin response as a function of anxiety. *J. abnorm. soc. Psychol.*, 1952, 47, 615–23. *92.*

BLEULER, E. *Affektivität, Suggestibilität, Paranoia.* Halle: C. Marbold, 1906. *135.*

BLEULER, E. *Dementia praecox or the group of schizophrenias.* New York: Int. Univ. Press, 1950. *186.*

BLUM, G. S. *Psychoanalytic theories of personality.* New York: McGraw-Hill, 1953. *8.*

BONIN, G., GARAL, H. W., & MCCULLOCH, W. S. The functional organization of the occipital lobes. *Birl. Symposia*, 1942, 7, 165–92. *175.*

BOOR, W. DE. *Pharmakopsychologie und Psychopathologie.* Berlin: Springer, 1956. *223.*

BOWDITCH, H. P., & WARREN, J. S. The kneejerk and its physiological modification. *J. Physiol.*, 1890, 11, 25–64. *177.*

BRAND, H. (Ed.) *The study of personality,* New York: J. Wiley & Sons, 1954. *75, 77, 190.*

BRENGELMANN, J. C. Figurrekonstruktion: Grösse und Variabilität der Grösse von Reproduktionen als Bestimmer der Extraversion-Introversion. *Mschr. Psychiat. Neurol.*, 1955, 130, 209–33. *187.*

BRENGELMANN, J. C. Positionseffekte und ihre Beziehung zur Extraversion und Psychose. *Arch. Psychiat. & Neurol.*, 1955, 193, 526–43. *187.*

BRENGELMANN, J. C. Figurkonstruktion: Rotationsfehler und Rotationsvariabilität als Indikatoren der Persönlichkeit, vorzüglich der Psychose. *Fol. Psychiat., Neurol., Neurochir., Neerl.*, 1956, 59, 230–54. *187.*

BRENGELMANN, J. C. Figurrekonstruktion: Psychose und Bewegungsausdruck. *Wiener Arch. Psychol., Psychiat. & Neurol.*, to appear. *187.*

BRENGELMANN, J. C. Grösse und Veränderung der Grösse von Reproduktionen als Mass des Bewegungsausdrucks. *Ztschr. f. diag. Psychol., u. Persönlichkeitsf.*, 1955, 3, 23–33. *187.*

BRENGELMANN, J. C. Der visuelle Objekterkennungstest. *Ztsch. f. exper. u. angew. Psychol.*, 1953, 1, 422–52. *18.*

BRENGELMANN, J. C., & PINILLOS, J. L. Le test de reconstruction de figures. *Rev. de psychol. appl.*, 1954, 4, 187–202. *18.*

BRENGELMANN, J. C., & PINILLOS, J. Bilderkemung als Persoenlichkeitstest *Zsch. f. exper. u. angew. Psychol.*, 1953, 1, 480–500. *18.*

BRENNER, MAY. Continuous stimulation and apparent movement. *Amer. J. Psychol.*, 1953, 66, 494–5. *171.*

BRENNER, MAY. An experimental investigation of apparent movement. London: Ph.D. Thesis, 1953. *171, 174.*

BRENNER, M. W. The effects of brain damage on the perception of apparent movement. *J. Personality*, 1956, 25, 202–12. *171.*

BRILL, N. Q., & BEEBE, G. W. A follow-up study of war neuroses. Washington: Medical monograph, 1955. *266.*

BROADBENT, D. E. The twenty dials test under quiet conditions. Cambridge: Appl. Psychol. Unit Rep. No. 130, 1950. *128.*

BROADBENT, D. E. The twenty dials and twenty lights test under noisy conditions. Cambridge: Appl. Psychol. Unit Rep. No. 160, 1951. *128*.

BROADBENT, D. E. Classical conditioning and human watch-keeping. *Psychol. Rev.*, 1953, 60, 331–9. *128*.

BROADBENT, D. E. Inhibition and extraversion. *Quarterly Bull., Brit. Psychol. Soc.*, 1956, 29, 13. *128*.

BROADHURST, A. Some variables affecting speed of mental functioning in schizophrenics. University of London: Ph.D. Thesis, 1956. *268*.

BROADHURST, P. L. Determinants of emotionality in the rat. I. Situational factors. *Brit. J. Psychol.*, 1957, 48, 1–12. *98*.

BROADHURST, P. L. Determinants of emotionality in the rat. II. Antecedent factors. To appear, 1957. *98*.

BROADHURST, P. Emotionality in the rat: a study of its determinants, inheritance and relation to some aspects of motivation. London : Ph.D. Thesis, 1956. *95*.

BROCK, L. G., COOMBS, J. S., & ECCLES, J. C. The recording of potentials from motor neurones with an intracellular electrode, *J. Physiol.*, 1952, 117, 431–60. *191*.

BROWN, J. S., & JACOBS, A. The role of fear in the motivation and acquisition of responses. *J. exper. Psychol.*, 1949, 39, 743–59. *210*.

BRUNSWICK, E. The conceptual framework of psychology. *International Encyclopedia of Unified Science 1*. No. 10. Chicago: University of Chicago Press, 1952. *76*.

BUCHWALD, A. E., & YAMAGUCHI, H. G. The effect of change in drive level on habit reversal. *J. exper. Psychol.*, 1955, 50, 265–8. *101*.

BUGALSKII, I. P. On one of the tasks of the psychoneurological dispensary. *Zh. Nevropat. Psikhat.*, 1952, 52, 65–6. *268*.

BUMKE, O. *Lehrbuch der Geisteskrankheiten*. Munich, 1948. *202, 205*.

BUTLER, J. M. Prospects and perspectives in psychotherapeutic theory and research. In: *Learning theory, personality theory, and clinical research*. New York: J. Wiley & Sons, 1954. *85*.

BYKOV, R. M. New data on the physiology and pathology of the cerebral cortex. Communication to the 19th Internat. Physiol. Congress, Montreal, 1953. *269*.

CAIN, P. A. Individual differences in susceptibility to monotony. Ph.D. dissertation, Cornell Univ., 1942. (Quoted by Ryan, T. A., *Work and effort*. New York: Ronald, 1947.) *134*.

CALVIN, A. D., CLIFFORD, L. T., CLIFFORD, B., BOLDEN, L., & HARVEY, J. Experimental validation of conditioned inhibition. *Psychol. Rep.*, 1956, 2, 51–6. *277*.

CANESTRARI, R. Sindromi psichiatriche e rigidita percettiva. *Riv. experimentale di Freniatria*, 1957, 81, 1–10. *28*.

CARL, G. B., & TURNER, J. B. The effects of benzedrine sulphate on performance in a comprehensive psychometric examination. *J. Psychol.*, 1939, 8, 165–216. *239*.

CARL, G. B., & TURNER, J. B. A further report on benzedrine sulphate (amphetamine sulphate): Psychophysical effects, and supplementary results from a fifth experimental group. *J. gen. Psychol.*, 1940, 22, 105–91. *239*.

CARLSON, V. R. Individual differences in the recall of word-association test words. Ph.D. Thesis. Johns Hopkins Univ., 1953. Quoted by Eriksen & Daniels, 1955. *216*.

CASTANEDA, A., & PELERMO, D. S. Psychomotor performance as a function of amount of training and stress. *J. exper. Psychol.*, 1955, 50, 175–9. *101*.

CATTELL, R. B. Second-order personality factors in the questionnaire realm. To appear, 1957. *J. consult. Psychol. 32.*

CATTELL, R. B., SAUNDERS, D. R., & STILL, G. F. The sixteen personality factor questionnaire. I.P.A.T., 1602, Coronado Dr., Champaign, Ill., 1949. *32*.

CHENEY, R. H. Comparative effect of caffein per se and a caffeine beverage (coffee) upon the reaction time in normal young adults. *J. Pharmacol. & Exp. Therap.*, 1935, 53, 304–13. *239*

CHENEY, R. H. Reaction time behaviour after caffeine and coffee consumption. *J. exper. Psychol.*, 1936, 19, 357–69. *239*.

CHERRY, E. C., SAYERS, B. MCA., & MARLAND, PAULINE M. Experiments on the complete suppression of stammering. *Nature, Lond.*, 1955, 176, 874–5. *268*.

CHERRY, C., & SAYERS, B. H. Experiments upon the total inhibition of stammering by external control, and some clinical results. *J. psychosom. Res.*, 1956, 1, 233–46. *268*.

CHILD, I. L. Personality. *Annual Rev. of Psychol.*, 1954, 5, 149–70. *100*.

CHYATTE, C. The relation of cortical potentials to perceptual functions. *Genet. Psychol. Monogr.*, 1954, 50, 189–266. *198*.

CLARIDGE, G. S. Factors affecting the motivation and performance of imbeciles. London: Ph.D. Thesis, 1956. *128*.

COHEN, B. D., KALISH, H. I., THURSTON, J. D., & COHEN, E. Experimental manipulation of verbal behavior. *J. exper. Psychol.*, 1954, 47, 106–10. *213*.

COHN, R. The occipital alpha rhythm: a study in phase variations. *J. Neurophysiol.*, 1948, 11, 31–7. *198*.

CRONBACH, L. J., & MEEHL, P. E. Construct validity in psychological tests. *Psychol. Bull.*, 1955, 52, 281–302. *261*.

CROSBY, H. O. Essential enuresis: successful treatment based on physiological concepts. *Med. J. Australia*, 1950, 2, 533–43. *268*.

CROZIER, W. J. The study of living organisms. In: Murchison, C. (Ed.), *The foundations of experimental psychology*. Worcester: Clark Univ. Press, 1929, 45–127. *77*.

CRUTCHFIELD, R. S. Conformity and character. *Amer. Psychologist*, 1955, 10, 191–8. *214*.

CULLER, E. Nature of the learning curve. *Psychol. Bull.*, 1928, 742–3. *79*.

CULLER, E. A. Observations on direct cortical stimulation in the dog. *Psychol. Bull.*, 1938, 35, 687–8. *43*.

CULLER, E., & GIRDEN, E. The learning curve in relation to other psychometric functions. *Amer. J. Psychol.*, 1951, 64, 327–49. *79*.

CUTHBERTSON, R. G., & KNOX, J. G. G. The effect of analeptics on the fatigued subject. *J. Physiol.*, 1947, 106, 47–58. *239*.

DARROW, C. W., & HEATH, L. C. Reaction tendencies relating to personality. In: *Studies in the dynamics of behavior.* (Ed. Lashley, R. S.) Chicago: Univ. of Chicago Press, 1932. *92*.

DARROW, W. Psychological effects of drugs. *Psychol. Bull.*, 1929, 26, 527–45. *223.*

DAVIDSON, J. A., & DOUGLASS, E. Nocturnal enuresis: a special approach to treatment. *Brit. Med. J.*, 1950, 1345–7. *268.*

DAVIS, D. R. Neurotic predisposition and the disorganization observed in experiments with the Cambridge Cockpit. *J. Neurol., Neurosurg., & Psychiat.*, 1946, 9, 119–24. *135.*

DAVIS, D. R. *Pilot error—some laboratory experiments.* London: H.M.S.O., 1948. *135.*

DAVIS, D. R. The disorder of skill responsible for accidents. *Quart. J. Exper. Psychol.*, 1949, 1, 136–42. *136.*

DAVIS, D. R. Increase in strength of a secondary drive as a cause of disorganization. *Quart. J. exper. Psychol.*, 1948, 1, 22–8. *136.*

DE, B. A study of the validity of the word association technique for the differentiation of normal and abnormal persons. Univ. of London, Ph.D. Thesis, 1953. *268.*

DEESE, J., LAZARUS, R. S., & KEENAN, J. Anxiety, anxiety-reduction, and stress in learning. *J. exper. Psychol.*, 1953, 46, 55–60. *101.*

DELGADO, H. Curso di psychiatrica. Lima: Santa Maria, 1953. *202.*

DENNIS, W. Spontaneous alternation in rats as an indicator of the persistence of stimulus effects. *J. comp. Psychol.*, 1939, 28, 305–12. *56.*

DENNY, M. B., FRISBY, N., & WEAVER, J. Rotary pursuit under alternate conditions of distributed and massed practice. *J. exper. Psychol.*, 1955, 49, 48–54. *71.*

DETHERAGE, B. H., & BITTERMAN, M. E. The effect of satiation on stroboscopic movement. *Amer. J. Psychol.*, 1952, 65, 108–9. *171.*

DODGE, R. The law of relative fatigue. *Psychol. Rev.*, 1917, 24, 89–113. *67.*

DODGE, R. Theories of inhibition. *Psychol. Rev.*, 1928, 33, 106–22, 167–87. *67, 192.*

DODGE, R. *Human Variability.* New Haven: Yale Univ. Press, 1931. *67.*

DODGE, R. The protective wink reflex. *Amer. J. Psychol.*, 1913, 24, 1–7. *177.*

DUNCAN, C. P. On the similarity between reactive inhibition and neural satiation. *Amer. J. Psychol.*, 1956, 69, 227–35. *150.*

DUNCKER, K. Some preliminary experiments on the mutual influence of pains. *Psychol. Forsch.*, 1937, 21, 311–26. *176.*

DUNLAP, K. *Habits, their making and unmaking.* New York: Liveright, 1932. *277.*

EBBINGHAUS, H. *Memory.* New York: Teachers Coll., 1913 (original: 1885). *78.*

ECCLES, J. C. *The neurophysiological basis of mind.* Oxford: Clarendon Press, 1953. *191.*

ELLIS, D. S. Inhibition theory and the effort variable. *Psychol. Rev.*, 1953, 60, 383–92. *55.*

ELSBERG, C., & SPOTNITZ, H. The neural components of light and dark adaptation and their significance for the duration of the foveal dark adaptation process. *Bull. Neurol. Inst.*, N.Y., 1938, 7, 148–59. *170.*

ENROTH, C. The mechanism of flicker and fusion studied on single retinal elements in the dark-adapted eye of the cat. *Acta Physiologica Scandinavica*, 1952, 27, Suppl. 100. *195.*

ERIKSEN, C. W. Individual differences in defensive forgetting. *J. exper. Psychol.*, 1952, 44, 442–6. *216*.

ERIKSEN, C. W. Psychological defences and 'ego-strength' in the recall of completed and incompleted tasks. *J. abnorm. soc. Psychol.*, 1954, 49, 45–50. *28, 216*.

ERIKSEN, C. W. Subception: fact or artifact? *Psychol. Rev.*, 1956, 63, 74–80. *213*.

ERIKSEN, C. W. Some personality correlates of stimulus generalization under stress. *J. abnorm. soc. Psychol.*, 1954, 49, 562–6. *216*.

ERIKSEN, C. W., & DAVIDS, A. The meaning and clinical validity of the Taylor anxiety scale and the hysteria-psychasthenia scale from the M.M.P.I. *J. abn. soc. Psychol.*, 1955, 50, 135–7. *32, 216*.

ERIKSEN, C. W., & KUETHE, J. L. Avoidance conditioning of verbal behavior without awareness: a paradigm of repression. *J. abnorm. soc. Psychol.*, 1956, 53, 203–9. *28, 216*.

EVANS, C. L. In: *Recent advances in physiology*, 4th Ed. Philadelphia: Blakiston, 1930. *228*.

EYSENCK, H. J. Types of personality—a factorial study of 700 neurotics. *J. ment. Sci.*, 1944, 90, 851–61. *27*.

EYSENCK, H. J. *Dimensions of Personality*. London: Kegan Paul, 1947. *9, 14, 26, 28, 103, 137, 200*.

EYSENCK, H. J. The effects of psychotherapy: an evaluation. *J. consult. Psychol.*, 1952, 16, 319–24. *8, 85, 265, 266*.

EYSENCK, H. J. *The scientific study of personality*. London: Routledge & Kegan Paul, 1952. *8, 9, 15, 17, 22, 33, 88, 103, 138, 267*.

EYSENCK, H. J. *The structure of human personality*. London: Methuen, 1953. *15, 26, 28, 31, 32, 88, 160, 197, 206, 261*.

EYSENCK, H. J. The logical basis of factor analysis. *Amer. Psychol.*, 1953, 8, 105–14. *152*.

EYSENCK, H. J. La rapidité du fonctionnement mental comme mesure de l'anomalie mentale. *Rev. de Psychol. appl.*, 1953, 3, 367–77. *18, 268*.

EYSENCK, H. J. *Uses and abuses of psychology*. London: Pelican, 1953. *18, 251, 280*.

EYSENCK, H. J. *Psychology of politics*. London: Routledge & Kegan Paul, 1954. *28, 214, 217*.

EYSENCK, H. J. *Psychology and the foundations of psychiatry*. London: H. K. Lewis, 1955. *259 f*.

EYSENCK, H. J. Psychiatric diagnosis as a psychological and statistical problem. *Psychol. Reports*, 1955, 1, 3–17. *17*.

EYSENCK, H. J. A dynamic theory of anxiety and hysteria. *J. ment. Sci.*, 1955, 101, 28–51. *229*.

EYSENCK, H. J. Cortical inhibition, figural after-effect, and the theory of personality. *J. abnorm. soc. Psychol.*, 1955, 51, 94–106. *28, 250, 153, 155*.

EYSENCK, H. J. Review: Rogers & Dymond, Psychotherapy and personality. *Brit. J. Psychol.*, 1955, 46, 237–8. *267*.

EYSENCK, H. J. Review of French: Kit of selected tests for reference aptitude and achievement factors. *Psychometrika*, 1955, 20, 168–9. *131*.

EYSENCK, H. J. Reminiscence, drive and personality theory. *J. abn. soc. Psychol.*, 1956, 53, 328–33. *28, 125, 153, 254*.

EYSENCK, H. J. The inheritance of extraversion-introversion. *Acta Psychol.*, 1956, 12, 95–110. *28, 279.*

EYSENCK, H. J. The questionnaire measurement of neuroticism and extraversion. *Rivista di Psicologia*, 1956, 50, 113-40. *28, 31, 120, 126, 214.*

EYSENCK, H. J. 'Warm-up' in pursuit rotor learning as a function of the extinction of conditioned inhibition. *Acta Psychol.*, 1956, 12, 349–70. *62, 126, 154, 253.*

EYSENCK, H. J. A new method in psychotherapy. *Medical World*, 1957, 86, 333–6. *259 f.*

EYSENCK, H. J. *Sense and Nonsense in Psychology*. London: Pelican Books, 1957. *260, 267.*

EYSENCK, H. J. Drugs and Personality: 1. Theory and methodology. *J. ment. Sci.*, 1957, 103, 119–31. *229.*

EYSENCK, H. J. Personality tests: 1950–1955. In: Fleming, G. W. T. H. (Ed.) *Recent progress in Psychiatry*. London: J. & A. Churchill, 1957. *89, 103, 148, 260.*

EYSENCK, H. J., & AIBA, S. Drugs and Personality: 5. The effects of stimulant and depressant drugs on the suppression of the primary visual stimulus. *J. ment. Sci.*, to appear, 1957. *241.*

EYSENCK, H. J., CASEY, S., & TROUTON, D. S. Drugs and Personality: 2. The effect of stimulant and depressant drugs on continuous work. *J. ment. Sci.*, 1957, to appear. *241.*

EYSENCK, H. J., GRANGER, G. W., & BRENGELMANN, J. C. *Perceptual processes and mental illness*. Maudsley Monograph Series, 1957. London: Chapman & Hall. *18, 148.*

EYSENCK, H. J., & HIMMELWEIT, H. T. An experimental study of the reactions of neurotics to experiences of success and failure. *J. gen. Psychol.*, 1946, 35, 59–75. *28.*

EYSENCK, H. J., HOLLAND, H., & TROUTON, D. S. Drugs and Personality: 3. The effects of stimulant and depressant drugs on visual after-effects. *J. ment. Sci.*, 1957, to appear. *241.*

EYSENCK, H. J., HOLLAND, H., & TROUTON, D. S. Drugs and Personality: 4. The effects of stimulant and depressant drugs on the rate of fluctuation of a reversible perspective figure. *J. ment. Sci.*, 1957, to appear. *241.*

EYSENCK, H. J., & PRELL, D. The inheritance of neuroticism: an experimental study. *J. ment. Sci.*, 1951, 97, 441, 465. *279.*

EYSENCK, S. B. G. A dimensional analysis of mental abnormality. Ph.D. Thesis, Univ. of London, 1955. *22.*

EYSENCK, S. B. G. Neurosis and psychosis: an experimental analysis. *J. ment. Sci.*, 1956, 102, 517–29. *22.*

EYSENCK, S. B. G. An experimental study of psychogalvanic reflex responses of normal, neurotic and psychotic subjects. *J. psychosom. Res.*, 1956, 1, 258–72. *154.*

FARBER, I. E. Response fixation under anxiety and non-anxiety conditions. *J. exper. Psychol.*, 1948, 38, 111–31. *210.*

FARBER, I. E. Anxiety as a drive state. In: Jones, M. R. (Ed.): Nebraska Symposium on Motivation. Nebraska: Univ. of Nebraska Press, 1954. *100.*

FARBER, I. E., & SPENCE, K. W. Complex learning and conditioning as a function of anxiety. *J. exper. Psychol.*, 1953, 45, 120-5. *101.*

FISHER, R. A. The statistical utilization of multiple measurements. *Ann. Eug.*, 1938, 8, 376-86. *17.*

FISHER, R. A. Use of multiple measurements in taxonomic problems. *Ann. Eug.*, 1936, 7, 179-88. *16.*

FOULDS, G. A. Temperamental differences in maze performance. *Brit. J. Psychol.*, 1951, 42, 209-17; 1952, 43, 33-41. *28, 200.*

FOULDS, G. A. A method of scoring the T.A.T. applied to psychoneurotics. *J. ment. Sci.*, 1953, 99, 235-46. *28.*

FOULDS, G. A. The ratio of general intellectual ability to vocabulary among psychoneurotics. *Internat. J. Soc. Psychiat.*, 1956, 1, 5-12. *28, 200.*

FRANKS, C. M. An experimental study of conditioning as related to mental abnormality. Ph.D. Thesis, Univ. of London, 1954. *115.*

FRANKS, C. M. A conditioning laboratory for the investigation of personality and cortical functioning. *Nature*, 1955, 175, 984-5. *115.*

FRANKS, C. M. Recidivism, psychopathy and personality. *Brit. J. Delinquency*, 1956, 6, 192-201. *214.*

FRANKS, C. M. Conditioning and personality; a study of normal and neurotic subjects. *J. abn. & soc. Psychol.*, 1956, 52, 143-50. *28, 115.*

FRANKS, C. M. The Taylor scale and the dimensional analysis of anxiety. *Rev. Psychol. appl.*, 1956, 6, 35-44. *88, 93.*

FRANKS, C. M. Personality factors and the rate of conditioning. *Brit. J. Psychol.*, 1957, 48, 119-26. *28, 120.*

FRANKS, C. M. Effect of food, drink and tobacco deprivation on the conditioning of the eyeblink response. *J. exp. Psychol.*, 1957, 53, 117-20. *93.*

FRANKS, C. M., & LAVERTY, S. G. Sodium amytal and eyelid conditioning. *J. ment. Sci.*, 1955, 101, 654-63. *233.*

FRANKS, C. M., SOUIEF, M. I., & MAXWELL, A. E. A factorial study of certain scales from the MMPI and the STDCR. To appear, 1957. *32, 123.*

FRANKS, C. M., & TROUTON, D. S. The effects of stimulant and depressant drugs upon conditioning in man. To appear, 1957. *233.*

FRANKS, C. M., & WILLETT, R. A. Algumas sugestoes subre a canduta delinquente. *Rev. de Psicologia norm. e. pat.*, 1954, 2, 3-10. *214.*

FRANKS, C. M., & WITHERS, W. C. R. Photoelectric recording of eyelid movements. *Am. J. Psychol.*, 1955, 68, 467-71. *40.*

FRASER, R. The incidence of neurosis among factory workers. M.R.C. Industrial Health Res. Board Report No. 90. H.M.S.O., 1947. *21.*

FREEMAN, E., & JOSEY, W. E. Quantitative index to memory impairment. *Arch. neurol. Psychiat.*, 1949, 62, 794-7. *164.*

FREEMAN, G. L., & WONDERLIC, E. F. Periodicity of performance. *Amer. J. Psychol.*, 1935, 47, 149-51. *65.*

FRIEDL, F. G. Anxiety and cortical alpha in normal subjects. Studies in Psychol. & Psychiat., Cath. Univ. Amer., 1954, 9, No. 2. *197.*

FURNEAUX, D. Some speed, error and difficulty relationships within a problem solving situation. *Nature*, 1952, 170, 37-8. *17.*

FURNEAUX, D. Manual of Nufferno Speed Tests. *Nat. Found. Educ. Res.*, 1955. *18, 132.*

BIBLIOGRAPHY AND AUTHOR INDEX

FURNEAUX, D. Manual of Nufferno Level Tests. *Nat. Found. Educ. Res.*, 1955. *18, 132.*

GAIER, E. L. Selected personality variables and the learning process. *Psychol. Monogr.*, 1952, 66, No. 17. *101.*

GALLESE, G. J. Spiral after-effect as a test of organic brain damage. *J. Clin. Psychol.*, 1956, 12, 254–8. *164.*

GALLI, A. On the perception of apparent movement produced by various sensory stimuli. Publ. Univ. Cathol. S. Cuore, 1931, 5, 79–122. (Quoted by Brenner, M.)

GANTT, W. H. *Experimental basis for neurotic behavior.* London: Hoeber, 1944. *78.*

GANTT, W. H. The conditioned reflex function as an aid in the study of the psychiatric patient. In: *Relation of psychological tests to psychiatry.* Hoch, P. V., & Zubin, J. (Eds.) New York: Grune & Stratton, 1950. *146.*

GARNER, W. R., HAKE, H. W., & ERIKSEN, C. W. Operationism and the concept of perception. *Psychol. Rev.*, 1956, 63, 149–59. *149.*

GASTAUT, H., ROGER, A., CORRIOL, J., & NAQUET, R. Etude electrographique du cycle d'excitabilité cortical. *E. E. G. Clin. Neurophysiol.*, 1951, 3, 401–28. *198.*

GERARD, M. The psychogenic tic in ego development. In: Freud, A. (Ed.): *Psychoanalytic study of the child.* Vol. 2, New York: Inter. Univ. Press. Inc., 1946. *275.*

GILES, G. H. *The practice of orthoptics.* London: Hammond, 1945. *19.*

GILLILAND, A. R., & NELSON, D. The effects of coffee on certain mental and physiological functions. *J. gen. Psychol.*, 1939, 21, 339–48. *239.*

GLANZER, M. The role of stimulus satiation in spontaneous alternation. *J. exper. Psychol.*, 1953, 45, 387–93. *56.*

GLANZER, M. Stimulus satiation: an explanation of spontaneous alternation and related phenomena. *Psychol. Rev.*, 1953, 60, 257–69. *56.*

GLEITMAN, H., NACHUIRAS, J., & NEISSER, U. The S.R. reinforcement theory of extinction. *Psychol. Rev.*, 1954, 61, 23–33. *277.*

GOLDSTEIN, K. *After-effects of brain injuries in war.* New York: Grune & Stratton, 1942. *178.*

GOLDSTEIN, K., & SCHEERER, M. Abstract and concrete behaviour. *Psychol. Monogr.*, 1941, 53, No. 2. *178.*

GOLDSTONE, S. Flicker fusion measurements and anxiety level. *J. exper. Psychol.*, 1955, 49, 200–2. *196.*

GOODMAN, L. S., & GILMAN, A. *The pharmacological basis of therapeutics.* New York: Macmillan, 1955. *229.*

GORDON, S. Some effects of incentives on the behaviour of imbeciles. London: Ph.D. Thesis, 1953. *128.*

GORDON, W. M., & BERLYNE, D. E. Drive-level and flexibility in paired associate nonsense-syllable learning. *Quart. J. exp. Psychol.*, 1954, 6, 181–5. *101.*

GRAHAM, C. H. Behaviour and the psychophysical methods: an analysis of some recent experiments. *Psychol. Rev.*, 1952, 59, 62–70. *176.*

GRAHAM, C. H., & GRANIT, R. Inhibition, summation and synchronization of impulses in the retina. *Amer. J. Physiol.*, 1931, 98, 664–73. *176.*

291

GRANGER, G. W. Personality and visual perception: a review. *J. ment. Sci.*, 1953, 99, 8–43. *18, 148.*

GRANGER, G. W. The night visual ability of psychiatric patients. *Brit. J. physiol. Opt.*, 1954, 11, 238–44. *166.*

GRANGER, G. W. Dark adaptation in neurotic patients. *J. ment. Sci.*, 1955, 101, 354–62. *166.*

GRANGER, G. W. Dark adaptation time in neurotic patients. *Brit. J. physiol. Opt.*, 1956, 13, 234–41. *166.*

GRANGER, G. W. Effect of psychiatric disorders on visual thresholds. *Science*, 1957, 125, 500–1. *166.*

GRANGER, G. W. Night vision and psychiatric disorder: a review of experimental studies. *J. ment. Sci.*, 1957, 103, 48–79. *166.*

GRANGER, G. W. Eysenck's theory of anxiety and hysteria, and the results of visual adaptation experiments. To appear. *Acta Psychologica*, 1957. *166, 176, 193, 194.*

GRANGER, G. W. Retinal inhibition and visual perception. To appear, 1957. *166.*

GRANIT, R. *Sensory mechanisms of the retina.* London: Oxford Univ. Press, 1947. *192 f.*

GRANIT, R. Sight and the physiology of the retina. *Acta Psychol. Fenn.*, 1951, 1, 21–9. *192, 194, 195.*

GRANIT, R. *Receptors and sensory perception.* New Haven: Yale Univ. Press, 1955. *192 f.*

GRANIT, R., MUNSHERLIGELM, A., & FEVI, U. The relation between concentration of visual purple and retinal sensitivity to light during dark adaptation. *J. Physiol.*, 1939, 96, 31–44. *170.*

GRANIT, R., & RIDDELL, R. A. The electrical responses of light and dark-adapted frog's eyes to rhythmic and continuous stimuli. *J. Physiol.*, 1934, 81, 1–28. *170.*

GRAVELY, A. Perceptual tests in personality research. Ph.D. Thesis, Univ. of London, 1950. *196.*

GRAY, M. G., & TROWBRIDGE, G. B. Methods for investigating the effects of drugs on psychological functions. *Psychol. Rev.*, 1942, 5, 127–48. *223.*

GREENSPOON, J. J. The reinforcing effect of two spoken sounds on the frequency of two responses. *Amer. J. Psychol.*, 1955, 68, 409–16. *213.*

GRICE, G. R., & REYNOLDS, B. Effect of varying amounts of rest on conventional and bilateral transfer 'reminiscence'. *J. exper. Psychol.*, 1952, 44, 247–52. *56.*

GROSS, O. *Die cerebrale Sekundärfunktion.* Leipzig: 1902. *197.*

GUTHRIE, E. R. *The psychology of learning.* (Rev. Ed.) New York: Harper, 1952. *213.*

HAIG, C. The course of rod dark adaptation as influenced by the intensity and duration of pre-adaptation to light. *J. gen. Physiol.*, 1941, 24, 735–51. *166, 169.*

HALL, C. S. Emotional behavior in the rat. I. Defecation and urination as measures of individual differences in emotionality. *J. comp. Psychol.*, 1934, 18, 385–403. *98.*

HALL, J. Some conditions of anxiety extinction. *J. abnorm. soc. Psychol.*, 1955, 51, 126–32. *210.*

HAMILTON, M. The personality of dyspeptics. *Brit. J. med. Psychol.*, 1950, 23, 182–98. *17, 19.*

HANVIK, L. J. A note on rotations in the Bender-Gestalt test on predictors of EEG abnormalities in children. *J. clin. Psychol.*, 1953, 9, 399. *180.*

HANVIK, L. J., & ANDERSSEN, A. L. The effect of focal brain lesions on recall and on the production of rotations in the Bender-Gestalt test. *J. consult. Psychol.*, 1950, 14, 197–8. *180.*

HAUTY, G. T., & PAYNE, R. B. Mitigation of work decrement. *J. exper. Psychol.*, 1955, 49, 60–7. *239.*

HEAD, H. *Studies in neurology.* London: Oxford Univ. Press, 1920. *183.*

HEAD, A., & HOLMES, G. Sensory disturbances from cerebral lesions. *Brain*, 1911, 34, 102–254. *178.*

HEBB, D. O. *The organization of behaviour.* New York: John Wiley & Sons, 1949. *190.*

HEBB, D. O. The role of neurological ideas in psychology. *J. Person.*, 1951, 20, 39–55. *190.*

HEBB, D. O. The distinction between 'clinical' and 'instrumental'. *Canad. J. Psychol.*, 1956, 10, 165–6. *209.*

HECHT, S., HAIG, C., & CHASE, A. M. The influence of light adaptation on subsequent dark adaptation of the eye. *J. gen. Physiol.*, 1937, 20, 831–49. *166, 169.*

HECHT, S., HAIG, C., & WALD, G. The dark adaptation of retinal fields of different size and location. *J. gen. Physiol.*, 1935, 19, 321–37. *168.*

HEILITZER, F., AXELROD, H. S., & COWEN, E. L. The correlates of manifest anxiety in paired associate learning. *J. Personality*, 1956, 24, 463–74. *101.*

HENDERSON, B. K., *Psychopathic states.* New York: Norton & Co., 1939. *200.*

HENDERSON, B. K. & GILLESPIE, A. *Textbook of psychiatry.* Oxford: Med. Publ., 1947. *203.*

HERING, E. *Zur Lehre vom Lichtsinne.* Vienna: 1878. *49.*

HERON, W. T., & SKINNER, B. F. The effects of certain drugs and hormones on conditioning and extinction. *Psychol. Bull.*, 1937, 34, 741–2. *238.*

HEYMANS, C. *Gesammelte kleinere Schriften zur Philosophie und Psychologie.* Haag, 1927. *176.*

HEYMANS, G., & WIERSMA, E. Beitrage zur speziellen Psychologie auf Grund einer Massenuntersuchung. *Zfachr. f. Psychol.*, 1909, 51, 1–72. *172.*

HILDEBRAND, H. P. A factorial study of introversion-extraversion. To appear, *Brit. J. Physiol.*, 1957–58, *28. 200.*

HILDEBRAND, H. P. A factorial study of introversion-extraversion by means of objective tests. Ph.D. Thesis, Univ. of London, 1953. *28, 200.*

HILGARD, E. A. *Theories of learning.* New York: Appleton Century Crafts, 1956. *35, 71.*

HILGARD, E. R. Reinforcement and inhibition of eyelid reflexes to light and sound. *Science*, 1931, 74, 638. *177.*

HILGARD, E. R., JONES, L. V., & KAPLAN, S. J. Conditioned discriminations as related to anxiety. *J. exper. Psychol.*, 1951, 42, 94–9. *91, 92.*

HILGARD, E. R., & MARQUIS, D. *Conditioning and learning.* New York: Appleton Century Crafts, 1940. *206.*

HILL, D., & PARR, G. *Electroencephalography.* London: MacDonald, 1950. *198.*

HIMMELWEIT, H. T. The intelligence-vocabulary ratio as a measure of temperament. *J. Personality*, 1945, 14, 93–105. *28, 200.*

HIMMELWEIT, H. T. Speed and accuracy of work as related to temperament. *Brit. J. Psychol.*, 1946, 36, 132–44. *28.*

HIMMELWEIT, H. T. A comparative study of the level of aspiration of normal and neurotic persons. *Brit. J. Psychol.*, 1947, 37, 41–59. *28, 200.*

HOLLAND, H. C. Some determinants of seen after-movement on the Archimedes spiral. To appear, 1957. *164.*

HOLLAND, H. C. The Archimedes spiral. *Nature*, 1957, 179, 432–433. *164.*

HOLLINGWORTH, H. L. The influence of alcohol. *J. abnorm. soc. Psychol.*, 1923–4, 18, 207–37, 311–33. *223.*

HOLLINGWORTH, H. L. The influence of caffeine on mental and motor efficiency. *Arch. of Psychol.*, 1912, 22, 1–166. *223.*

HOTELLING, H. The generalization of 'student's' ratio. *Ann. math. Statist.*, 1931, 2, 360–8. *16, 158.*

HOTELLING, H. Relation between two sets of variates. *Biometrika*, 1936, 28, 321–77. *17.*

HOVLAND, C. I., & KURTZ, K. H. Experimental studies in rote learning theory: IV. Influence of work-decrement on verbal learning. *J. exper. Psychol.*, 1951, 42, 265–72. *56.*

HOYT, C. Test reliability obtained by analysis of variance. *Psychometrika*, 1941, 6, 153–60. *156.*

HUDSON, B. B. One-trial learning in the domestic rat. *Genet. Psychol. Monogr.*, 1950, 41, 94–146. *213.*

HUGHES, J. B., SPRAGUE, J. L., & BENDIG, A. W. Anxiety level, response alternation, and performance in serial learning. *J. Psychol.*, 1954, 38, 421–6. *101.*

HULL, C. L. The influence of caffeine and other factors on certain phenomena of rote learning. *J. gen. Psychol.*, 1935, 13, 249–64. *228.*

HULL, C. L. *et la. Mathematico-deductive theory of rote learning.* New Haven: Yale Univ. Press, 1940. *35.*

HULL, C. L. *Principles of behavior.* New York: Appleton, Century Crafts 1943. *35, 146.*

HULL, C. L. The place of innate individual and species differences in a natural-science theory of behaviour. *Psychol. Rev.*, 1945, 52, 55–60. *78, 113.*

HULL, C. L. *Essentials of behavior.* New Haven: Yale Univ. Press, 1951, *35, 113.*

HULL, C. L. *A behavior system.* New Haven: Yale Univ. Press, 1952. *35, 113.*

IRION, A. L., & GUSTAFSON, L. M. 'Reminiscence' in bilateral transfer. *J. exper. Psychol.*, 1952, 43, 321–3. *56.*

ISCHLONDSKY, V. E. *Neuropsyche und Hirnrinde.* 2 vols. Berlin: Urban und Schwarzenberg, 1930. *49, 176.*

ISCHLONDSKY, V. E. *Brain and behaviour.* London: H. Kimpton, 1949. *49, 176.*

JAFFE, R. Kinaesthetic after-effects following cerebral lesions. *Amer. J. Psychol.*, 1954, 67, 668–76. *159.*

JAFFE, R. Tactile adaptation disturbances in lesions of the nervous system. *A.M.A. Arch. of Neurol. & Psychiat.*, 1955, 73, 57–65. *160.*

JOHNSON, W. (Ed.) *Stuttering in children and adults.* Minneapolis: Univ. of Minnesota Press, 1955. *268.*

JONES, E. The pathology of dyschiria. *Rev. Neurol. & Psychiat.,* 1909, 7, 499–599. *178.*

JONES, G. The application of conditioning and learning techniques to the treatment of a psychiatric patient. *J. abnorm. soc. Psychol.,* 1956. *52, 269, 414–19.*

JONES, L. Explorations of experimental situations and spontaneous recovery in stuttering. In: Johnson, W., *Stuttering in children and adults. 268.*

JORDAN, F. *Character as seen in body and parentage.* London: Kegan Paul, 1890. *28.*

JUNG, C. G. *Psychologische Typen.* Zürich: Rascher, 1921. *28.*

KAHN, E. *Psychopathic personalities.* Yale Univ. Press, 1931. *201.*

KENDALL, M. G. *The advanced theory of statistics.* London: Griffin, 1946. *16.*

KENDALL, M. G. Factor analysis. *J. Roy. stat. Soc.,* 1950, 12, 60–73. *152.*

KENDLER, H. H. Reflections and confessions of a reinforcement theorist. *Psychol. Rev.,* 1951, 58, 368–74. *209.*

KESSEN, H., & KIMBLE, G. A. 'Dynamic systems' and theory construction. *Psychol. Rev.,* 1952, 59, 263–8. *190.*

KIMBLE, G. A. An experimental test of a two-factor theory of inhibition. *J. exper. Psychol.,* 1949, 39, 15–23. *59.*

KIMBLE, G. A. Transfer of work inhibition in motor learning. *J. exper. Psychol.,* 1952, 43, 391–2. *56.*

KIMBLE, G. A., & SHATEL, R. B. The relationship between two kinds of inhibition and the amount of practice. *J. exper. Psychol.,* 1952, 44, 355–9. *59.*

KLEEMEIER, L. B., & KLEEMEIER, R. S. Effects of benzedrine sulphate (amphetamine) on psychomotor performance. *Amer. J. Psychol.,* 1947, 60, 89–100. *239.*

KLEIN, G. S., & KRECH, D. The problem of personality and its theory. *J. Person.,* 1951, 20, 2–24. *77, 190.*

KLEIN, G. S., & KRECH, D. Cortical conductivity in the brain injured. *J. Person.,* 1952, 21, 118–48. *155, 159, 160.*

KOCH, E. Clark L. Hull. In: *Modern learning theory.* New York: Appleton Century Crafts, 1954. *55, 114.*

KOGAN, N. Authoritarianism and regression. *J. abnorm. soc. Psychol.,* 1956, 53, 34–7. *216.*

KÖHLER, W. *Dynamics in psychology.* New York: Liveright, 1940. *150, 216.*

KÖHLER, W., & DINNERSTEIN, D. Figural after-effects in kinesthesis. In: *Miscellany psychologica* (Albert Michotte). Louvain: Institut Superieur de Philosophie, 1947. *155.*

KÖHLER, W., & FISHBACK, J. The destruction of the Muller-Lyer illusion in repeated trials: I. An examination of two theories. *J. exper. Psychol.,* 1950, 40, 267–81. *150, 255.*

KÖHLER, W., & FISHBACK, J. The destruction of the Muller-Lyer illusion in repeated trials: II. Satiation patterns and memory traces. *J. exper. Psychol.,* 1950, 40, 398–410. *255.*

KÖHLER, W., & WALLACH, H. Figural after-effects. *Proc. Amer. Phil. Soc.,* 1944, 88, 265–357. *150, 190.*

KONORSKI, J. *Conditioned reflexes and neurone organization.* Cambridge: Univ. Press, 1940. *190.*

KRAEPELIN, E. *Psychiatrie.* Leipzig: Barth, 1904. *205.*

KRAFFT-EBING, R. V. Lehrbuch der Psychiatrie. Stuttgart: Enke, 1906. *202, 204.*

KRECH, D. Dynamic systems as open neurological systems. *Psychol. Rev.*, 1950, 57, 345–61. *190.*

KRECH, D. Dynamic systems, psychological fields and hypothetical constructs. *Psychol. Rev.*, 1950, 57, 283–90. *190.*

KRUGMAN, H. E. Flicker fusion frequency as a function of anxiety reaction: an exploratory study. *Psychosom. Med.*, 1947, 9, 269–72. *196.*

L'ABATE, L. Transfer and manifest anxiety in paired-associate learning. *Psychol. Rep.*, 1956, 2, 119–26. *101.*

LANDIS, C. An annotated bibliography of flicker fusion phenomena covering the period 1740–1952. Ground Forces National Res. Council, 1953. *239.*

LANDIS, C. Determinants of the critical flicker fusion threshold. *Physiol. Rev.*, 1954, 34, 259–86. *239.*

LASHLEY, K. S. *Brain mechanisms and intelligence.* Chicago: Univ. of Chicago Press, 1929. *145.*

LAVERTY, S. G., & FRANKS, C. M. Sodium amytal and behaviour in neurotic subjects. *J. Neurol., Neurosurg., & Psychiat.*, 1956, 19, 137–43. *233, 239.*

LAZARUS, R. S., & MCCLEARY, R. A. Autonomic discrimination without awareness: a study of subception. *Psychol. Rev.*, 1951, 58, 113–22. *213.*

LAZARUS, R. S., DEESE, J., & HAMILTON, R. Anxiety and stress in learning: the role of intraserial duplication. *J. exper. Psychol.*, 1954, 47, 111–14. *101.*

LE BEAU, J. *Psycho-chirurgie et functions mentales.* Paris: Massan et Cie, 1954. *32.*

LE BEAU, J., & PETRIE, A. Etudes psychologiques des changements de la personalité produite par des operations préfrontales selectives. *Rev. de Centre de Psychol. Applique*, 4, No. 1, 1956. *32.*

LEHMANN, A. Preliminary report on a device for the objective measurement of the negative after-image phenomenon. *Science*, 1950, 112, 199–201. *243.*

LEPLEY, W. M. Serial reactions considered as conditioned reactions. *Psychol. Monogr.*, 1934, 46, No. 205. *146, 228.*

LETESTU, S. Note sur l'analyse discriminatoire. *Experientia*, 1948, 4, 22–3. *17.*

LITTMAN, R. A., & ROSEN, G. Molar and molecular. *Psychol. Rev.*, 1950, 57, 58–65. *76.*

LIVSON, N. H., & KRECH, D. Dynamic systems, rote learning, and retroactive inhibition. *J. Personal.*, 1955, 24, 2–19. *153.*

LOWENFELD, J., RUBENFELD, S., & GUTHRIE, G. M. Verbal inhibition in subception. *J. gen. Psychol.*, 1956, 54, 171–6. *213.*

LUBIN, A. Some contributions to the testing of psychological hypotheses by means of statistical multivariate analysis. Univ. of London: Ph.D. Thesis, 1951. *16, 17.*

LUBIN, A. Linear and non-linear discriminating functions. *Brit. J. Psychol.*, Stat. Sec., 1950, 3, 90–103. *16, 19.*

LUCAS, J. The interaction effects of anxiety, failure and intraserial duplication. *Amer. J. Psychol.*, 1952, 65, 166–73. *101.*

LYKKEN, D. T. A study of anxiety in the sociopathic personality. *J. abnorm. soc. Psychol.*, 1957, to appear. *122.*

LYTHGOE, R. J. The mechanism of dark adaptation: a critical résumé. *Brit. J. Ophthal.*, 1940, 24, 21–43. *170.*

MAAS, O. Fall von linksseitiger Apraxie mit bemerkenswerter Sensibilitätsstörung. *Neurol. Zeutrabl.*, 1910, 29, 962–7. *178.*

McCLEARY, R. A., & LAZARUS, R. S. Autonomic discrimination without awareness: an interim report. *J. Person.*, 1949, 18, 171–9. *213.*

MACCORQUODALE, K., & MEEHL, P. E. On a distinction between hypothetical constructs and intervening variables. *Psychol. Rev.*, 1948, 55, 95–107. *53.*

MCDOUGALL, W. *Outline of abnormal psychology.* London: Methuen, 1926. *224.*

MCDOUGALL, W. The chemical theory of temperament applied to introversion and extraversion. *J. abnorm. soc. Psychol.*, 1929, 24, 293–309. *224.*

MCGEOCH, J. A., & IRION, A. L. *The psychology of human learning.* New York: Longmans, Green & Co., 1952. *35, 67, 71.*

MACKINNON, D. V. The structure of personality. In: Hunt, J. McV. (Ed.) *Personality and the behaviour disorder.* New York: Ronald, 1944. *76.*

MACKWORTH, H. Researches in the measurement of human performance. M.R.C. Special Report No. 268. London: H.M.S.O., 1948. *128, 241.*

MAGARET, A. Clinical methods in psychodiagnostics. *Ann. Rev. of Psychol.*, 1952, 3, 283–320. *264.*

MAILLAUX, N. M., & NEUBERGER, M. The work curves of psychotic individuals. *J. abnorm. soc. Psychol.*, 1941, 36, 110–14. *65.*

MALMO, R. B. Eccles' neurophysiological model of the conditioned reflex. *Canad. J. Psychol.*, 1954, 8, 125–9. *191.*

MALMO, R. B., & AMSEL, A. Anxiety-produced interference in serial rote learning with observations on rote learning after partial frontal lobectomy. *J. exper. Psychol.*, 1948, 38, 440–54. *146.*

MANDLER, E., & SARASON, S. B. A study of anxiety and learning. *J. abnorm. soc. Psychol.*, 1952, 47, 166–73. *102.*

MARTIN, B., & KUBLY, D. Results of treatment of enuresis by a conditioned response method. *J. consult. Psychol.*, 1955, 19, 71–3. *268.*

MARX, M. H., & EDERSTRAM, H. G. The effect of repeated pentobarbital administration on learning. *J. comp. Psychol.*, 1950, 43, 420–35. *239.*

MAUDSLEY, H. *Responsibility in mental disease.* London: Haig & Co., 1896. *201.*

MAUDSLEY, H. *The pathology of mind.* New York: Appleton & Co., 1899. *201.*

MAY, M. Experimentally acquired drives. *J. exper. Psychol.*, 1948, 38, 66–77. *210.*

MEAD, L. C. The effects of alcohol on two performances of different intellectual complexity. *J. gen. Psychol.*, 1939, 21, 3–23. *239.*

MEIGE, H., & FEINDEL, E. *Tics and their treatment.* London: Appleton, 1907. *277.*

MERCIER, C. *Textbook of insanity.* London: Macmillan & Co., 1902. *201.*

MEYER, M. The psychological effects of drugs: a review. *Psychol. Bull.*, 1922, 19, 173–82. *223.*

MEYER, V. Critique of psychological approaches to brain damage. *J. ment. Sci.*, 1957, 103, 90–109. *145*.

MILLER, D. R. Responses of psychiatric patients to threat of failure. *J. abnorm. soc. Psychol.*, 1951, 46, 378–87. *28, 200*.

MILLER, J. G. Autonomic discrimination without awareness. *Amer. J. Psychol.*, 1939, 52, 562–78. *213*.

MILLER, N. E. Learnable drives and rewards. In: Stevens, S. S. (Ed.) *Handbook of experimental psychology*. London: Wiley & Sons, 1951. *86, 101*.

MILLER, N. E. Comments on multiple-process conceptions of learning. *Psychol. Rev.*, 1951, 58, 375–81. *209*.

MILLER, N. E., & DOLLARD, J. *Social learning and imitation*. New Haven: Yale Univ. Press, 1941. *55*.

MILLER, N. E., & DOLLARD, J. *Personality and psychotherapy*. New York: McGraw-Hill, 1950. *77, 82*.

MILLER, S., & KONORSKI, J. Sur une forme particulière des reflexes conditionnels. *C. R. Soc. Biol.*, Paris, 1928, 99, 1155–7. *206*.

MONTAGUE, E. K. The role of anxiety in serial rote learning. *J. exper. Psychol.*, 1953, 45, 91–6. *101*.

MONTGOMERY, K. An experimental investigation of reactive inhibition and conditioned inhibition. *J. exper. Psychol.*, 1951, 41, 39–51. *56*.

MONTGOMERY, K. C. A test of two explanations of spontaneous alternation. *J. comp. physiol. Psychol.*, 1952, 45, 287–94. *56*.

MORSIER, G. DE, & FELDMAN, H. Le traitement biologique de l'alcoolisme chronique par l'apomorphine. *Ann. med. Psychol.*, 1949, 107, 454–82. *268*.

MOTE, F. A., & RIAPELLE, A. J. The effect of varying the intensity and the duration of pre-exposure upon subsequent dark adaptation in the human eye. *J. comp. physiol. Psychol.*, 1953, 46, 49–55. *166, 169*.

MOWRER, O. H. A stimulus-response analysis of anxiety and its role as a reinforcing agent. *Psychol. Rev.*, 1939, 46, 553–65. *101*.

MOWRER, O. H. *Learning theory and personality dynamics*. New York: Ronald, 1950. *77, 82, 104, 206*.

MOWRER, O. H. Enuresis—a method for its study and treatment. In: *Learning theory and personality dynamics*, 340–417. *268*.

MOWRER, O. H. Two-factor learning theory in summary and comment. *Psychol. Rev.*, 1951, 58, 350–4. *209*.

MOWRER, O. H. *Psychotherapy: theory and research*. New York: Ronald, 1953. *82*.

MOWRER, O. H. Two-factor learning theory reconsidered, with special reference to reconditioning, reinforcement and the concept of habit. *Psychol Rev.*, 1956, 63, 114–28. *209*.

MOWRER, O. H., & JONES, H. G. Extinction and behavior variability as functions of effortfulness of task. *J. exp. Psychol.*, 1943, 33, 369–86. *55*.

MOWRER, O. H., & LAMOREAUX, R. R. Fear as an intervening variable in avoidance conditioning. *J. comp. Psychol.*, 1946, 39, 29–50. *210*.

MUNDY-CASTLE, A. C. The electro-encephalogram in relation to temperament. *Acta Psychol.*, 1955, 11, 397–411. *197*.

MUNDY-CASTLE, A. C. The relationship between primary–secondary function and the alpha rhythm of the electro-encephalogram. *J. Nat. Inst. Personnel Res.*, 1955, 6, 95–102. *197*.

MUSSEN, P. H., & CONGER, J. J. *Child development and personality*, New York: Harper & Bros., 1956. *221.*

MYERSON, A. Neuroses and neuropsychoses: the relationship of symptom groups. *Amer. J. Psychiat.*, 1936, 93, 263–301. *10.*

NELSON, E. H. An experimental investigation of intellectual speed and power in mental disorders. Univ. of London, Ph.D. Thesis, 1953. *268.*

NEWBURGER, M. The relative importance of homogeneity and difficulty in the development of mental fatigue at two different levels of intelligence. *J. appl. Psychol.*, 1942, 26, 81–93. *65.*

NICHOLLS, E. G. The relation between certain personality variables and the figural after-effect. Ph.D. Thesis, Univ. of London, 1955. *154, 158.*

NUNBERG, H. On the physical accompaniments of association processes. In: Jung, C. G., *Studies in word association*. London: Heinemann, 1918. *135.*

OPPENHEIM, A. A study of social attitudes of adolescents. Univ. of London, Ph.D. Thesis, 1956. *221.*

OPPENHEIM, N. Kurze Mitteilung. *Neurol. Zentralb.*, 1885, 23, 529–33. *178.*

OSGOOD, G. E. *Method and theory in experimental psychology.* New York: Oxford Univ. Press, 1953. *35, 57, 71, 193.*

OSGOOD, G. E., & HEYER, A. W. A new interpretation of figural after-effects. *Psychol. Rev.*, 1951, 59, 98–118. *190.*

OSLER, S. F. Intellectual performance as a function of two types of psychological stress. *J. exper. Psychol.*, 1954, 47, 115–21. *101.*

PATTERSON, A., & ZANGWILL, O. L. Recovery of optical orientation in the post traumatic confusional state. *Brain*, 1944, 67, 54–68. *185.*

PAVLOV, I. P. *Conditioned reflexes.* London: Oxford Univ. Press, 1927. *107, 183, 190.*

PAVLOV, I. P. *Selected works.* Moscow: Foreign Language Publishing House, 1955. *107.*

PAYNE, R. B., & HAUTY, G. T. The pharmacological control of work output during prolonged tasks. *USAF Sch. Aviat. Med. Prog. Rep.*, 1953, No. 21–1601–004 (Rep. No. 2). *239.*

PAYNE, R. B., & HAUTY, G. T. The effects of experimentally induced attitudes upon task proficiency. *J. exper. Psychol.*, 1954, 47, 267–73. *239.*

PAYNE, R. B., & HAUTY, G. T. Effect of psychological feedback upon work decrement. *J. exper. Psychol.*, 1955, 50, 343–51. *239.*

PETRIE, A. *Personality and the frontal lobes.* London: Routledge & Kegan Paul, 1952. *32, 280.*

PETRIE, A. A comparison of the psychological effects of different types of operations on the frontal lobes. *J. ment. Sci.*, 1952, 48, 226–319. *32.*

PETRIE, A. A comparison of the personality changes after (1) pre-frontal selective surgery for the relief of intractable pain and for the treatment of mental cases, and (2) cingulectomy and topectomy. *J. ment. Sci.*, 1953, 99, 53–61. *32.*

PETRIE, A., & LE BEAU, J. Psychologic changes in man after chlorpromazine and certain types of brain surgery. *J. clin. exper. Psychopath.*, 1956, 17, 170–9. *32.*

PHILIP, B. R. Studies in high speed continuous work: I. Periodicity. *J. exper. Psychol.*, 1939, 24, 499–510. *65.*

PHILPOTT, S. J. F. Fluctuations in human output. *Mon. Suppl. Brit. J. Psychol.*, 1932, 17. *65.*

PHILPOTT, S. J. F. Fluctuations in mental output. *Quart. Bull. Brit. Psychol. Soc.*, 1950, 2, 1–19. *65.*

POFFENBERGER, G. T. Drugs. *Psychol. Bull.*, 1914, 11, 408–21. *223.*

POFFENBERGER, G. T. Drugs. *Psychol. Bull.*, 1916, 13, 434–6. *223.*

POFFENBERGER, G. T. Drugs. *Psychol. Bull.*, 1917, 14, 408–11. *223.*

POFFENBERGER, G. T. Drugs. *Psychol. Bull.*, 1919, 16, 291–8. *223.*

POFFENBERGER, G. T. The effects of continuous mental work. *Amer. J. Psychol.*, 1927, 39, 283–96. *65.*

POPPELREUTER, W. Zur Psychologie und Pathologie der optischen Wahrnehmung. *Ztschr. f.d. ges. Neurol. u. Psychiat.*, 1923, 83, 26–89. *178.*

POSTMAN, L. The history and present states of the law of effect. *Psychol. Bull.*, 1943, 44, 489–563. *51.*

PRICE, A. C., & DEABLER, H. L. Diagnosis of organicity by means of the spiral after-effect. *J. consult. Psychol.*, 1955, 19, 299–302. *164.*

RAMOND, C. K. Anxiety and tasks as determiners of verbal performance. *J. exper. Psychol.*, 1953, 46, 120–4. *101.*

RAO, C. R. Tests with discriminant functions in multivariate analysis. *Sankhya*, 1946, 7, 407–14. *17.*

RAO, C. R. Utilization of multiple measurements in problems of biological classifications. *J. Roy. statist. Soc.*, B., 1948, 10, 159–203. *17.*

RAO, C. R. Tests of significance in multivariate analysis. *Biometrika*, 1948, 35, 58–79. *17.*

RAO, C. R., & SLATER, P. Multivariate analysis applied to differences between neurotic groups. *Brit. J. Psychol.*, *Stat.*, *Sect.*, 1949, 2, 17–29. *17, 19.*

RAZRAN, G. Conditioning and perception. *Psychol. Rev.*, 1955, 62, 83–95.

REES, L., & EYSENCK, H. J. A factorial study of some morphological and psychological aspects of human constitution. *J. ment. Sci.*, 1945, 91, 8–21. *160.*

REESE, W. G., DOSS, R., & GANTT, W. H. Autonomic responses in differential diagnoses of organic and psychogenic psychoses. *A.M.A. Arch. of Neurol. & Psychiat.*, 1953, 70, 778–93. *146.*

REIFENSTEIN, E. G., & DAVIDOFF, E. The psychological effects of benzedrine sulphate. *Amer. J. Psychol.*, 1939, 52, 56–64. *223.*

RESTLE, F., & BEECROFT, R. S. Anxiety stimulus generalization and differential conditioning: a comparison of two theories. *Psychol. Res.*, 1955, 62, 433–7. *92.*

REUNING, H. A new flicker apparatus and its application to the measurement of temperament. *J. Nat. Inst. Personnel Res.*, 1955, 6, 44–54. *198.*

RIDDOCH, G. Visual discrimination in homonymous half fields. *Brain*, 1955, 78, 376–98. *178.*

RITCHIE, B. F. Can reinforcement theory account for avoidance? *Psychol. Res.*, 1951, 58, 382–6. *209.*

ROBACK, A. G. *The psychology of character.* London: Kegan Paul, 1931. *26.*

ROBACH, G. S., KRASNO, L. R., & ING, A. C. Effect of analytic drugs on the comnifacient effect of seconal and antihistamines as measured by the flicker fusion threshold. *J. appl. Physiol.*, 1952, 4, 516–74. *239.*

ROBINSON, E. S. Principles of work decrement. *Psychol. Rev.*, 1926, 33, 123–34. *67.*

ROBINSON, E. S., Work of the integrated organism. In: Murchison, C. (Ed.) *Handbook of general experimental psychology.* Worcester: Clark Univ. Press, 1934. *61, 67.*

ROBINSON, E. S., & BILLS, A. G. Two factors in the work decrement. *J. exper. Psychol.*, 1926, 9, 415–43. *65.*

ROCKWAY, M. R. Bilateral reminiscence in pursuit rotor learning as a function of amount of first-hand practice and length of rest. *J. exper. Psychol.*, 1953, 46, 337–44. *56.*

ROGERS, C. R., & DYMOND, R. F. *Psychotherapy and personality change.* Chicago: Univ. of Chicago Press, 1954. *267.*

ROSANOFF, A. J. *Manual of psychiatry.* New York: Wiley & Sons, 1938. *203.*

ROSENBAUM, A. Stimulus generalization as a function of experimentally induced anxiety. *J. exper. Psychol.*, 1953, 45, 35–43. *92.*

ROSVOLD, J. E., MINSKY, I. F., SARASON, I., BRANSOME, E. D., & BECK, L. W. A continuous performance test of brain damage. *J. consult. Psychol.*, 1956, 20, 343–50. *147.*

ROY, S. M. P-statistics or some generalizations in the analysis of variance appropriate to multivariate problems. *Sankhya*, 1939, 4, 381–96. *17.*

RUBENFELD, S., LOWENFELD, J., & GUTHRIE, G. M. Stimulus generalization in subception. *J. gen. Psychol.*, 1956, 177–82. *213.*

RUSHTON, W. A. H., & COHEN, R. R. Visual purple level and the course of dark adaptation. *Nature*, 1954, 173, 301–2. *170.*

SADLER, W. S. *Theory and practice of psychiatry.* London: Kimpton, 1936. *202, 204.*

SAMPSON, H., & BINDRA, D. 'Manifest' anxiety, neurotic anxiety, and the rate of conditioning. *J. abnorm. soc. Psychol.*, 1954, 49, 256–9. *125.*

SARASON, I. Effect of anxiety, motivational instruction, and failure on serial learning. *J. exper. Psychol.*, 1956, 51, 253–60. *102.*

SAUCER, R. T., & DEABLER, H. L. Perception of apparent motion in organics and schizophrenics. *J. consult. Psychol.*, 1956, 20, 385–9. *171.*

SCHIFF, E., DONGASS, C., & WELCH, L. The conditioned PGR and the EEG as indicators of anxiety. *J. abnorm. soc. Psychol.*, 1949, 44, 549–52. *91.*

SCHILDER, P. *The image and the appearance of the human body.* London: Routledge, 1935. *178.*

SCHLOSBERG, H. The relationship between success and the laws of conditioning. *Psychol. Rev.*, 1937, 44, 379–94. *206.*

SCHOENFELD, W. N. An experimental approach to anxiety, escape and avoidance behavior. In: Hoch, P. H., & Fabian, J. (Eds.) *Anxiety.* New York: Grune & Stratton, 1950. *210.*

SCHOUTEN, Z. F., & ORNSTEIN, L. S. Measurements of direct and indirect adaptation by means of a binocular method. *J. opt. Soc. Amer.*, 1939, 29, 168–82. *176, 193.*

SEASHORE, R. H., & JOY, G. C. The effects of analeptic drugs in relieving fatigue. *Psychol. Monogr.*, 1953, 67, No. 15. *239.*

SEITZ, C. G., & BARMACK, J. E. The effects of 10 mgs. of benzedrine sulphate and low oxygen tension on the span of attention for letters and other factors. *J. Psychol.*, 1940, 10, 241–8. *239.*

SETTLAGE, O. The effect of sodium amytal on the formation and elicitation of conditioned reflexes. *J. comp. Psychol.*, 1936, 22, 339–43. *238.*

SEWARD, G. H., & SEWARD, J. P. Alcohol and task complexity. *Arch. Psychol.*, 1936, No. 206. *239.*

SEWARD, J. P. Hull's system of behavior: an evaluation. *Psychol. Rev.*, 1954, 61, 145–59. *257.*

SHAGASS, C. The sedation threshold. *EEG. Clin. Neurophysiol.*, 1954, 6, 221–5. *227, 234.*

SHAGASS, C. Sedation threshold: a neurophysiological tool for psychosomatic research. *Psychosom. Med.*, 1956, 18, 410–19. *234.*

SHAGASS, C. A measurable neurophysiological factor of psychiatric signifi-cance. *Electroencephalography and clinical neurophysiology*, 1957, 101–8. *234.*

SHAGASS, C., & NAIMAN, J. The sedation threshold, manifest anxiety, and some aspects of ego function. *A.M.A. Arch. of Neurol. & Psychiat.*, 1955, 74, 397–406. *234.*

SHAGASS, C., & NAIMAN, J. The sedation threshold as an objective index of manifest anxiety in psychoneurosis. *J. psychosom. Res.*, 1956, 1, 49–57. *234.*

SHAGASS, C., NAIMAN, J., & MIFALIK, J. An objective test which differentiates between neurotic and psychotic depression. *A.M.A. Arch. of Neurol. & Psychiat.*, 1956, 75, 461–71. *234.*

SHAPIRO, M. B. Experimental studies of a perceptual anomaly. I. Initial experiments. *J. ment. Sci.*, 1951, 97, 90–110. *180.*

SHAPIRO, M. B. Experimental studies of a perceptual anomaly. II. Con-firmatory and explanatory experiments. *J. ment. Sci.*, 1952, 98, 605–17. *180.*

SHAPIRO, M. B. Experimental studies of a perceptual anomaly. III. The testing of an explanatory theory. *J. ment. Sci.*, 1953, 99, 394–409. *180.*

SHAPIRO, M. B. A preliminary investigation of the effects of continuous stimulation on the perception of 'apparent motion'. *Brit. J. Psychol.*, 1954, 45, 58–67. *171.*

SHAPIRO, M. B. An experimental investigation of an anomaly in the perform-ance of the block design test. London: Ph.D. Thesis, 1956. *145, 180.*

SHAPIRO, M. B., & BEECH, R. Effects of psychiatric disorder on the reproduc-tion of designs by drawing. To appear: Maudsley Monograph Series, 1958. *180, 185.*

SHAPIRO, M. B., & NELSON, E. H. An investigation of the nature of cognitive impairment in co-operative psychiatric patients. *Brit. J. Med. Psychol.*, 1955, 28, 239–56. *268.*

SHEFFIELD, F. D. The contiguity principle in learning theory. *Psychol. Rev.*, 1951, 5, 362–7. *209.*

SHELDON, W. H. *The varieties of human physique.* New York: Harper, 1940. *160.*

SHELDON, W. H. *The varieties of temperament.* New York: Harper, 1942. *160.*

SHERRINGTON, C. *The integrative action of the nervous system.* London; 1906. *49.*

SHIELDS, J. Twins brought up apart. To appear, 1957. *279.*

SHOBEN, E. J. Psychotherapy as a problem in learning theory. *Psychol. Bull.*, 1949, 46, 366–92. *212, 265.*

SHOCK, N. W. Some psychophysiological relations. *Psychol. Bull.*, 1939, 36, 447–76. *223.*

SIDOWSKI, J. B. Influence of awareness of reinforcement upon verbal conditioning. *J. exper. Psychol.*, 1954, 48, 355–60. *213*.

SIMONSON, G., & ENZER, E. The effect of amphetamine (benzedrine) sulphate on the state of motor centers. *J. exper. Psychol.*, 1941, 29, 517–23. *239*.

SKINNER, B. F. *The behaviour of organisms*. New York: Appleton Century Crafts, 1938. *206*.

SMITH, D. G. P., & DAYGAR, A. I. Verbal satiation and personality. *J. abnorm. soc. Psychol.*, 1956, 52, 323–6. *216*.

SMITH, K. The statistical theory of the figural after-effect. *Psychol. Rev.*, 1952, 59, 401–2.

SMITH, K. R. Visual apparent movement in the absence of neural interaction. *Amer. J. Psychol.*, 1948, 61, 73–8. *175*.

SOLOMON, R. L. The influence of work on behavior. *Psychol. Bull.*, 1948, 45, 240. *57*.

SOLOMON, R. L., NAMIN, L. J., & WYNNE, L. C. Traumatic avoidance learning: the outcome of several extinction procedures with dogs. *J. abnorm. soc. Psychol.*, 1953, 48, 291–302. *210*.

SOLOMON, R. L., & WYNNE, L. C. Traumatic avoidance learning: the principles of anxiety conservation and partial irreversibility. *Psychol. Rev.*, 1954, 61, 353–85. *210*.

SPEARMAN, C. *Abilities of men*. London: Macmillan, 1927. *195*.

SPENCE, K. W. Theoretical interpretations of learning. In: Stevens, S. S. (Ed.) *Handbook of experimental psychology*. New York: John Wiley & Sons, 1951. *88*.

SPENCE, K. W. Mathematical formulations of learning phenomena. *Psychol. Rev.*, 1952, 59, 152–60. *88*.

SPENCE, K. W. Learning and performance in eyelid conditioning as a function of intensity of the UCS. *J. exper. Psychol.*, 1953, 45, 57–63. *88*.

SPENCE, K. W. *Behavior theory and conditioning*. New Haven: Yale Univ. Press, 1956. *88*.

SPENCE, K. W., & BEECROFT, R. S. Differential conditioning and level of anxiety. *J. exper. Psychol.*, 1954, 48, 399–403. *92*.

SPENCE, K. W., & FARBER, I. E. Conditioning and extinction as a function of intensity of anxiety. *J. exper. Psychol.*, 1953, 45, 116–19. *88, 89*.

SPENCE, K. W., & FARBER, I. E. The relation of anxiety to differential eyelid conditioning. *J. exper. Psychol.*, 1954, 47, 127–34. *92*.

SPENCE, K. W., FARBER, I. E., & MCFAUN, H. H. The relation of anxiety (drive) level to performance in competitional and non-competitional paired-associate learning. *J. exper. Psychol.*, 1956, 52, 296–305. *88, 89*.

SPENCE, K. W., FARBER, I. E., & TAYLOR, E. The relation of electric shock and anxiety to level of performance in eyelid conditioning. *J. exper. Psychol.*, 1954, 48, 404–8. *88, 89*.

SPENCE, K. W., & TAYLOR, J. A. Anxiety and strength of the UCS as determiners of the amount of eyelid conditioning. *J. exper. Psychol.*, 1951, 42, 183–8. *88, 89*.

SPENCE, K. W., & TAYLOR, J. A. The relation of conditioned response strength to anxiety in normal, neurotic and psychotic subjects. *J. exper. Psychol.*, 1953, 45, 265–72. *88, 89*.

SPENCE, K. W., TAYLOR, J., & KETCHEL, R. Anxiety (drive) level and degree of competition in paired-associates learning. *J. exper. Psychol.*, 1956, 52, 306–10. *88, 89.*

SPRAGG, S. D. S. The effects of certain drugs on mental and motor efficiency. *Psychol. Bull.*, 1941, 38, 354–63. *223.*

STANDLEE, L. S. The Archimedes negative after-effect as an indication of memory impairment. *J. consult. Psychol.*, 1953, 17, 317. *164.*

STEINBERG, H. Selective effects of an anaesthetic drug on cognitive behaviour. *Quart. J. exper. Psychol.*, 1954, 6, 170–80. *239.*

STEINBERG, H. Some effects of depressant drugs on behaviour. Ph.D. Thesis, Univ. of London, 1954. *239.*

STEINBERG, H., & SUMMERFIELD, A. Effects of nitrous oxide on learning and retention. *Bull. Brit. Psychol. Soc.*, 1955, 6, 6–7. *239.*

STELLAR, E. The physiology of motivation. *Psychol. Rev.*, 1954, 61, 5–22.

STIGLER, R. Metacontrast: IX Congress Int. de Phys. Groningen, 1913, Arch. Intern. de Phys., 1913, XIV, I, 78. *176.*

STRAUSS, A. A., & LEHTINEN, L. G. *Psychopathology of the brain-injured child.* New York: Grune & Stratton, 1947. *186.*

STRONGIN, E. I., & WINDSOR, A. L. The antagonistic action of coffee and alcohol. *J. abnorm. soc. Psychol.*, 1935, 30, 301–13. *239.*

SWITZER, S. A. The effect of caffeine on experimental extinction of conditioned reactions. *J. gen. Psychol.*, 1935, 12, 78–94. *238.*

SWITZER, S. A. The influence of caffeine upon 'inhibition of delay'. *J. comp. Psychol.*, 1935, 19, 155–75. *238.*

SYLVESTER, J. D., & LEVERSEDGE, L. A. Conditioning techniques in the treatment of writer's cramp. *Lancet*, 1955, 1, 1147–9. *268.*

TAFFEL, C. Anxiety and the conditioning of verbal behavior. *J. abnorm. soc. Psychol.*, 1955, 51, 496–501. *213.*

TAYLOR, J. A. The relationship of anxiety to the conditioned eyelid response. *J. exper. Psychol.*, 1951, 41, 81–2. *88, 89.*

TAYLOR, J. A. A personality scale of manifest anxiety. *J. abnorm. soc. Psychol.*, 1953, 48, 285–90. *88.*

TAYLOR, J. A. Drive theory and manifest anxiety. *Psychol. Bull.*, 1956, 53, 303–20. *88, 91, 100.*

TAYLOR, J., & SPENCE, K. W. The relationship of anxiety level to performance in serial learning. *J. exper. Psychol.*, 1952, 44, 61–6. *101.*

TEUBER, H., & WEINSTEIN, S. Ability to discover hidden figures after cerebral lesions. *A.M.A. Arch. of Neurol. & Psychiat.*, 1956, 76, 369–79. *145.*

THIRMANN, J. Conditioned reflex treatment of alcoholism. *New Engl. J. Med.*, 1949, 241, 368–70, 406–10. *268.*

THOMPSON, G. N., & BIELINSKI, B. Improvement in psychoses following conditioned reflex treatment for alcoholism. *J. nerv. ment. Dis.*, 1953, 117, 537–63. *268.*

THOMPSON, L. C. The influence of variations in the light history of the eye upon the course of its dark adaptation. *J. Physiol.*, 1949, 109, 430–8. *170.*

THORNDIKE, E. L. Animal intelligence. *Psychol. Rev. Monogr. Suppl.*, 2, No. 8, 1898. *51.*

THORNDIKE, E. L. *Animal intelligence.* New York: Macmillan, 1911. *51.*

THORNDIKE, E. L. The curve of work. *Psychol. Rev.*, 1912, 19, 105–94. *61.*

THORNDIKE, E. L. *The fundamentals of learning.* New York: Teachers College, 1932. *51.*

THORNDIKE, E. L. *Selected writings from a connectionistic psychology.* New York: Appleton Century Crafts, 1949. *51.*

THORNTON, G. R., HOLDER, H. G. O., & SMITH, E. L. The effect of benzedrine and caffeine upon performance of certain psychomotor tasks. *J. abnorm. soc. Psychol.*, 1939, 34, 96–113. *239.*

THURSTONE, L. L. The relation between learning time and length of tasks. *Psychol. Rev.*, 1930, 37, 44–53. *79.*

THURSTONE, L. L. The learning function. *J. gen. Psychol.*, 1930, 3, 469–93. *79.*

TINTNER, G. Some formal relations in multivariate analysis. *J. Roy. statist. Soc.*, B., 1950, 12, 95–101. *16*

TIZARD, B. A theoretical and experimental study of the relations between higher mental processes and brain integrity. Ph.D. Thesis, University of London, 1956. *145.*

TODD, J. W. Reactions to multiple stimuli. *Arch. Psychol.*, 1912, 3, No. 25. *177.*

TOLMAN, G. C. Retroactive inhibition as effected by conditions of learning. *Psychol. Monogr.*, 1917–18. *238.*

TOLMAN, G. C. *Purposive behaviour in animals and men.* New York: Appleton Century Crafts, 1932. *52.*

TOLMAN, G. C. Principles of performance. *Psychol. Rev.*, 1955, 62, 315–26. *52.*

TREADWELL, G. Motor reminiscence and individual personality differences. B.A. Thesis, University of Belfast, 1956. *126.*

TRENT, G. C. Narcosis and visual contour clarity. *J. gen. Psychol.*, 1947, 36, 65–78. *239.*

TROTTER, J. R. The physical properties of bar-pressing behaviour and the problem of reactive inhibition. *Quart. J. exper. Psychol.*, 1956, 8, 97–106. *55.*

TROUTON, D. S., & MAXWELL, A. E. The relation between neurosis and psychosis. *J. ment. Sci.*, 1956, 102, 1–21. *12.*

TUKEY, J. W. Dyadic anova, an analysis of variance for vectors. *Hum. Biol.*, 1949, 21, 67–110. *17.*

TURNER, W. R., & CARL, G. P. Temporary changes in effect and attitude following ingestion of various amounts of benzedrine sulphate. *J. Psychol.*, 1939, 8, 415–82. *239.*

VANNER, W. B. The effects of alcohol on two maze habits of albino rats. *Psychol. Bull.*, 1933, 30, 616. *239.*

VENABLES, P. H. A study of motor and autonomic responses to experimentally induced stress in an industrial setting. London: Ph.D. Thesis, 1953. *139.*

VENABLES, P. H. Change in motor response with increase and decrease in task difficulty in normal industrial and psychiatric patient subjects. *Brit. J. Psychol.*, 1955, 46, 101–10. *139.*

VENABLES, P. H. Some findings on the relationship between GSR and motor task variables. *J. gen. Psychol.*, 1956, 55, 199–202. *139.*

VENABLES, P. H. Car-driving consistency and measures of personality. *J. appl. Psychol.*, 1956, 40, 21–4. *144*.

VENABLES, P. H., & TIZARD, J. Paradoxical effects in the reaction time of schizophrenics. *J. abnorm. soc. Psychol.*, 1956, 53, 220–4. *99, 109*.

VENABLES, P. H., & TIZARD, J. The effect of stimulus light intensity on reaction time of schizophrenics. *Brit. J. Psychol.*, 1956, 47, 144–6. *99, 109*.

VERNON, P. E. *Personality tests and assessments*. London: Methuen, 1953. *261*.

WALD, G. Area and visual threshold. *J. gen. Physiol.*, 1938, 21, 269–87. *168*.

WALD, G., & CLARK, A. B. Visual adaptation and chemistry of the rods. *J. gen. Physiol.*, 1937, 21, 93–105. *166*.

WALDFOGEL, S., FINESINGER, J. E., & VERZEANO, M. The effects of low oxygen on psychologic performance tests in psychoneurotic patients and normal controls. *Psychosom. Med.*, 1950, 12, 244–9. *239*.

WALLACE, J. A. The treatment of alcoholics by the conditioned reflex method. *J. Tenn. St. Med. Ass.*, 1949, 42, 125–8. *268*.

WARBURTON, F. W. An examination of Philpott's theory of the work curve by orthodox statistical techniques. *Brit. J. Psychol.*, 1957, to appear. *65*.

WARREN, N., & CLARK, B. Blocking in mental and motor tasks during a 65-hour vigil. *J. exper. Psychol.*, 1937, 21, 97–105. *65*.

WATERS, R. H. The law of effect as a principle of learning. *Psychol. Bull.*, 1934, 31, 408–25. *51*.

WELCH, L., & KUBIS, J. The effect of anxiety on the conditioning rate and the stability of the PGR. *J. Psychol.*, 1947, 23, 83–91. *91*.

WELCH, L., & KUBIS, J. Conditioned PGR (psychogalvanic response) in states of pathological anxiety. *J. nerv. ment. Dis.*, 1947, 105, 372–81. *91*.

WENAR, C. Reaction time as a function of manifest anxiety and stimulus intensity. *J. abnorm. soc. Psychol.*, 1954, 49, 335–40. *92*.

WENTINCK, E. A. The effects of certain drugs and hormones upon conditioning. *J. exper. Psychol.*, 1938, 22, 150–63. *238*.

WERNER, H. Studies in contour: Strobostereoscopic phenomena. *Amer. J. Psychol.*, 1940, 53, 418–22. *176*.

WERNER, H., & THUMA, A. A deficiency in the perception of apparent motion in children with brain injury. *Amer. J. Psychol.*, 1941, 55, 58–67. *171*.

WERTHEIMER, M. Experimentelle Studien über das Schauen von Bewegungen. *Ztschr. J. Psychol.*, 1912, 61, 161–212. *170*.

WERTHEIMER, M. The differential satiability of schizophrenic and normal subjects: a test of deductions from the theory of figural after-effects. *J. gen. Psychol.*, 1954, 51, 291–9. *160*.

WERTHEIMER, M. Figural after-effect as a measure of metabolic efficiency. *J. Person.*, 1955, 24, 56–73. *153, 160*.

WERTHEIMER, M. Theories and facts about individual differences in figural after-effects. Paper read at Chicago APA Meeting, 1956. *160, 216*.

WERTHEIMER, M., & WERTHEIMER, N. A metabolic interpretation of individual differences in figural after-effects. *Psychol. Rev.*, 1955, 61, 279–80. *160*.

WHITE, R. K. The case of the Tolman-Lewin interpretation of learning. *Psychol. Rev.*, 1943, 50, 157–86. *52*.

WHITING, E. F., & ENGLISH, E. P. Fatigue tests and incentives. *J. exper. Psychol.*, 1925, 8, 33–49. *66*.

WIERSMA, E. D. *Lectures on psychiatry*. London: H. M. Lewis, 1932. *198*.

WILKS, S. S. Certain generalizations in the analysis of variance. *Biometrika*, 1932, 23, 471–94. *16, 17.*

WILLETT, R. A. The effects of a stimulant and a depressant drug on the serial rote learning of nonsense syllables. To appear, 1957. *244.*

WILLIAMS, W. L., LUBIN, A., GIESEKING, C., & RUBENSTEIN, I. An experimental study of block design rotation in brain-injured and controls. *J. consult. Psychol.*, 1956, 20, 275–80. *180.*

WISCHNER, G. Stuttering behaviour and learning: a preliminary theoretical formulation. *J. Speech & Hearing Disorder*, 1950, 15, 324–35. *268.*

WOHLGEMUT, A. On the after-effect of seen movement. *Brit. J. Psychol. Monogr. Supplement 1*, 1911. *163.*

WOLF, E., & FISHER, M. J. Dark adaptation time and size of test-field. *J. oph. Soc. Amer.*, 1950, 40, 211–18. *168.*

WOLF, H. G., & GANTT, W. H. Caffeine sodiobenzoat, sodium isoamylethyl barbiturate, sodium bromide and chloral hydrate. Effect on the highest integrative functions. *Arch. Neurol. Psychiat.*, 1935, 33, 1030–57. *238.*

WOLPE, J. Need-reduction, drive-reduction, and reinforcement, a neurophysiological view. *Psychol. Rev.*, 1950, 57, 19–26. *272.*

WOLPE, J. Experimental neuroses as learned behaviour. *Brit. J. Psychol.*, 1952, 43, 243–68. *272.*

WOLPE, J. Objective psychotherapy of the neuroses. *S. Africa Med. J.*, 1952, 26, 825–9. *272.*

WOLPE, J. Reciprocal inhibition as the main basis of psychotherapeutic effects. *A.M.A. Arch. of Neurol. & Psychiat.*, 1954, 72, 205–6. *272.*

WRIGHT, W. D., & GRANIT, R. On the correlation of some sensory and physiological phenomena of vision. *Brit. J. Ophthal. Monogr. Suppl.*, 9, 1938. *193.*

WYATT, S., & LANGDON, J. N. Fatigue and boredom in repetitive work. M.R.C. Report, No. 77, H.M.S.O., 1937. *134.*

WYNNE, L. C., & SOLOMON, R. L. Traumatic avoidance learning: acquisition and extinction in dogs deprived of normal peripheral autonomic function. *Genet. Psychol. Monogr.*, 1955, 52, 241–84. *210.*

YATES, A. J. The validity of some psychological tests of brain damage. *Psychol. Bull.*, 1954, 51, 359–79. *33.*

YATES, A. J. Experimental studies of a perceptual anomaly. IV. The effect of monocular vision on rotation. *J. ment. Science*, 1954, 100, 975–9. *185.*

YATES, A. J. An experimental study of the block design rotation effect with special reference to brain damage. Ph.D. Thesis, Univ. of London, 1954. *180, 185.*

YATES, A. J. The rotation of drawings by brain-damaged patients. *J. abnorm. soc. Psychol.*, 1956, 53, 178–81. *180, 185.*

YATES, A. J. The application of learning theory to the treatment of tics. *J. abnorm. soc. Psychol.*, to appear, 1957. *268, 273.*

YERKES, R. M. Inhibition and reinforcement of reaction in the frog *Rana clamitans. J. comp. Neurol. & Psychol.*, 1904, 14, 124–37. *177.*

YERKES, R. M., & DODSON, J. D. The relation of strength of stimulus to rapidity of habit formation. *J. comp. Neurol. & Psychol.*, 1908, 18, 459–82. *94.*

BIBLIOGRAPHY AND AUTHOR INDEX

YOUNG, P. T. *Motivation of behavior.* New York: Wiley & Sons, 1936. *94.*

YOUNG, P. T. The role of hedonic processes in the organization of behavior. *Psychol. Rev.*, 1952, 59, 249–62. *95.*

ZWAARDEMAKER, H., & LANE, L. J. Über ein Studium relativer Unerregbarbeit als Ursache des intermittierenden Charakters des Lidschlagreflexes. *Zentlb. Physiol.*, 1900, 13, 325–9. *177.*

308

SUBJECT INDEX

SUBJECT INDEX

Pleasure principle, 207
Politics, Psychology of, 219
Porteus Maze Test, 29
Postulate of individual differences, 114
Practice, massed *vs.* spaced, 44, 67
Pre-excitatory inhibition, 243
Primary drives, 82
Principal components, 22
Projection tests, 148
Protective inhibition, 109
Pseudo-conditioning, 40
Psychasthenia, 26
Psychiatry, classical, 7, 10
Psychiatry, dynamic, 8
Psychoanalysis, 7, 256
PGR conditioning, 91, 116, 123
PGR scoring, 154
Psychology, 73
Psychopathy, 28, 81, 122, 200
Psychosis, 10, 15, 22, 25, 180
Psychotherapy, 8, 85, 265 f.
Psychoticism, 33
Pursuit rotor, 68

Questionnaires, 31

Reaction time test, 109
Reaction types, 135
Reactive inhibition, 50, 59, 60
Reality principle, 208
Reciprocal inhibition, 272
Recovery, spontaneous, 44
Refractory period, 64
Reinforcement theory, 36, 86
Reminiscence, 56, 68, 125, 149
Repression, 28, 215
Retardation, 14
Retroactive inhibition, 153
Reversible perspective, 244
Rorschach Test, 28
Rorschach, validity of, 260

Saliva, 45
Sanguine, 26, 109
Satiation, 149, 175
Science, function of, 7
Score pattern analysis, 132
Secondary function, 215
Sedation, 229
Sedation threshold, 28, 228, 234
Selective breeding experiment, 90
Semi-tendinosus muscle, 43
Sense of humour, 28
Sensory after-effects, 163

Serial position effect, 146, 245
Single-trial conditioning, 213
Slutzky-Yule effect, 65
Sociability, 28, 214
Socialism, 218
Sociology, 73
Sociopathy, 122
Sodium amytal, 234, 242 f.
Spatial inhibition, 47, 174, 194
Stammering, 268
Static Ataxia Test, 23
Stimulus generalization, 45
Stimulus-intensity dynamism, 53
Stimulus theory of inhibition, 57
Stress reactions, 28
Strychnine, 229
Subception, 263
Suggestibility Test, 29
Super-ego, 84
Sympathectomy, 210
Syndrome, 8

s^t_R, 53, 59
Tactile adaptation effects, 160
Temporal inhibition, 47, 149, 174, 194
Temporal inhibition, law of, 46
Tender-mindedness, 219
Thematic Apperception Test, 28
Theory, definition of, 250
Tics, 268, 273 f.
T-maze, 101
Tough-mindedness, 219
Transfer, 66
Tsai-Partington pathways test, 56
Twenty-dials test, 128
Two-factor theory of learning, 206
Typological postulate, 117

Unconscious motivation, 265

V, 53, 59
Values, 220
Variate scores, 20
Verbal conditioning, 213
Vigilance, 128

W, 55, 56, 59
w, 53, 55, 59
Watch-keeping, 128
Word Association Test, 23, 267
Work decrement, 61, 128, 147, 242
Writer's cramp, 268

Yerkes-Dodson law, 94 f.
Y maze, 95

311